MW01044757

Selfless Insight

The MIT Press
Cambridge, Massachusetts
London, England

Selfless Insight

Zen and the Meditative Transformations of Consciousness

James H. Austin, M.D.

MIT Press books may be purchased at special quantity discounts for business or sales promotional use. For information, please e-mail special_sales@mitpress.mit.edu or write to Special Sales Department, The MIT Press, 55 Hayward Street, Cambridge, MA 02142.

This book was set in Palatino and Frutiger on 3B2 by Asco Typesetters, Hong Kong and was printed and bound in the United States of America.

Library of Congress Cataloging-in-Publication Data

Austin, James H., 1925–
Selfless insight : Zen and the meditative transformations of consciousness / James H. Austin.
    p. cm.
Includes bibliographical references and index.
ISBN 978-0-262-01259-1 (hardcover : alk. paper) 1. Meditation—Zen Buddhism. 2. Zen Buddhism—Psychology. 3. Consciousness—Religious aspects—Zen Buddhism. I. Title.
BQ9288.A95 2009
294.3'4435—dc22   2008026983

10 9 8 7 6 5 4 3 2 1

Also by James H. Austin

Zen-Brain Reflections (2006)
Chase, Chance, and Creativity (2003)
Zen and the Brain (1998)

To my early teachers Nanrei Kobori-Roshi, Myokyo-ni, and Joshu Sasaki-Roshi, for inspiration; and to all those whose contributions to Zen, and to the brain, are reviewed in these pages.

Your true self is free from beauty and ugliness, free from God and evil.
When you manifest yourself as emptiness, at that moment, you are free
from everything.

Joshu Sasaki-Roshi (1907–)

Contents in Brief

Contents in Detail

Chapters Containing Testable Hypotheses

It is better to know some of the questions than all of the answers.

James Thurber (1894–1968)

The outcome of any serious research can only be to make the two questions grow where only one grew before.

Thorstein Veblen (1857–1929)

These chapters suggest potential correlates between brain functions, meditative training, and the phenomena of alternate states of consciousness.

List of Figures

List of Tables

Preface

Familiarity with the workings of the emotional household is the first step in the training.

Irmgard Schloegl (Myokyo-ni) (1921–2007)[1]

Certitude is not the test of certainty.

Oliver Wendell Holmes, Jr. (1841–1935)

This is a book of words about Zen. Neither our usual English words nor the old Sanskrit and Sino-Japanese words make it easy to understand where contemporary Zen is coming from. Could new words clarify this situation, at least with regard to the emotional household in which we live every day?

Two new words did enter the English language in 2006. One word was "truthiness." It helps to recall that Stephen Colbert introduced this word during his *Comedy Central* television program. He used it in a tongue-in-cheek context to refer to a *slippery* truth, one that "comes from the gut, not from books." Viewers understand that Colbert employs satire in his make-believe act as an archconservative. He mostly *pretends* to hold an opinion that his visceral emotions have told him is true. Therefore, his emotional "truthiness" is neither real, nor true, but patently *false*. These layers of falsity aside, Merriam-Webster, the dictionary publisher, still declared "truthiness" to be its word of the year for 2006.

So truthiness is only what *seems* to be true. It is not *really* true. Can this new word serve a useful function on these pages? It can, if we allow its usage to remind us of the source of the most troublesome workings in our emotional household. They arise from exaggerated, error-prone conditionings in our emotional brain. Often, the more our ideas and opinions seem to shine with the veneer of certainty, the more likely it is that we are being deceived. Let that sobering fact remind us: Zen comes from a direction oriented toward a different value system. In any search for existential truth, the emphasis in Zen will fall on *clear, objective, insightful comprehension*, not on visceral emotionality, as the major avenue. Do such insights necessarily convey "ultimate truth?" No, because Zen also practices skepticism, and uncertainties abound. All insights must run the gauntlet of doubt, like other beliefs. Ultimate truth remains eternally elusive.

The second new word of the year came from the American Dialect Society. In 2006, its new word was "plutoed." The choice was influenced by the earlier official decision of the International Astronomical Union to exclude Pluto as a planet. For decades, we had grown up confident in the belief system that when the trio of Uranus, Neptune, and Pluto came together, Pluto was just as much a planet as the others, only smaller. However, professional astronomers had just rejected that belief. So how did this dialect society define their new word? To pluto is "to demote or devalue someone or something."

Humans had survived a previous belief-shattering experience of astronomical proportions. Their planet Earth had once undergone a similar demotion. Before that, earthlings had felt grounded in the certainty that they occupied the very center of the whole universe. All other planets had seemed to revolve around *them*, as did the Sun itself! (Of course, in ignorance and arrogance, they had first positioned themselves at the hub.) After Copernicus (1473–1543) overturned that premise of truthiness, people awakened to a stark new reality: the Sun was the true center of the solar system. In one stroke, Earth was no longer at the axial hub of a geocentric universe. Even Mercury and Venus deserved a place in line before their own planet in this heliocentric system.

So we now have this second new word, "plutoed," to remind us what Zen awakening means. It means that Selfhood's old fictions have been devalued. Indeed, "Selfless" occurs in the title of this book because selflessness is the pivotal fact when the emotional household undergoes a spring cleaning and consciousness shifts toward insight-wisdom.

Part I begins by revisiting the Zen emphasis on paying *attention*, a major theme in earlier volumes. We will discover many subtleties in our networks of attention. They enable us to direct attention voluntarily—from the "top down"—or reflexly—from the "bottom up"—and to focus it either internally or externally.

Part II returns to a second major Zen theme, the origins and nature of our private *Self-consciousness*. We are programmed to distinguish our personal Self (inside) from that other world "out there" in the environment. Meditative training cultivates attention. As it begins to reprogram attention, the results become the prelude to key issues considered in part III: How can meditation train a calm, mindful awareness in general, come to a one-pointed mode of attention during the absorptions, lead the trainee toward more selfless behavior in daily life and then finally to let go of all Self-centered physiological biases and enter the deeper states of *kensho-satori*?

In part IV, we take up a topic of universal human importance: the nature of *insight* in general. Insights are key ingredients in the lengthy process of creative intuition. Recent research hints how ordinary insights that instantly unveil so much can also strike anonymously.

Part V inquires: Do similar principles of ordinary insight extend into the extraordinary realms of *insight-wisdom*? Notably, the special insights celebrated in Zen flash in selflessly, fearlessly, timelessly, and they illuminate existential issues with stark objectivity.

Part VI considers how meditative training can favorably influence the normal developmental trajectory of emotional maturity.

Part VII briefly reviews and updates selected topics of research.

Page xvi lists chapters that contain testable hypotheses. For the reader's convenience, helpful background information on many topics herein is cross-referenced (using brackets) to earlier pages in the two preceding books in this series: *Zen and the Brain* [ZB:] and *Zen-Brain Reflections* [ZBR:].

Zen is no simple topic. Neither is the brain. In my role as a secular guide to the ways these two topics are interrelated, I invite you to read slowly, skim when appropriate, and to refer often to the figures, tables, glossary, and mondo summaries at the end of each part.

Acknowledgments

I'm indebted to Barbara Murphy and Tom Stone at MIT Press for encouraging me to write a slender sequel to the earlier books. My thanks again go to Katherine Arnoldi Almeida for her skilled editorial assistance, and to Yasuyo Iguchi for her artistic skill in designing the cover and icons.

I'm especially grateful to Lauren Elliott for her ongoing patience and skill in deciphering my handwriting on multiple drafts of her excellent typing, and for helping to keep the manuscript organized as it expanded. Many thanks also to Kathleen Knepper, James W. Austin, Scott W. Austin, and Lynn A. Manning for their valued assistance in reviewing and commenting on the manuscript. I also thank Scott Greathouse for his artistic skill in bringing the figures to fruition and Betty March for preparing two earlier tables.

In recent years, I have been privileged to share in the inestimable bounties of regular Zen practice with our sangha at Hokoku-an, led by Seido Ray Ronci, in the activities of the Show-Me Dharma, led by Virginia Morgan, and in those of the Maui Zendo, led by Patti Gould. Gassho to all!

By Way of Introduction

If you make subjective, personalized judgments about events in the past and present but have not been through the process of refining and purifying your insight, you are doing a sword dance without having first learned how to handle a sword.

Master Fa-yen Wenyi (885–958)[1]

This happens to be the fourth volume in a long quest to understand the nature of creative insight. My original biases were what you might expect from someone raised as a Unitarian, trained to be a clinical neurologist, who then tried to solve clinical problems by pursuing them into the research laboratory. I began Zen training late. During these last three decades, I have been learning how to handle a sword poised at the cutting edge of both Zen and the neurosciences. Every year, I've stumbled across new examples illustrating that these two large fields are mutually illuminating.

The Path of Zen is a Buddhist Path. It is viewed here as an inspired human product, neither divine in origin nor esoteric. It can be traced back to the ancient yoga practices, which then evolved over millennia. The word *Zen* encapsulates its history. When Buddhism spread north from India into China, its teachings were influenced by the established cultures of Taoism and Confucianism. There, in China, the old Sanskrit term for meditation (*dhyana*) would change into *Ch'an*. Still later, when the Ch'an practice of meditation entered Japan, the word would be pronounced *Zen*.

My quest has spanned an era of unprecedented progress in neuroscience research. Every month or so, new developments help us envision how meditation trains attention, how our notions of Self are rooted in interactive brain functions, and how extraordinary states arise that can help us live more harmoniously and selflessly. This is an exciting time. A whole new field is taking shape.

Part I
On the Varieties of Attention

Each of us literally chooses, by his way of attending to things, what sort of universe he shall appear to himself to inhabit.

William James (1842–1910)

S   S
S   S
S S S S S
S   S
S   S

1

Training Attention

Ordinary man to Zen Master Ikkyu: "Master, please write the maxims exemplifying the highest wisdom."

Ikkyu immediately writes the ideogram "Attention," with his brush.

The man asks, "Will you please add something more?"

Ikkyu now writes, twice: "Attention. Attention."

The man remarks, with an edge, "There's really not much depth or subtlety here."

Ikkyu then writes the same ideogram three times: "Attention. Attention. Attention."

The man now demands: "What does that word 'Attention' *mean*, anyway?"

Ikkyu replies: "Attention means attention."[1]

The cultivation of attentional stability has been a core element of the meditative traditions throughout the centuries, producing a rich collection of techniques and practices.

B. Alan Wallace[2]

As the mind becomes clearer, it becomes more empty and calm, and as it becomes more empty and calm, it grows clearer.

Master Sheng-yen[3]

Attention is basic. It exemplifies a universal form of biological wisdom. Ancient yogic traditions emphasized the art of training attention long before Ikkyu (1393–1481). Subsequent generations rediscover the simple principle: a simple way to begin to cultivate attention is to focus it on the in-and-out movements of one's breathing. As meditation practices evolved, the several Buddhist practices addressed attention in two mutually reinforcing ways. These two generic categories are *concentrative* meditation and *receptive* meditation [ZBR:30].

Table 1 summarizes the two approaches. At the start of any one period, the meditator usually concentrates on the breath. Thereafter, during the next 20 to 40 minutes, shifts occur more or less spontaneously between the two styles of meditation as an expression of covert cycles and rhythms over which the meditator can choose to superimpose degrees of voluntary control.

Concentrative meditation, having begun by directing one's intentions, continues to direct attention in a more focused and exclusive manner. Receptive meditation often follows, cultivating a sustained awareness that is more unfocused, open, and all-inclusive. Readers interested in how different traditions vary these

Table 1
The Attentive Art of Meditation

Receptive Meditation	Concentrative Meditation
A more effortless, sustained attention, *un*focused and inclusive	A more effortful, sustained attention, focused and exclusive
A more open, universal, bare awareness	A more deliberate, one-pointed attention
It expresses involuntarily modes of global monitoring and bottom-up processing	It requires voluntary, top-down processing
More other-referential	More Self-referential
May shift into intuitive, insightful modes	May evolve into absorptions
A bare, choiceless awareness	Paying attention

Note the overlaps between receptive modes of meditation, the ventral attention system outlined in table 4, and the allocentric processing stream outlined in table 7.

major themes are referred to a forthcoming authoritative review by Lutz and colleagues.[4] It cannot be overemphasized that a prerequisite for *any* form of meditative practice is a solid foundation of calmness based on a simplified, ethical lifestyle (*shila*) [ZBR:29–40].

Zen traditions alternate both styles of regular, *open*-eyed meditation, emphasizing an attentive posture, frequent interviews with one's teacher, daily life practice, and meditative retreats. Daily life practice (*shugyo*) means that you pay close, mindful attention to events during both your ordinary housekeeping and garden varieties of activity, as well as to your personal relationships. Zen traditions encourage practitioners to remain fully aware in the present *now*, avoiding the two extremes: one being "monkey-mind" wandering, the other being sluggish meditation. Zen tends not to dwell on the intricacies of lists often used in other Buddhist traditions, is wary of words, and steers clear of theological speculations.[5,6]

Levels along the Path of Attentional Training

The early Indian Buddhists drew on ancient practices that had progressively refined attention through some eight or more successive levels [ZB:473–478]. The first four stages unfold as the meditator begins to concentrate on a material object or concept. The early texts refer to the next four phases as the "formless" levels. During these, the meditator develops further refinements of both one-pointedness and equanimity. On balance, these steps can be conceptualized as an intensive approach that continues to refine *concentrative* meditation on the path of the absorptions.

Along this path toward the absorptions, several trajectories converge subtly. At other times, these would usually describe diverging mental phenomena. Now, however, their vectors begin to cross in ways that seem paradoxical. For example, when we usually choose both to intensify and to focus attention, we invest a high degree of effort into each of these two acts. In contrast, when we settle down to become deeply relaxed, we then tend to slide in the opposite direction—toward drowsiness and low levels of attentional vividness.[7]

Not so along this path of the absorptions. As a result of the underlying calming that occurs, internal thoughts and emotions no longer prove distracting during the four higher levels described in Indo-Tibetan traditions. Yet, even though the next most refined mental field might sometimes be called "dwelling in tranquility," the utter "stillness" at its center can become infused with a hyperawareness now vivid in its intensity.[8]

Zen tends toward a less structured approach. During Zen retreats, the receptive mode of meditation also tends to settle into an early foundation of calmness, which then evolves toward phases combining both mental alertness and physical relaxation. Gradually, recurrent waves of one-pointed attention *superimpose themselves spontaneously* on this entry phase of tranquility. As these waves become more sustainable, they can occasionally evolve into transient states that reach spontaneous peaks of attentional vividness.

The Zen view of the relationship between the two meditative approaches is traceable as far back as the pre-Ch'an period when the term "silent illumination" was used by the Chinese monk Seng-Chao (378–414) [ZBR:330]. The phrase refers to aspects of a practice that blended a form of concentrative meditation carried to the phase of stillness with an openly aware form of receptive meditation that could evolve into insights of various sizes.[9] At this writing, we still await a comprehensive functional magnetic resonance imaging (fMRI) study that monitors a large group of advanced Zen meditators while they engage in very carefully defined, 30- to 40-minute intervals characteristic of the spontaneous flexibility that occurs in their daily meditation, with no other tasks being required.

Quiet Periods, and So-Called Cessations of Experience

Meditators following various traditions sometimes report other unusual episodes. These appear to represent variations on the theme of the absorptions. For example, during one of these episodes, a meditator might sit quietly absorbed for several hours [ZBR:321–322]. Uncommon episodes lasting this long await a detailed, first-person description of their internal form and content.[10]

Jack Kornfield's teacher, Mahasa Sayadaw, was in the Theravada Buddhist tradition. He taught that the "first taste of Nirvana" came in the form of a cessation of experience.[11] It was a particular kind of cessation, said to arise out of the "deepest state of concentration and attention." When it occurs, "the body and mind are dissolved, the experience of the ordinary senses ceases," and "perfect equanimity prevails." In the course of their intensive meditative practices, Kornfield estimated that "perhaps 3% of the trainees" at that time could have had such a "stream entry" experience. The words used to describe such a state suggest that it resembles other states on the path of the absorptions [ZB:469–518, 589–592; ZBR:315–322, 334–335]. The phenomena are impressive, and serve to motivate meditators to continue their quest. To what degree and for how long might an individual trainee's brain be permanently changed by one substantial cessation experience? This remains an open question, but the emphasis in Zen remains on the long path that leads beyond toward selfless insight.

Perceptual Effects in Monks during Training in One-Pointed Attention

Highly trained Tibetan monks have been studied both during and after their periods of one-pointed meditation.[12] The test technique was simple: use display goggles to present a different image of parallel lines to each eye: horizontal lines to the right eye; vertical lines to the left eye. Normal subjects rapidly switch attention back and forth between the two stationary images. First the version from one eye dominates, then the other. This normal condition of spontaneous alteration is called "perceptual rivalry."

However, *during* their five-minute test periods of one-pointed meditation, 3 of the 23 monks reported complete perceptual stability of the image from one eye or the other. During such periods of perceptual stabilization, the visual percepts being experienced often differed subtly from the actual line patterns.

After undergoing periods of one-pointed meditation for various lengths of time, half of the monks also reported that during the intervals of visual stabilization, their episodes when one eye assumed perceptual dominance lasted much longer than usual.

Perceptual rivalry tests have implications not only for how long attention can be sustained on a simple scene but also for how effectively it resists being *disengaged*. An incidental finding was of interest: the separate practice of a compassion type of meditation did *not* change the normal rate of perceptual rivalry. Inducing compassion during meditation has other interesting social, as well as laboratory, correlates [ZBR:48–50, 269–270].

Three Months of Meditative Training Improves the "Attentional" Blink

If you see two separate numbers that arrive *less* than half a second apart, you often fail to detect the second number. Although this normal failure is called a "blink," it represents a defect of *attention*, not a failure of vision caused by closing the eyelids. Slagter and colleagues studied the brain potentials of 17 experienced practitioners at the beginning and end of a 3-month Vipassana retreat.[13] The retreat was rigorous: the practitioners meditated 10 to 12 hours a day.

They, and their controls, would see the first number (e.g., 3) followed by the second number (e.g., 9). The second number could be either "hard" to detect or "easy" to detect. A hard second number was a number that came only 336 ms later. Note that this interval is often much too short for the stimulus to be detected. In contrast, the easy number could come 672 ms later. This interval is long enough to be detectable. All practitioners improved their accuracy. They detected more of the hard numbers at the end of their retreat than they did at the beginning. However, only 16 of 23 controls did so.

Electroencephalograms monitored the subjects' event-related potential (ERP) responses. These ERP data showed that when the practitioners *successfully* identified *both* their first (hard) number *and* their second (easy) number, they accomplished this feat with *lower* corresponding amplitudes of their P400 potentials.

What does it mean when the practitioners have *lower* ERP amplitudes during their successful detection of the first number? The authors interpreted this to mean that their subjects' greater processing efficiency enabled them to *retain* more "attentional resources." These resources in reserve could then be devoted toward the successful detection of the second number, whether it was easy or hard. This could explain why the practitioners also had fewer "blinks" of attention when the second number arrived, and why they could then detect *more* of the hard numbers than did their controls.

Limitations on the Effectiveness of Short-Term Alertness Training

Healthy seniors trained in a 5-week program of the relaxation response (RR) show significant improvement in their reaction times on a simple test of attention, but not on more complex tasks of attention or factual memory.[14]

Functional MRI monitored the responses of seven brain-damaged neurological patients whose visuospatial neglect had lasted for more than 3 months.[15] Three weeks of computerized alertness training improved their visual performance. It also increased the fMRI signals within parts of the attentional network on both sides of the brain. These regions included their frontal cortex, anterior cingulate gyrus, precuneus, cuneus, and angular gyrus. Four weeks after training ended, however, most temporary improvements had returned to baseline, even though a few increased fMRI signals lingered. When the visuospatial neglect is caused by chronic, major structural brain disease, computerized training approaches seem limited in their effectiveness.

2

Meditating Mindfully at the Dawn of a New Millennium

> The setting: Jon Kabat-Zinn is asking Morinaga Soko-Roshi how it is possible to introduce hospital patients in the West to the benefits of mindful meditative practice when they resist hearing about the Buddha and the Asian religious context of his teachings.
> The Roshi answers: "Throw out Buddha, throw out Zen."[1]

Zen meditation taps practical, everyday roots. Many early benefits of a meditative approach need no elaborate religious or philosophical belief system. Some benefits evolve over a period as short as 2 months when subjects fully commit themselves to an ongoing practice of daily meditation. Herbert Benson made similar observations after he introduced his Western subjects to a "simple, non-cultic" technique of passive meditation called the "relaxation response" [ZB:78–83]. Its methods combined a mental device and a passive attitude that resulted in a decrease in muscle tone.

What Does Mindfulness Mean?

Kabat-Zinn's 8-week program of mindfulness training, now widely introduced and studied, is called "mindfulness-based stress reduction" (MBSR) [ZBR:56–57]. He views MBSR as a "family" of practices. They do not "*de*-contextualize Buddhist meditation practice," but "*re*-contextualize it creatively," enabling it to become more "American without denaturing it." What does it mean to be mindful? He comments that in the "internal experience of mindfulness, you comprehend what it is."[2] One example, elegant in its simplicity, is the actual tasting of a single raisin, *deeply*, as each trainee's introduction to acute, explicit, delicious perception. Because mindfulness is multifaceted, its internal experience can vary from person to person. As Zen trainees shift back and forth during concentrative and receptive modes of meditation, they have ample opportunity to witness each rising and falling of different aspects of their own mental experience.

Ruth Baer based her recent analysis of mindfulness on descriptions of how a variety of normal subjects experience mindfulness internally when they are (more or less) "just sitting."[3] Their mental experience includes:

- Acting with greater awareness. This implies that the subjects are neither being distracted nor are they acting solely on "automatic pilot."
- Experiencing internal and external events nonjudgmentally.

- Noting an experience, but not reacting to it.

- Identifying mind states and describing them silently with words.

- Simply observing sensations that arise in the body, noticing feelings and thoughts, while attending to each of them with awareness.

When students made progress in the first three of these areas, they tended to experience less psychological suffering. Among the subgroup of subjects who had already meditated in the past, this fifth factor of simple "observation" and noticing tended to correlate more with the first four. It was also associated with a greater openness to experience in general. Simply being mindful of bodily sensations and feelings was a practice highly recommended by the Buddha in an early sutra (*Anguttara Nikaya* I, 21). While noticing per se would not be a helpful prescription for a patient who is a hypochondriac, simple noticing can be adaptive in a *meditative* population, because in this instance it is tempered by the meditator's nonjudgmental attitude.

Some styles of meditation add a silent labeling to whatever emotion the meditator happens to be experiencing. During fMRI monitoring, this affect labeling was studied as one task. The control task was simply to label which gender was associated with a person's first name.[4] In response to these experimental tasks, the general disposition toward mindfulness was associated with a widespread prefrontal increase in fMRI signals. Moreover, affect labeling was associated with a bilateral decrease in amygdala signals when compared with the gender-labeling control condition. Self-reports that suggested greater degrees of mindfulness correlated with greater decreases in the amygdala signals.

Jain and colleagues recently compared the benefits of only a 1-month course of mindfulness meditation with the benefits of simple body relaxation.[5] Their subjects were 83 students who were suffering from various kinds of psychological distress. Each technique enhanced positive mood and reduced distress. Mindfulness meditation appeared the more effective in reducing distractive and ruminative thoughts and behaviors.

Kristeller's recent review suggests that the 8-week MBSR program is probably efficacious in different patient populations suffering from a wide variety of disorders.[6] For purposes of rigorous scientific research, those on a waitlist are no longer regarded as an adequate control group. Future studies will benefit from the inclusion of an *active* control group, one designed to test for expectation effects, demand characteristics, and the role of inspiring teachers. Preliminary results from such an active control group indicate that normal subjects report non-specific improvements in global stress and depression after they become involved in, and motivated by, an inspiring program of intervention called "Wellbeing."[7]

Zen looks to a much longer-term commitment. The discussion later in part I will explain that an extended mindfulness approach goes on to include more than a detached attentiveness that registers bare perception, and that notices without elaboration. It will also become a practice that trains a more implicit mode of meta-awareness. This includes the capacity of attention to recollect (*sati*), to *disengage gently and to keep returning* to the main topic at hand.

The meditator who persists in a regular training program for much longer than 8 weeks discovers that mindfulness gradually expands its basic functions of increasing mental clarity into moments that tap into other worthwhile functions. These key psychological domains include introspection, self-analysis, various degrees of intuition, and an incremental ethical character change [ZBR:641–653]. Zen traditions use a variety of long-range approaches to retrain the *I-Me-Mine*, to defuse its overreactivities, and to redeploy more fruitfully the energies thus released. Those meditators who continue to go on retreats and who persist for years on the Zen Way discover that it evolves into an endless process of reprogramming and personal transformation. Formal sitting meditation involves at least ten different aspects [ZBR:31–32]. It proves difficult to ascribe the long-term benefits of mindfulness to a single physiological mechanism, because the various aspects interact in concert.[8,9]

Meanwhile, Soko-Roshi's terse response in the epigraph sounds a welcoming note to all potential meditators: You can choose to lower the sights on your "spiritual quest," and avoid being consumed by theological complexities. Robert Aitken-Roshi also observes, in his personal collection of excellent gathas, that the simple act of entering the shower can serve to remind us to "cleanse this body of Buddha and go naked into the world."[10]

James Ford blends his practices as a Unitarian-Universalist minister with those of an experienced Zen teacher. His recent book provides a useful survey of the various schools of contemporary Zen in North America.[11] He perceives that a "liberal Buddhism" is emerging in the West. His pages also include a practical section for any seeker, entitled "What to look for when looking for a Zen teacher."

The early rigorous monastic approaches to Zen training continue to evolve among lay practitioners in the cultural diversity of the West. One newly developing variety was first called "Neo Zen."[12] It has more recently been described as a kind of "New Buddhist Psychology."[13] From this perspective, our sense of Self begins as a narrative construction of fiction. Only when our earlier egocentric constructs are *de*constructed can the requisite *re*structuring begin. Then the whole framework of our personality can be transformed along more fruitful lines using different priorities [ZBR:5–6].

It is no accident that the reader will find *restructuring* and *transformation* to be terms that recur in these pages. We return to them not only in relation to the psychophysiological basis of insight (part IV) but also in the context of personality development (parts V and VI).

3

Meditation: "JUST THIS"

Meditation practice is a crucial tool for Buddhist studies because the Wisdom spoken of in Buddhism is really only accessible to a settled and focused mind.

Andrew Olendzki[1]

Align your body, assist the inner power. Then it will gradually come on its own.

Chinese Taoist text, fourth century B.C.E.[2]

First Principles

Zen meditation is a relaxed attentive state, a *passive activity*. Both aspects are important. The intervals spent in quiet meditation are designed gradually to calm the overactive mind, to clarify its perceptions, *and* to open up its spontaneous receptivities. It will be on this basic foundation—*the settled mind*—that the deep "inner power" of our intuitive skills will gradually ripen. Later, this innate capacity can slowly mature in the direction of insight-wisdom and genuine compassion.

Meditation is a time to *be* and to open up, not a time to *do*. Beginning meditators try much too hard. They're not alone. Meditative researchers tend to push their subjects to perform tasks. However, back on the cushion in the meditation room after the preliminary phase of concentration, most Zen approaches sooner or later involve one's settling down, and then gravitate toward one's passive *letting go* of discursive thoughts. This gradual process leads to an *emptying* of Self-referential mental activities and to an *opening up* to more universal themes [ZB:141–145]. In Christian meditative traditions, the term *kenosis* refers to a similar ancient process. No mysterious purpose is involved in either case. The intent is to empty the personal Self of its overconditioned egocentric preoccupations.[3]

The wandering of my own mind during meditation led me to improvise a simple-minded home remedy [ZBR:33–37]. Its first stage exemplifies intention: it involves saying the word "JUST" silently, during each inbreath. Then, during each successive breathing out, the numbers from one to ten are counted silently. This process continues for a variable period. In the background, down in the lower abdomen, is a simple awareness of the in-and-out movements of breathing.

The next stage involves saying the word "THIS," while breathing in. It is again followed by each silent number from one to ten while breathing out. Later, all the number counting fades and drops out. At this point, "JUST" returns to reoccupy the whole inbreath, leaving "THIS" to shift over to occupy the entire outbreath. Now, a silent "JUST THIS" remains throughout each in-and-out cycle of breathing. Later, it, too, dissolves into the breathing movements of the lower abdomen and vanishes like any other concept.

Of course, "JUST THIS" is a temporary expedient. It signifies that *only this* precious moment exists, within the whole world of awareness. At this moment, there's nothing more to strive for, nothing more to attain. This is it, right *now*.

Ancient Fingers Pointing toward "JUST THIS"

Although "JUST THIS" became a new evocative phrase for me, it turned out that comparable phrases were already present in China during the Tang dynasty (618–907). Ch'an master Daowu (748–807) advised his trainees to "Live in an un-fettered manner, in accord with circumstances. Give yourself over to everyday mind, because there is nothing sacred to be realized outside of *this*."[4]

Another early Ch'an master who used "just this" was Yunyan Tansheng (784–841). Later, Yantou Quanho (827–887) would say: "If you want to know the last word, it is 'just this!' "[5] In Japan, the exclamation "shako" (this) points directly toward genuine reality.

Whatever "just this" might have stood for in its ancient context, it can continue to serve as an elastic phrase, usefully applied in any era to point toward a beginning breath, toward a last word, or to whatever event occupies each present moment between our first breath and what will be our terminal exhalation . . .

Coda

Having completed this chapter in April, I was fascinated to discover in July 2007 that Morinaga Soko-Roshi (1925–1995) had made a contemporary reference to "just this," and that he had trained in the Rinzai tradition at Daitokuji in Kyoto. The autobiographical account of his odyssey, just translated and published post-humously, has an interesting subtitle that was also applicable in my case: "An On-going Lesson in the Extent of My Own Stupidity."[6]

Soko-Roshi's first use of "just this" is with reference to the equanimity of any "person who exerts himself or herself with dignity, without worrying about results and without giving in to disappointment." He believes that any such person is practicing the essence of the Zen Way. He regards the full expression of their quiet innate competence—"just this"—as the true form and measure of "human well-being." In the final farewell sentence of his autobiography, Soko-Roshi expresses the earnest hope that his readers will be stimulated to "live each and every instant with great care, aware that *just this* is the great dynamic, lively dancing life."

What is the meaning of the phrase "Living Zen?" We might define it as expressing with equanimity and compassion *just this* mindful attention to every present moment of daily life. This means remaining fully in touch with an event as an explicit matter of fact while gradually becoming less self-consciously aware of one's underlying implicit sense of awareness. Chapter 4 considers how both processes can coincide.

Different Styles of Meditation

Meditation is not monolithic. Its passive activities represent an unusual admixture: purposefulness and letting go, attention and nonattachment, self-discipline and spontaneity, introspection and extrospection, settling down in quiet solitude as the prelude to bringing your internal calmness and clarity out to engage the disquietude of the unsettled world at large.

When Cahn and Polich recently reviewed the literature on meditation research as a whole, they concluded that the "Central nervous system function is clearly affected by meditation, but the specific neural changes and differences among practices are far from clear."[7] Moreover, with regard to the various research techniques used, they also stated that "None of the approaches has yet isolated or characterized the neurophysiology that makes explicit how meditation induces altered experiences of self."

Ospina and colleagues concluded that "future research on meditation practices must be more rigorous in the design and execution of studies, and in the analysis and reporting of results."[8]

Responding to both critiques, in the following pages we first explore new research findings relevant to meditative attention, then turn to brain-mapping research that identifies separate facets of the Self. Subsequent chapters slowly reassemble isolated parts of this large jigsaw puzzle. To what purpose? To develop a simpler, coherent understanding of how the ancient Path of transformation leads toward rare states of consciousness. These enlightened states enter experience directly as *selfless insight-wisdom*. This brief awakening sets the stage for the person to go on to live more objectively and compassionately within the world at large.

4

Neurologizing about Attention

> Pay attention and quiet your mind as soon as you get up in the morning.
>
> Ch'an Master Yuan-Wu (1063–1135)

Awareness, Alerting, Attention

Unaware creatures dropped out of the gene pool eons ago. Human survivors invented the term *awareness* to describe the way they remain in a wary, watchful state. Zen traditions emphasize an open, bare awareness during receptive meditation. Down at this lowest level, while awareness registers a weak stimulus as a faint sensory intrusion, the brain still remembers to return to its online condition of noticing, even though its awareness may have lapsed for a while. At levels farther along on the sensory spectrum, we start experiencing a stimulus as a more refined *perception*. Awareness implies just these purely sensate phases of receptivity.

In contrast, attention *stretches toward* something. Its higher levels of alertness represent a more "heads-up" attitude. Both attention and alertness express dynamic, selective, *orienting* properties. Attention has so many facets[1] that researchers in this larger field now publish over two thousand articles a year![2] This chapter selects highlights from this vast database and discusses techniques that enable researchers to test how efficiently meditation trains attention. We start with impulses that travel much faster than you can blink—so fast that only specialized techniques can detect them. Don't expect to digest all the latest fast-paced research in this chapter. Move on when it becomes too daunting.

Stimuli Elicit Event-Related Potentials

Electrodes on the scalp detect the brain's electrical responses to stimuli. These event-related potentials (ERPs) are waveforms that are deflected upward or downward [ZBR:190–191]. Paying more attention to external stimuli causes the peaks and valleys of these ERP responses to arrive sooner and changes their shape.

How does our brain register a bare visual percept?[3] Suppose you are an astute observer, straining to detect the arrival of a faint gray dot close to your threshold for perception. Only your correct "hits" show up in the first wave of "visual awareness negativity." This peaks over your posterior *temporo-occipital* leads at 200 to 300 milliseconds (ms) after the stimulus begins. This first negative wave correlates with your explicit, correct perception of the bare stimulus (with your so-called *phenomenal* consciousness). A positive wave comes later. It peaks at *parietal* lobe sites, and it doesn't arrive until after 400 to 500 ms. This later positive wave is associated with your higher-level, feature-detection forms of visual discrimination (with your "*reflective* consciousness").

The earliest half of that first negative wave (130 to 200 ms) is too "hard-wired" to be influenced by your trying to pay attention. But its later half (at 200 to 260 ms) can be influenced slightly. In contrast, the whole later positive wave is obviously "soft-wired." It is an index of how accurately you have been consulting your memory stores to decide whether or not you had just correctly identified the stimulus.

Meanwhile, other aspects of visual processing have also been unfolding down in the occipital and temporal lobes. They may take some 60 to 80 ms or so to flow forward along the whole lower visual stream. However, this ventral flow of impulses does not alone make us *fully* conscious of the visual percept. Not until impulses *descend* from the higher levels of the cortex back *down* to reach the earlier visual association areas do the recent theories suggest that we can "see" complex patterns *consciously*.

Yet, hints of such *recurrent* impulses begin as soon as 100 ms after the stimulus starts. (Note that this means that they might already be making *silent* contributions to events even before the first ERP wave of visual awareness negativity begins.) Moreover, after these initial recurrent activations reenter the occipital region, still later waves of recurrent interactions then spread over multiple parietal and frontal attention areas. These *global* processes sponsor our more sophisticated levels of *reflective* consciousness. Now the percept registers in our memory bank. Now it can also become a conscious event that we can report to someone else. Bare awareness unfolds through these three phenomenal, recurrent, and reflective steps as it emerges into full conscious perception.

Changes in Event-Related Potentials during Introspection

Suppose you volunteer to be a subject during a thought experiment. All you have to do is engage in an internally oriented, Self-centered act of introspection. But notice: You are *not* being asked to direct your attention *outward*, say to focus it on an apple *out there* on a plate. Instead, your task is to turn your attention around, to focus on your own *interior* state. Your goal is to answer this question: "How am *I experiencing* the apple, in this present moment?"

The researchers had a difficult question of their own: Do people change their brain potentials when they shift into this *intro*spective mode?[4] They finally settled on only certain moments, the times when the subjects indicated they had *already* entered into the introspective mode, and were focusing on *just this* internal experience of visual perception.

Two things happened at this point: (1) The subjects' first negative waveform (N1) arrived slightly earlier than before, and (2) their late positive waveform (P500) also increased in amplitude. These results suggested that active introspection might have two chances to influence perception, both in its early *preconscious* phase (N1) and during those later stages (P500) when the event could go on to register in memory.

So what? The ERP findings are relevant to Zen meditative training, because its approach follows this same dual path toward insight: being both mindfully aware and occasionally introspective [ZB:125–129]. The findings may relate to a key question: Why do some sensory stimuli trigger kensho's insights, and only at certain times? The ERP data suggest a testable hypothesis: Perhaps such sensory triggers might be more effective when they strike at particular times—say, when the more fully trained meditators happen to be engaged in either a no-thought awareness or in a more introspective mode of consciousness.

In the next section, we consider how the early and later *gamma waveforms* in the EEG respond to an auditory stimulus. Note that these brain waves are also recorded high up on the surface of the *scalp*, far from the brain beneath. Even so, sensitive techniques are now able to show that the subjects' mode of attention heightens brain responses as early as the first tenth of a second after researchers deliver a sound stimulus. Do the subjects' recognize the *quality* of the sensory trigger? This split-second decision can also shape slightly later stages of the gamma EEG response from the underlying brain.

Stimuli Elicit Two Phases of Gamma Wave Responses in the EEG

Gamma waves are fast. They cycle up and down some 30 to 100 times a second. In general, an auditory stimulus event prompts two different phases of gamma responses during the first half-second [ZBR:44–47]. The brain's initial responses, termed *evoked* responses, are more hard-wired. The delayed responses come much later. They are called *induced* responses.[5] They suggest that the person is now matching the sound against similar, earlier patterns that were stored in the (reflective) expectations of long-term memory (see table 2).

During the first 300 ms after a stimulus, scalp recordings show that the *height* of the gamma waves can rise to a peak four to seven times each second. These rhythms correlate with the rates of the *theta* phase of spontaneous EEG oscillations [ZBR:42–43]. Why? Perhaps during visual perception, the fast gamma rhythms that are localized to the more posterior sensory regions could be serving our immediate perceptual needs. In contrast, the slower rhythmical theta oscillations that are more widespread could be involved in processing other interactions within the frontal cortex that help to link sites separated by longer distances.[6]

Table 2
Two Types of Event-Related Gamma Wave Responses

	Evoked Responses	Induced Responses
Origin	Directly related to the immediate processing of a sensory stimulus	Related more to cognitive discriminations involved in memory processing; not strictly phase-locked to the stimulus
Nature	Correlate with object-selective attention and with sensory matching	Correlate with the way the matching information is used in subsequent cortical processing
Onset	Start within the first 100 ms of the stimulus (e.g., P50, N100 potentials)	Begin later, at around 200 ms after the stimulus, and continue (e.g., P200, N400)
Location	More focal and related to sensory modality	Much more widespread
Effect of not recognizing the identity of the stimulus	Negligible	Larger P200 amplitudes occur when auditory stimuli are *not* recognized
Effect of recognizing the stimulus	Neglible	Larger N400 amplitudes occur when auditory stimuli are recognized with the aid of long-term memory

From D. Lenz, J. Schadow, S. Thaerig, et al. What's that sound? Matches with auditory long-term memory induced gamma activity in human EEG. *International Journal of Psychophysiology* 2007, 64:31–38.

Sequences during Top-Down Visual Attention

Slower EEG waveforms in the theta, alpha, and beta frequencies correlate with simpler kinds of top-down processing. During visual experiments, researchers can provide a visual cue. It serves notice: Heads up! Get ready to pay more intensive attention! Networks over the lateral frontoparietal cortex consume much of the time it takes to process the cues themselves.[7]

Some circuits along the midline also participate during the sequences of attention-orienting. For example, the negative ERP wave in the medial frontal regions starts at around 400 ms after the cue. Subsequent waves then appear in parietal regions, and reappear much later back in the visual cortex at around 800 to 900 ms. This sequence suggests that when we first orient attention voluntarily in response to a visual cue, the medial frontoparietal regions then signal the visual cortex in ways that influence what we will register next in vision.

The lateral frontal cortex also influences perception. Direct stimulation of the right frontal eye field (FEF in figure 1) enhances perception in the peripheral visual fields while decreasing it simultaneously in the central zone.[8] Refer to figures

Table 3
Frontal and Parietal Aspects of Paying Visual Attention

Region Tested	General Functions	Comment
Lateral orbitofrontal cortex (BA 11)	Processing negative rewards	Is active during negative reward at the stage when the switch is being implemented
Medial orbitofrontal cortex (R, L) (BA 12)	Processing positive rewards	Is active during positive feedback, but plays no direct role in switching attention
Ventrolateral prefrontal cortex (R, L) (BA 45)	Switching attention [e.g., from buildings (parahippocampal place area) to faces (fusiform face area)]	Occupies this pivotal executive position at the termination of the ventral visual stream
Dorsolateral prefrontal cortex (BA 46)	Involved more generally in the search for a visual solution	Plays a higher coordinating role
Posterior parietal cortex (R, L) (BA 40)	Contributes a multimodal spatial context	Is active when prior stimulus-response patterns must be changed into new patterns

After A. Hampshire and A. Owen. Fractionating attentional control using event-related fMRI. *Cerebral Cortex* 2006; 16:1679–1689. The article itself cites X-, Y-, and Z coordinates, not BA regions which are provisionally suggested above.

1, 2, and 3 in the next two chapters to see which of the various discrete regions of the cortex are located on the lateral or medial aspects of the hemispheres.

Different Frontal Lobe Contributions to Paying Attention

In the laboratory, task-oriented researchers tend to assign meditators tasks to perform during experiments. However, on the cushion and out in the world at large, meditators shift their attention flexibly, on *their* own time. Recently, fMRI scans monitored normal subjects while they were left alone. Now, *they* could choose which strategies to use when they shifted attention in response to various stimuli.[9] This is a sensible way to proceed, because it mimics the spontaneous way we human beings normally shift attention. Different frontal lobe regions make distinctive contributions. Table 3 summarizes the pertinent findings.

The *ventrolateral* prefrontal cortex plays a key executive role. This is in keeping with its pivotal anatomical position near the front end of the ventral visual stream. In contrast, the *dorsolateral* prefrontal cortex is involved in our more deliberate process of *searching* for a visual solution. In addition, the lateral orbital frontal cortex also participates when negative messages are being processed (part VII). In each of these distinctive frontal functions, the parietal lobe is a coparticipant. The posterior parietal cortex in the region around the supramarginal gyrus (BA 40) contributes some of its spatial context to the message.

Different Responses in the Medial and Lateral Parts of the Frontal Polar Cortex

Different thought processes activate different parts of our prefrontal cortex. Whenever we "mentalize," the frontal pole (BA 10) shows relatively short reaction times, on both its medial and lateral sides. Suppose, however, that the immediate task requires us to reach back into our ongoing working *memory*. Now the faster reactions (at 300 ms) occur first in the medial region, and only later in the lateral region (not until 450 ms).[10] Why? A meta-analysis of some 104 neuroimaging studies provides an answer. This medial side of our polar cortex is the more responsive during lower-level thinking tasks. At these times, we need quickly to orient attention out toward the *external* environment. In contrast, the lateral part of BA10 deliberates longer over more complex decisions. These help *switch* our attention back and forth, between thought processes oriented outward toward an external stimulus and the internal thoughts that arise independently of events in the environment.

Magnetoencephalography Documents Foresight: The Orbital-Frontal Connection

Sensitive magnetoencephalography (MEG) and fMRI studies now show that our frontal lobe is much more forward-looking than we had realized from the standard EEG (see also chapter 52). Even as messages conveying object recognition are relaying forward through the temporal lobe, coarse images of low spatial frequency have already been relayed up from the medial pulvinar as far as the left posterior orbital frontal gyrus.[11] This crude visual information provides an "initial guess." It develops in this frontal gyrus some 50 to 85 ms before MEG signals peak back in the fusiform gyrus of the right temporal lobe.

Suppose that the visual stimulus happens to be a picture of an elephant. Not until 250 and 300 ms after this animal image is first presented does the right fusiform gyrus activity reach its maximum. The evidence suggests that this orbital frontal region—the one which receives major input from our amygdala—already has a preview of the event horizon. Instantly, it can provide the top-down feedback that alerts and enhances the refined responses of our posterior occipital and temporal visual areas to messages that might soon be reaching them.

Semivoluntary Shifting of Mental Sets

Attention is malleable. We can intensify it, shift it either voluntarily or involuntarily. We can soften it, diffuse it. We can deploy global attention toward tangible external objects, or to their intangible attributes. We can direct attention internally to retrieve items that we have stored in memory. We can sustain attention by infusing a component of motivation, either from the top-down (by intention) or by much more subtler means related to our habitual ongoing attitudes.

During *successful* shifts of attention, the medial prefrontal cortex and the anterior cingulate gyrus play an active role.[12] Some fMRI evidence suggests that we can improve our task performance when we co-activate both the *ventral medial* prefrontal cortex and the *rostral* anterior cingulate gyrus. What functions could this ventral medial prefrontal cortex be contributing? Wager and colleagues suggest that it plays a twofold role: (1) helping to update the motivational relevance of stimuli, and (2) relaying these signals about relevance in ways that influence how the dorsal lateral prefrontal cortex represents and helps process the pending task. In turn, this dorsal lateral region could help in two ways by (1) maintaining goal-directed types of information, and (2) representing the more general rules and abstract categories that are pertinent to our behavior.

People differ. Who shifts attention most efficiently? The most efficient are those fortunate subjects who learn to accomplish the job with the least expenditure of energy. (Chapter 8 discusses this principle in greater detail.) These subjects accomplish an assigned task at the *lower* operating levels of activation of their ventral medial and anterior cingulate regions. Of course, during successful shifts, other regions will share in the attentive and processing efforts required. These contributions come from such sites as the right ventral anterior insula, the left intraparietal sulcus, and the left precuneus.

Many studies suggest that the anterior cingulate tends to monitor cognitive conflicts at the level of their competing *responses*.[13] However, certain tasks involve stimuli that conflict with one another in their visual-*emotional* content. In these instances, our responses activate the *more caudal* portions of this anterior cingulate cortex.[14]

The Executive Control of Auditory Spatial Attention

Wu and colleagues studied the auditory responses of 13 subjects in their early twenties, using the technique of event-related fMRI.[15] Their subjects listened carefully, straining to detect a faint sound. This target stimulus could appear in either the left side or the right side of the auditory space, and in only some of the trials. The subjects received voice cues of two types. One type said "left" or "right." The second type instructed the subjects *not* to orient attention to either side. In general, during this task of auditory spatial orienting, the cues activated regions that were located slightly more superiorly and medially than those sites which responded to cues during visuospatial attention.

Does the Front of the Thalamus Influence Attention?

Barrett and colleagues, in Heilman's group at the University of Florida show that the front of the thalamus contributes to our attentive skills.[16] They studied a 52-year-old woman whose infarct damaged the *left* anterior and dorsal medial thalamic nuclei (see figure 6). Fortunately, she knew that when she drove her car, she tended to head toward people and cars on the *right* side of the road.

Behavioral tests confirmed that she had an abnormal and asymmetrical bias. She *over*attended to items located in the distant extrapersonal space on her *right* side. The authors review evidence showing that certain regions on one side of the brain, gathered into one circuit, can normally bias our attention toward that *same* side of the environment. Among these biasing regions are the anterior and medial dorsal thalamic nuclei (as well as the dorsolateral frontal lobe, and the retrosplenial cortex.) In their patient, therefore, whose damage to the front of her thalamus occurred on the *left* side, attention was biased (pushed/pulled) to head toward the *right* side of space, *opposite* the side of her lesion. The authors conclude that some attentional systems could be preferentially "obedient" to *far* extrapersonal space, reasoning on evolutionary grounds that "this is the region where threatening or novel relevant stimuli first appear." Chapter 23 discusses the significance of this visual principle from the standpoint of the visual stimuli that can trigger kensho.

In Summary

Attention is a complex associative function. It relies on expectant interactive networks, poised to provide integrated top-down and bottom-up information. Readers might think: If I've been attending for a lifetime already, why do I need further training? And mind-wandering meditators may wonder: What's in this new research for me?

5

On Remaining Attentive while We Meditate

> Time flies like an arrow, so waste no energy on trivial matters. Be attentive! Be attentive!
> Master Daito Kokushi (1283–1337) (founder, Daitoku-ji monastery)

Not until you try to meditate do you really understand the problem. Then you discover how much your mind tends to wander. Gradually, the truth dawns:

meditation does train one's attentive faculties. With continued practice, your discursive mind stops wandering so far down so many unfruitful paths. Finally, in moments of awesome perceptual clarity, bare awareness opens spontaneously and becomes thought-free. At least for a while...

The next chapters review recent research into how meditators learn to be more attentive. These pages highlight only a tiny sample of worldwide research. Some articles are selected because they provide tantalizing glimpses of how our brains change when we *try* to "pay attention." Others are included for precisely the opposite reason. Subsequent chapters provide hints about another attribute of long-term training: how their practice of attention can enable meditators to become more self*less*.

Read slowly. No topics reviewed will be easy to grasp. Gradually, you may discover something interesting: attention and selflessness differ physiologically, yet they tend to interact in complementary ways, like yin and yang. Meanwhile, whenever you find your own attention waning, return to Master Daito's injunction: Be attentive!

Lapses and Recoveries of Attention

We've observed that the brain is constantly changing, from one millisecond to the next. Some functions increase, some decrease. Research that measures these underlying shifts—up or down—in the balances between excitation and inhibition can help understand how mental phenomena arise. A recent report from Duke University contains information relevant to all meditative traditions. It describes how changes in the normal brain are responsible for not only *lapses* of attention but also for the *recoveries* from such lapses.[1] Weissman and colleagues studied 16 young adults during a challenging visual task. They monitored their subjects' standard response times as well as fMRI signals.

The subjects' assigned task seemed straightforward. They had to decide: Was a big letter made up of many identical small letters, or of many different small letters? For example, a given **H** might be large because it was composed of 11 small letter *H*s. Alternatively, the **H** could be large because it was made up of 11 small letter *S*s (as in the icon of part I). Therefore, these subjects first needed to pay active, acute, highly selective visual attention. Next, in order to signal their choice, they had to press one of two buttons.

They possessed the basic youthful skills, and their overall accuracy remained high (97%). Even so, on occasion they paused and responded slowly. These slow response times suggested that brief lapses of attention had undermined their skills. Why did their attention wane? Equally important: After each lapse, what physiological change helped the subjects recover their mental focus? First a slight digression, followed by an explanation.

The figures below begin to point toward some answers. Why does the terrain look familiar? Because the lobes are indeed the same old brain "continents" you have seen elsewhere before. However, some of their major landmarks have labels that are less familiar. In this new millennium, when the artists' arrows point to these gyri and sulci, the labels often represent names from the newer "functional anatomy," not from the old topography.[2] No acronym needs to be memorized. However, you might encounter these terms again in the daily papers, magazines, or on TV, because the media increasingly display similar "brain-mapping" images.

After this preamble, let us use a question-and-answer approach to probe the results in this article from Duke.

- What made the researchers sure that their subjects' attention really had lapsed? Slow reaction times were only one of several lines of evidence. Thus, fMRI signals *had already fallen* in certain locations just *before* each such lapse of attention and slow response time. Three relevant regions showed these decreased signals. Two decreases were on the *right* side. They occurred in the *right* inferior frontal gyrus (IFG) and in the *right* middle frontal region. Decreases also occurred in the anterior cingulate cortex (ACC) on *both* sides of the brain. (See figures 1 and 2.)

Normally, these two right frontal regions help us point to, access, and retrieve the specific immediate memory functions we need to address an urgent problem. They help us meet immediate working goals and to update our responses appropriately. Moreover, one of the (multiple) functions of the anterior cingulate cortex is to monitor conflict situations and to detect errors. Therefore, it is especially significant to find that lapses were associated with *decreased* fMRI signals in each of these three "executive" regions. This evidence suggests that key "top-down" functions in the front part of the subjects' brains had not been fully *prepared*—just *before* each lapse and slow response—to help focus attention on the working tip of its impending visual task. (Similar regions and similar considerations will arise once again in part IV, when we explore what happens during the prelude to insights.)

- Did the subjects' lack of "executive readiness" have any secondary sensory consequences in the back of the brain, where their visual cortex is located? Indeed, fMRI signals were also reduced in the lower part of this occipital cortex, on both sides. This confirmatory evidence also suggested that—just *before* their attention waned—the quality of visual processing had itself already been compromised, back at the initial level when it first contributes to coarse *visual perception*.

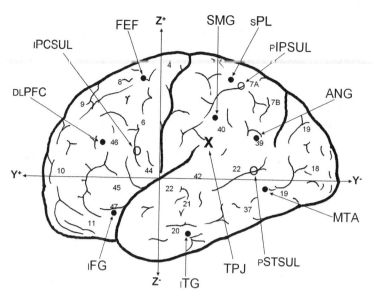

Figure 1   Lateral view of the left hemisphere
Starting at the left, in the frontal lobe: ɪFG, inferior frontal gyrus; DɪPFC, dorsolateral prefrontal cortex; ɪPCSUL, inferior precentral sulcus; FEF, frontal eye field; SMG, supramarginal gyrus; sPL, superior parietal lobule; PIPSUL, posterior intraparietal sulcus; ANG, angular gyrus; MTA, middle temporal area; PSTSUL, posterior superior temporal sulcus; TPJ, temporoparietal junction; ɪTG, inferior temporal gyrus.

Y+ and Y− are on an anteroposterior line. Z+ and Z− are on a dorsal-ventral line. Both lines represent the standardized planes used to localize discrete brain sites in terms of their three-dimensional coordinates. The small numbers refer to Brodmann's areas [ZBR:146–148]. The open circles indicate cortical regions on the banks of a sulcus.

- Were the subjects' slower reaction times linked to any other evidence of local deficiencies? Yes, but this gets tricky. Why? *Because it is normal for certain brain regions to become deactivated during more effortful tasks.* (We expand on this crucial point in part II.) Among these other potentially impaired sites was the right precuneus (PRECUN). In this instance, what was the evidence that the right precuneus was impaired? It *failed to show its expected decrease in signals.* This fact suggests a different localized deficiency. Moreover, the observations are in accord with this important general principle: to achieve an optimum, efficient level of performance, we must *skillfully integrate our patterns of increased brain activation with those of deactivation.*

- Could the brain have started to adjust for these lapses even *during* that *same* trial in which reaction times were slow? Yes, fMRI signals did *increase* in several *different* prefrontal, lateral parietal, and anterior cingulate regions during these slow

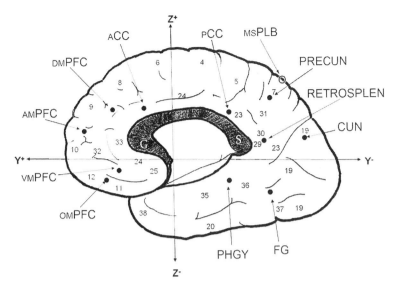

Figure 2 Medial view of the right hemisphere

This view represents the inside surface of the right side of the brain. Starting at the left, in the frontal lobe: oMPFC, orbital medial prefrontal cortex; vMPFC, ventral medial prefrontal cortex; aMPFC, anterior medial prefrontal cortex; dMPFC, dorsal medial prefrontal cortex; aCC, anterior cingulate cortex; pCC, posterior cingulate cortex; msPLB, medial superior parietal lobule; PRECUN, precuneus; RETROSPLEN, retrosplenial cortex; CUN, cuneus; FG, fusiform gyrus; PHGY, parahippocampal gyrus. The dark curved area in the center is the corpus callosum. G refers to its genu; S refers to its splenium. The vertical and horizontal planes are shown intersecting at their zero point, the anterior commissure.

response trials. One normal role of these different sites is to engage in "supervisory" efforts, the kinds we use to reduce distractions during higher-order tasks of visual processing. Thus, in a given slow-response trial, such local increases could be interpreted as ways to "compensate" for the subjects' other difficulties in choosing between the two alternatives.

- What happened on the *next* trial, the one immediately *after* attention had lapsed in that previous, slower trial? How did the brain adjust then? During this next trial, certain right-sided regions did show *increased* fMRI signals. These two active regions were the *right* temporoparietal junction (TPJ) and the *right* inferior frontal gyrus (iFG). (Note that this iFG region had shown *reduced* signals during the earlier lapse.)

The subjects' performance also improved during this next trial, in keeping with the local increases in right-sided signals. These observations, plus other lines of evidence (soon to be cited in the discussion of figure 3), support the following interpretation: These two regions—the TPJ and the IFG—both on the right side, normally help sponsor our automatic *reorienting* of attention toward salient events. They enter into that quick general process of recovery from a brief lapse of attention. This normal recovery process is a "bottom-up" function. It *helps our attention return to refocus on the task.* Researchers interested in measuring how meditation evolves longitudinally would benefit by incorporating many of the aspects of this Duke study into their experimental design.

The TPJ region is shown as a large X here in figure 1. Later, in figure 3 (see chapter 7) it will be shown as a large red area in the right hemisphere. There it will be suggested that its several functional roles can draw on adjacent regions of the (right) supramarginal and superior temporal gyrus that deactivate during a visual search, yet activate as the fresh target is detected.[3]

A recent behavioral study did use a similar global/local letters test to see whether prior meditation would enhance the orientational aspects of attentional processing.[4] The Stroop task was used to test for executive processing (based on the subjects' need to inhibit their incorrect responses). Efficient performance correlated with how many minutes were spent meditating each day, not with the total numbers of hours of practice.

A Take-Home Message for Meditators

Learn to be much more patient with yourself. Every mind wanders. It is a normal phenomenon. Remember: We're talking about a regular *practice* of meditation. Practice means you're not perfect. Implicit in the phrase, "regular practice" is a subtle, dynamic, fringe benefit. During long-range training, you're practicing a gentle art. You are learning to *return* to your original focus—*time after time after time*—whenever your attention strays. Through trial and error, you're *developing the habit of returning* to that original focus, whether it had been narrow or open, intense or soft.

So, develop a more lenient, nonjudgmental attitude toward this autonomous, bottom-up faculty of attention. Why? Because *its innate capacity is to return.* It is learning to reengage itself, to shift subconsciously. Allow room for this natural compensatory process to develop. Give it time to become strengthened as it evolves. This how *your brain keeps repeatedly training itself, involuntarily.* Do not think of lapses as a series of shortcomings or "failures" on your part. Instead, you are learning how to delegate attentional functions in a more skillful other-relational direction. As you become more proficient, the question then becomes, Are you gradually learning to place more trust in what you then more openly perceive?

6

Perceiving Clearly

> The faculty of voluntarily bringing back a wandering attention, over and over again, is the very root of judgment, character, and will.
>
> William James (1842–1910)

Can we trust what we perceive? William James pointed to another attribute of attention: it helped augment the "clearness of all that we perceive or conceive." Meditators discover that the more they train attention, the more it seems to enhance their *dual* sense of perceptual and conceptual clarity. The lastest ERP studies suggest that the perceptual aspects might arrive first, and the conceptual contributions might evolve later.

Irmgard Schloegl emphasized that such clear seeing doesn't blur unpleasant scenes. One still continues to see distinctions, warts and all. On the other hand, a greater objectivity can develop, because "in this clear seeing, there is no rush to judgment."[1] Research worldwide is starting to clarify both how greater degrees of mental clarity can evolve and how the older biased judgments and concepts that we had attached to scenes can be softened, suspended, or dissolved.

Our visual percepts arrive with varying degrees of clarity. Our visual judgments also come in shades of gray, not all in black and white. Mark Christensen and colleagues in Copenhagen studied these gradations.[2] Aided by fMRI, they monitored 13 normal subjects whose task it was to glimpse very simple line drawings. These were flashed briefly on a screen.

- Which particular set of three images did these Danish researchers use? The set would have elicited a smile—if not a roaring belly laugh—from Zen Master Sengai. Two centuries earlier in Japan, his fluid brushstrokes had rendered the very same symbols:

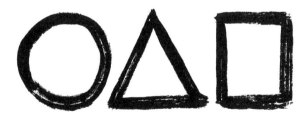

Given Sengai's sense of humor, which cryptic meanings had he encoded in this classic example of calligraphy? [ZB:414]. Generations thereafter have speculated at great length [ZBR:593]. No subjects in Copenhagen had this luxury. They had only a mere 33 to 100 ms to glimpse just one of these three potential images. These few milliseconds make the point: much of our so-called attention is *pre*attentive, reflexive, too fast for thought.

The subjects also had to make more than one decision while each image flashed past. Was this image (1) perfectly clear? Or, (2), perceived only vaguely? Or, (3), not perceived at all? To specify which perceptual choice they had selected, they then pressed a button with one of three fingers on the right hand.

- How clearly did their consciousness register each option? Clarity was not simply present or absent. Their conscious responses were *graded*. Moreover, linked with this spectrum of subjective clarity was a widely distributed network of fMRI signals. The posterior intraparietal sulcus (pIPSUL) and the fusiform gyrus (FG) were among the leading cortical regions that contributed to increasingly clear perception. These dorsal parietal lobe (pIPSUL) and ventral temporal lobe (FG) sites are crucial to the themes discussed in these pages. Check figures 1 and 2 to be sure you are clear where they are.

In Paris, Stanislas Dehaene and colleagues were reviewing related issues.[3] They adopted a three-level perspective. They suggested that when a visual stimulus first enters from the outside world, it would register at some lower levels, but only (1) *subliminally*. Next, its message might relay farther up, say, to some intermediate levels in the thalamus (a deep subcortical region shown later in figure 6). In the thalamus, the message may (or may not yet) become fully accessible for (2) *preconscious processing*. However, they too concluded that (3) *full consciousness* has no final access to the whole message, nor can it be *reported* verbally, until several more *recurrent* steps provide feedback *after* the next sequence carries the early impulses up to still higher, cortical levels.

- What do the French authors believe we require to achieve this full spectrum of conscious perception? First, a strong, adequate stimulus whose messages rise from the "bottom up." Next, an activation that reaches the higher levels of association cortex. Finally, that further amplification of attention which develops only after recurrent "top-down" messages descend from these same parietal, prefrontal, and anterior cingulate regions.

Koch and Tsuchiya, in Pasadena, California, take a different tack.[4] They point out that we can use preconscious processing to apprehend the *gist* of an entire scene in only 30 ms. Gist predictions occur much too quickly to be explained by the higher layers of our usual top-down attention. Moreover, even when subjects already fix their top-down attention selectively on a central task, they can still distinguish whether a brief secondary stimulus—a simple image glimpsed only in a flash out in the periphery—is the image of an elephant, or of a male or female face.

Gist mechanisms that serve the "objective" awareness of our phenomenal consciousness can detect fearful-face targets in as little as 17 ms. A more "subjective awareness" can yield discriminating impressions even though we glimpse the target for a mere 33 ms[5] [ZBR:379–380].

To Summarize

In the early milliseconds of the brain's preattentive responses, some perceptions arrive with surprising clarity. This perceptual clarity resembles insight, in the sense that it seems too fast and effortless to be accomplished by our ordinary processes of thought. Do some involuntary forms of "no-thought" attention normally exist that can be cultivated during long-term meditative training?

7

Network Systems Serving Different Forms of Attention

> We identify a bilateral dorsal attention system and a right-lateralized ventral attention system solely on the basis of spontaneous activity.
>
> Michael Fox and colleagues[1]

Imagine that you're famished. Then, nearby, you glimpse a round, red, shiny object. Your immediate impression: a red *apple*! Inside that first second, you guessed it was also ripe enough to eat. Attention is pivotal in shaping such "simple" decisions.

"Paying" close attention is more effortful than is allowing awareness to "open up." How do we either "pay" close attention narrowly or "open up" awareness more diffusely to these outside stimuli? Two simpler terms accurately describe the two ways. One way proceeds from the top down. It operates in a manner more intentional and voluntary. The other way is a bottom-up form. Its responses are more reflexive, automatic, subconscious.

The earlier chapters provided examples of how event-related potential (ERP) techniques, position emission tomography (PET) scans, and fMRI scans detect the ways the attentive brain responds to a wide variety of standardized external stimuli. In June 2006, Michael Fox and colleagues published another in the series of major articles from the group at Washington University in St. Louis. The report began with a cogent review of the lines of evidence that had led neuroscientists to recognize that our brain pays attention to outside stimuli in these two fundamentally different ways.

- In general, does some larger network of attention response systems interconnect several local regions? Yes. These larger attentional systems extend over the brain's convex *outer* cortical surface. Note how different this *lateral* distribution is (figure 3) when compared with the more *medial* distribution of the brain's most metabolically active regions. Their separate discussion is deferred to part III (see figure 5).

- What do these mostly lateral attention systems accomplish? At least four things, seamlessly:

  1. Some stay ready, on standby alert, to detect salient stimuli that can arrive, unexpectedly, from anywhere in the *external* environment.
  2. Some help us deliberately engage our attention *selectively* on the most relevant visual, auditory, and touch stimuli.
  3. Some then help us stay focused "on target," despite irrelevant distractions.
  4. Some are also poised to jog our memory, reminding us to return to the immediate task even though we keep drifting away from it.

- These several attributes of the larger attention system are distributed within the circuitry of its two major subdivisions. The purpose of table 4 is to summarize the two sets of their different responses.

  1. The *dorsal* attention network. The dorsal system is attuned to respond to prior external sensory *cues*. Please notice that it is represented equally on the right and on the left side of our brain. Each side has a particular preference: it is prepared to *search* the *opposite* side of its environment for further information. This *contra*lateral bias of its attention illustrates one meaning of the word "lateralized."

     Moreover, each side of this dorsal system reacts to these cues in a manner that is more top-down, voluntary, and intentional. Subtle cues alert us to tap into our higher-order functions, the kinds that we might draw on when we'd like to redirect our intentional responses more intelligently. Thus, one such prior cue might hint *where* this next stimulus might soon appear. Another might suggest *when* it might arrive, or perhaps even *what* this stimulus might actually be. Key modules in this dorsal system are the intraparietal sulcus (IPS) in its posterior part (pIPSUL) and the frontal eye fields (FEF). In a sense, these dorsal system functions might seem analogous to those of the cursor whose movements you control on the computer screen by the deliberate ways you decide to move the mouse by hand. You learned from long practice how to delegate these choices. They are now second nature. Long-term meditative practice develops similar habitual skills, often unstated, that evolve toward more efficient and effortless modes of top-down scanning.

  2. The *ventral* attention network. In contrast, this system is represented *mostly on the right side*. It is strongly "stimulus-driven." This means that it orients automatically to an external stimulus, especially when that stimulus seems

Table 4
Representations and Responses of the Dorsal and Ventral Attention Systems[a]

	Dorsal Attention System	Ventral Attention System
Anatomical Representation	Symmetrical, on both sides	Right-sided predominantly
Responds attentively to	Opposite side of the environment	Both sides of the environment, L > R
Modes of orienting	More "top-down," voluntary, and intentional	Strongly "stimulus-driven"; reflexive, automatic, "bottom-up"
Fluctuates spontaneously	Yes	Yes
Major modules	Intraparietal sulcus (IPS) Frontal eye field region (FEF)	Right temporoparietal junction (TPJ) Right ventrolateral frontal cortex (VFC)
Responds most actively to	Prior cues denoting "what-where-when"	Salient task-relevant targets in unexpected locations; fresh needs to disengage attention and to reorient it
Allied regions include	Supplementary motor cortex; area MT +	Angular gyrus (ANG)
"Executive overlap" that can integrate the two systems	Right prefrontal cortex; in the middle and inferior frontal gyrus (lesions here cause patients to be distractible and to perseverate)	

Adapted from M. Fox, M. Corbetta, A. Snyder, et al. Spontaneous neuronal activity distinguishes human dorsal and ventral attention systems. *Proceedings of the National Academy of Sciences U.S.A.* 2006; 103:10046–10051.
[a]The representations of these two attention systems are defined here by their *spontaneous*, intrinsic activity. The subjects are resting passively. Their eyes are either open and looking at a crosshair, are open in dim light, or are closed. No task is superimposed; no stimuli are being added.

significant, when it changes suddenly, or appears in an unexpected location. Its key modules are lower down: in the *right* temporoparietal junction (TPJ) and the *right* ventrolateral frontal cortex (VFC) (chapter 5). "Tight" programs determine its bottom-up styles of operation. In a sense, they operate in a manner comparable with that other cursor on your word processor. With no effort on your part, its programming enables it to drop down and return instantly to the left margin as soon as words run out of space at the end of the line on the right.

Neurologists have long observed that damage to one side of the brain caused their patients to neglect the opposite side of space and of their own body. Often, the results were not symmetrical. Right brain damage caused a more severe degree of inattention off to the patient's *left* side than did equivalent structural damage over on the left side of the brain. Why? One obvious explanation for this asymmetrical *clinical* neglect is this much stronger, predominantly *right*-sided *anatomical* lateralization of the ventral subdivision. In fact, this major right-sided anatomical representation and physiological predominance is the reason why the right side of the brain was selected to display, in figure 3, the intrinsic topography of this ventral attention network (see figure 3). Yet, even so, most circuits issuing from this right side still cross over the midline to connect with allied regions in the left hemisphere. This means that their total *physiological* reach enables them to attend also to the right side of our environment, not only to the left.

- What does the temporoparietal junction accomplish? A region this large has multiple over lapping functions. The right TPJ plays key roles in the way relevant stimuli drive the ventral network. When the dorsal voluntary network is already engaged, it acts as a "circuit breaker." This means that it disengages attention and enables it to shift toward the new, salient stimulus.[2]
- How do we normally harness our two big subdivisions in order to distribute multiple attentional skills appropriately within the whole, wide global scene? The collective fMRI evidence suggests that we often use the two yellow regions in the *right* frontal lobe—the inferior frontal gyrus (iFG) and the middle frontal gyrus (MFG)—to coordinate the two functional systems. We can choose which of the several styles of attentive focusing we need to engage, sustain, and readily update, with the aid of these and related high-level, flexible "executive" influences (chapter 5).

Serences and Yantis, at Johns Hopkins in Baltimore, report that one other small region becomes activated when we choose to shift and engage attention for a variety of more abstract, top-down reasons.[3] Figure 2 places this small region high on top of the medial superior parietal lobule (msPLB) on both sides of the midline.

Clearly, meditators have options to exercise a full range of these attentional attributes, because they are both practicing, learning, forgetting, relearning, and remembering to keep on training attention [ZBR:29–40, 61, 179–183].

Attending to "Real-Life" Complexities

You have probably noticed that researchers have been resorting to artificial stimuli in order to prompt most of the responses surveyed thus far. Objection: These responses in the laboratory are too far removed from our "real-life" situations. What bearing do such experiments have on the real-life, gritty events that we all (meditators included) must confront in daily life?

Golland, Malach, and colleagues report an alternative research approach.[4] The fact that this team at the Weizmann Institute in Israel chose a particular

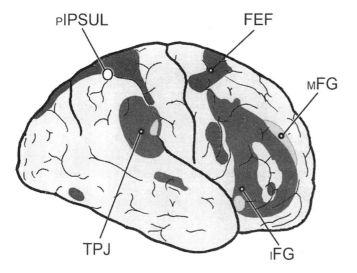

Figure 3   Lateral view of the right hemisphere
In this view, the frontal lobe is positioned on the viewer's right. The right hemisphere was chosen because the ventral ("bottom-up") subdivision of the attention system (shown in a shade of red) is distributed chiefly over the brain's right outer surface. In contrast, the dorsal ("top-down") subdivision (shown in blue) has an almost bilaterally symmetrical distribution. Both systems have only minimal medial representations (those of the ventral subdivision being represented superiorly only on the right side.) Note the two areas of overlap shown, in yellow, in the right inferior and middle frontal region. They may help coordinate the two subdivisions in ways that serve our global needs to pay attention to events on both sides of the environment.

Starting in the right frontal lobe: IFG, inferior frontal gyrus; MFG, middle frontal gyrus; FEF, frontal eye field; PIPSUL, posterior intraparietal sulcus; TPJ, temporoparietal junction (see similar distributions in figure 1). The unlabled red area in the temporal lobe is in a more anterior portion of the superior temporal sulcus (STS). The unlabled blue oval at the bottom left is in the posterior part of the middle temporal area (MTA). Its actual position is in the middle temporal gyrus, a site more superior than illustrations often suggest.

The topographical patterns represented here in schematic form are part of a larger attention network. Its fMRI signals not only increase quickly in response to conventional tasks, they also undergo slow spontaneous, coherent fluctuations of comparable amplitude. Accordingly, the figure is freely adapted both from the text and from figure 5 in M. Fox, M. Corbetta, A. Snyder, et al. Spontaneous neuronal activity distinguishes human dorsal and ventral attention systems. *Proceedings of the National Academy of Sciences U.S.A.* 2006; 103:10046–10051. See plate 1 for the color version of this figure.

Western movie to deliver "virtual reality" stimuli is an interesting sociological commentary. Their subjects viewed several dramatic 15-minute segments of the film *The Good, the Bad, and the Ugly*. A passive rest condition served as a control, during which the subjects closed their eyes for ten minutes.

- What happened during this "naturalistic" audiovisual stimulation? It prompted a conventional pattern of increased fMRI signals. They arose from "task-positive" responsive regions of cortex. Indeed, these responses were similar in many respects to the anticipations of that large *lateral* attention network just described above. As might be expected when viewing such a movie, this "extrinsic" network also included other visual regions: parts of the fusiform gyrus (FG) which respond to different faces, portions of the parahippocampal gyrus (PHGY) which respond to different places, and some nearby visual processing regions in the inferior occipital cortex as well (see figure 2).

- Did anything else occur? Yes. It was almost as though another system in the brain stayed casually indifferent to the mayhem being shown in this "spaghetti Western" film. In fact, other regions continued to pursue their own distinct pattern of *spontaneous* activity, much as they had during the separate eyes-closed resting control period. Which other regions? They were connected into an "intrinsic," largely *medial frontoparietal* network. As part III will explain, these *intrinsic* regions remained essentially *de*coupled from the brisk responses of the lateral attention network.

Commentary

This survey of recent research carries practical implications for readers interested in their own long-term approach to meditation and to alternate states of consciousness.

- Our brain normally engages a repertoire of top-down and bottom-up attention functions. Their operations maintain our immediate preattentive processing "online." They confer both focus and flexibility on our various resources of attention.
- Masters Ikkyu and Daito emphasized simple messages for their trainees: remember to exercise, mindfully, your many attentive functions as often as you can. They are mutually reinforcing.
- A corollary principle for everyone: allow your natural, automatic, attentional recovery functions to evolve spontaneously, nonjudgmentally.

What benefits come when you develop a variety of more proficient attentive skills?

8

The Implications of Training More Efficient Attentional Processing

> A focal state of attention is an emergent property of the whole system of attention, with no sharp divide between preattentive and attentive phases.
>
> S. Shipp[1]

Novices engage top-down levels of willfully supervised intention, whether it's their first try at chopsticks or at riding a bike. Later—after novice meditators make attentive practice a regular part of their daily meditative training—habitual responses evolve that become increasingly involuntary. More proficient meditators will delegate their attention toward automatic mechanisms and bottom-up physiological functions that arise nearer to the early, *pre*attentive core of mindfulness (see table 4). [ZB:278–281].

Preattentive Processing

What does *pre*attentive mean? Suppose you are now looking at a separate sheet of paper. Covering its whole surface are several printed letters of the alphabet. Most letters have straight lines. They are either green **X**s or brown **T**s. Scattered among them is a rare letter that curves. It is an **S**. You're not trying to think about an **S**. You don't care whether it's green or brown. Yet, instantly, each rare **S** "pops out" from this mixture. This *pop-out* process happens automatically. There's no charge for this **S**; you don't have to "pay" attention to it. It arrives courtesy of your normal preattentive mechanisms. They operate reflexly, in less than one twentieth of a second. Aided by parallel distributed processing and by an effortless processing capacity that seems almost unlimited, these hawk-eyed scanning mechanisms first encompass a very large field, then swoop down to grasp their target. Even so, further training can sharpen one's usual keen preattentive processing skills.

Recent Studies of the Pop-out Phenomenon

Sensitive MEG techniques have recently monitored the ordinary kinds of pop-out phenomena.[2] In adult human subjects, two mechanisms converge: (1) one response highlights just *this*, the focal point of visual attention; (2) this central response is suppressed throughout the adjacent zone that surrounds it. The net effect of this surrounding valley of inhibition is to heighten the epicenter and to emphasize its sharp central peak of excitability. Infants have an acute, well-developed pop-out phenomenon when they are only 3 months old,[3] further evidence of its intrinsic significance.

Many preattentive pop-out mechanisms are attributable to the pulvinar of the thalamus (see figure 6). [ZBR:175–176]. Once the pulvinar receives important messages from the superior colliculus directly and/or on their "fast track" relay via the lateral geniculate system, it forwards them instantly in to-and-fro interactions that sweep through the dorsal and ventral attention networks.[4] Why are the impulses that the pulvinar forwards through the ventral visual pathway such an essential part of this circuitry? (See also figures 4, 5, and 6.) Because these messages integrate the vital survival functions of the colliculi, the ventral pulvinar, and the primary visual cortex (BA 17) with those of the temporal lobe as far forward as its temporal pole (BA 38).

With respect to the inherent speed of subcortical processing, it is noteworthy that the most recent sensitive MEG techniques can now detect the first responses to fearful faces in the hypothalamus and thalamus a mere 15 ms after the face stimulus arrives, and show that some of the next relays arrive in the amygdala at only 25 ms![5] (chapter 52).

Potential Implications of Prolonged, Fast Processing

We usually think that the pop-out phenomenon is only a small, immediate event. Its "pop" is obviously self-limited in time. Its "out" seems restricted to one small target (like an **S**) in our visual field. Yet these intrinsic qualities merit a closer examination. After the pop-out phenomenon achieves its first, quick, overall scan, what creates that almost "tunnel vision–like" effect which sharply constricts its attentive field to one small spot occupied by the **S**? Inhibitory circuits at several levels normally provide ample spatial constraints on such visual processing.

But let us now suppose that a major physiological shift were to bypass the *dorsal* pulvinar. Suppose that the shift suspended any such constraints on the scope of the visual field. Now, the usual automatic properties intrinsic to a *preattentive* operation could become extended both in time and space. One can envision the resulting mental field opening wide, effortlessly unleashing parallel, distributed functions that seem of almost unlimited capacity. Part III will postulate that this combination of events might happen in the extraordinary state called kensho in Zen.

A major attribute of kensho is the *extended stability* of its sequences of enhanced visual processing. When these sequences are fully engaged during a substantial surge (prolonged for several seconds, not for an instant), novel, dynamic qualities can be infused. Such a moment has now been transformed into an *allocentric state of consciousness*. This state—led by preattentive mechanisms and prolonged by more openly attentive training—becomes even more impressive when it resonates with other meaningful associations flowing through the ventral visual pathway. For these reasons, the pulvinar's normal pivotal role in assigning instant salience will prove crucial as we continue to search in parts III and IV for the sources of kensho's quick, effortless, comprehensive grasp.

Meanwhile, why is it important to appreciate the fact that most sudden awakenings into kensho do *not* happen while one is seated in formal meditation?

Paying Mindful Attention: The Advantages of Extended Years of Practice

What is Zen practice in daily life? It is an attitude toward consciousness that employs a mindful introspective mode of attention to address the here and now on the long Path toward selfless insight-wisdom. This practice is not limited to a Sunday morning service once a week or to a short daily prayer. Living Zen continues off the cushion and continues to attend *actively*, acutely, objectively to each daily life event as it unfolds from one present moment to the next. As their practice ripens, experienced trainees tend to arrive at a calm clarity that helps to sponsor greater degrees of an ever-present, implicit mindful awareness. Could this make it any more likely that a "peak experience" will be more likely to happen when they further hone their attentional skills during a retreat?

Never easy to untangle and single out are all the mechanisms of brain plasticity that become embedded in such complex, longitudinal events. Meanwhile, several testable hypotheses are plausible: First, that training one's regular mindful attention sharpens a wide range of more *enduring* attentive skills, receptive as well as concentrative. Second, that some of their subtle physiological mechanisms—only a few of which are now known—are relevant to the sensitivities that enable triggers to prompt kensho's long-delayed arrival. Third, that several basic mechanisms of attention related both to circuit-breaking and stability could also facilitate the reactive shift toward an unusually prolonged, preattentive-like mode of enhanced allocentric processing. Interesting preliminary reports relating to such theories are arriving, based on serial, semilongitudinal measurements of a variety of meditators' attentive skills. To begin with four brief examples:

- Some long-term meditators report that they are starting to notice a relatively continuous state of 24-hour, "ever-present awareness." EEG measurements document this subjective impression [ZBR:184–187, 234–239]. The physiological implications of such an ever-present awareness are profound. They point to a subtle change in brain function: to a level and degree of ripened attentiveness that has evolved far beyond its explicit beginnings in the novice toward a more *implicit* form of ongoing, involuntary awareness. It will be of great interest to determine its other behavioral, ERP, and neuroimaging correlates. It is time to test the working hypothesis that bottom-up processing contributes attentional resources to ever-present awareness, and also to see if its refined form is comparable with that 360 degree expanded circumspatial awareness implied in the Japanese phrase *happo biraki*. It means "open on all sides" [ZB:496, 672].

- Our perceptual threshold for a barely conscious awareness can be detected. As cited in chapter 4, one way to do so is to use ERP to measure the early visual awareness negativity that peaks 200 to 300 ms after a visual stimulus [ZBR:185, 190–191].

- Another way to test attentiveness is to measure an increased processing *efficiency* that can follow meditative training. This enhanced efficiency is indexed during the entire "attentional blink" phenomenon. As discussed in chapter 1, this approach measures the P3B potential response to the first presentation of a visual target. It then compares it with the response to a second stimulus that follows it some 300 to 600 ms later.[6]

- Brefczynski-Lewis and colleagues at the University of Wisconsin recently studied long-term Buddhist meditators.[7] Their subjects' impressive hours of practice fell into two clusters. Experts in one of these two groups had each averaged an estimated 19,000 *total* hours of prior practice. (Calculations would translate this figure into the equivalent of some 2.2 *years* of continual meditative practice!) Those experts who were most experienced had each practiced for an estimated 44,000 hours (this figure would be equivalent to 5 *years* of continual meditative practice!) The most experienced meditators showed an "increased processing efficiency." When these virtuosos first shifted into each period of concentration meditation, they displayed a shorter "meditation start-up" increase in their initial fMRI responses. In contrast, the less experienced experts tended to have a more sustained but lesser total response.

Commentary

Our culture does not encourage such heroic levels of Olympian training. It is hard to retrain one's attention after many early years of habitual, mindless multitasking. It takes commitment. Whereas self-reports and anecdotal observations suggest that years of training in a monastic context make it more likely that "peak experiences" will then happen, statistical scientific proof has not yet been forthcoming.

Meanwhile, consider some crucial hypotheses that remain to be tested rigorously. Do *longitudinal* studies show that *individual* meditators are gradually transformed, both psychologically and physiologically, over the decades? Do they develop such changes as faster response times and gradually increasing processing efficiencies, in parallel with increases in sensitivity and responsivity (documented by ERP and MEG studies)? Do meditative trainees reveal increases and decreases in signals and certain network connectivities (as shown by fMRI scans), together with corresponding patterns of appropriate *decreases and increases* in metabolism that are detectable in PET scans? We turn next to recent short-term studies in meditators, both of novices and experts, that begin to address these key issues.

9

Studying Meditators' Brains

> Considering the diversity of meditation techniques, there is no simple answer to the question "What is being trained while meditating?"
>
> Hölzel, Ott, Hempel, et al.[1]

Earlier chapters have explained why it is difficult to isolate and understand all of the mechanisms underlying meditation. However, the discussions also offered one simplified answer to the question above: meditation trains both our top-down and bottom-up forms of attention. Confirming this view is the recent report by Jha and her colleagues at the University of Pennsylvania. They conducted an excellent behavioral study of how *prior* meditation had affected three different indices of attention.[2] Using standardized visual and spatial tasks on computer screens, they tested the reaction times and accuracies of three contrasting groups of subjects:

1. Seventeen advanced meditators (averaging 34 years of age and 5 years of prior meditative practice), both before and after their 30-day formal retreat. During this retreat, conducted mostly in silence, the meditators engaged in a concentrative/receptive form of meditation for 10 to 12 hours each day.

2. Seventeen naive MBSR students (averaging 24 years of age), both before and after their 8-week course of mindfulness-based stress-reduction training.

3. Seventeen controls who had not meditated before (averaging 22 years of age.)

Each subject's task was to respond to random sets of visuospatial problems presented on a computer screen. The subjects responded using the index finger of each hand. The task procedure included a central fixation point in the back-ground, various visual cues, and a line of five target arrows. The middle arrow (third in line) was the key: Was it pointing toward the left or toward the right?

Each problem set was designed to test for a particular category of attention. Table 5 summarizes the behavioral results both in relation to the three different subsystems of attention that were being tested for, and in the context of the two major forms of meditation that the subjects had been practicing.

Table 5
Relationships between Different Types of Attention and the Major Forms of Meditation

	The Dorsal Attention System for Top-Down Attention	The Ventral Attention System for Bottom-Up Attention
Anatomical representation (figure 3)	Symmetrical, mostly bifronto-parietal	Chiefly right frontal-parietal-temporal
Physiological orientation (table 3)	Each side responds to the opposite side of the environment	The right side attends to the right and left sides of the environment
Type of attentional activity (table 3)	More "executive" (voluntary, purposeful, higher-level)	More driven by stimuli to serve alerting needs ("watchful")
Implications for the form of meditation[a]	More involved during focused, concentrative meditation practices	More involved during openly receptive meditation practices
Three subsystems of attention	1. *Response* systems directed toward monitoring conflicting data, disregarding irrelevancy, and guiding relevant responses (e.g., PFC, anterior cingulate gyrus) 2. *Orienting* systems that help select sensory input; "tuning" at the level of perception (e.g., PIPSUL, FEF)	3. *Alerting systems*, ready and waiting to detect unknown stimuli from anywhere that have not yet arrived (e.g., right TPJ, VFC)

PFC, prefrontal cortex; TPJ, temporoparietal junction; VFC, ventral-frontal cortex; PIPSUL, posterior intra-parietal sulcus; FEF, frontal eye field.
Adapted from A. Jha, J. Krompinger, and M. Baime. Mindfulness training modifies subsystems of attention. *Cognitive, Affective, and Behavioral Neuroscience* 2007; 7:109–119.
[a] See also table 2 in ZBR, page 30.

Three findings were intriguing. Please note that the first two correlate with certain *top-down* attentional processing skills.

1. The advanced meditators already began, at *baseline*, with better performance skills referable to *their response systems*. These skills are revealed during tests that measure the person's ability to monitor conflicting information.

2. *After* their 8-week course, the MBSR participants showed improved performance skills referable to their *orienting systems*. These are the skills that fine-tune one's attention at an earlier, *perceptual* level.

The third finding correlated with *bottom-up* attentional processing skills. These are the skills that are expressed during a bare awareness that remains *open and alert to respond* to any stimulus (see table 1)

3. The advanced meditators appeared more skillful—*after* their retreat—in the performance of their *alerting systems*. They detected events efficiently and needed

no prior alerting cues to direct them either to the place or to the time when the next targets would appear.

Immediately prior meditation (whether it had continued for 30 days or 8 weeks) did not improve the subjects' (top-down) attentional performance skills in monitoring and responding to conflicting data. However, it deserves emphasis that the 30-day retreat did appear to enhance the advanced meditators' *bottom-up* receptive category of attentional skills. Indeed, both their shorter reaction times and greater accuracy confirmed that these meditators had improved their *alerting* performance skills. It is tempting to consider that highly intensive, concentrative meditation, being difficult to maintain for long periods, may evolve spontaneously toward the more subtle receptive forms of meditation, as suggested in the data.

Neuroimaging Studies of Meditating Brains

Brefczynski-Lewis and colleagues monitored expert meditators and controls with fMRI *while they were actually practicing* a one-pointed form of concentrative meditation.[3] Their 14 experts (average age 47) were recruited from two schools in the Tibetan Buddhist tradition. (The review by Lutz and colleagues clarifies the complex theoretical and practical aspects of various styles of Buddhist meditation.)[4]

All subjects were looking at a small dot on a gray screen. They were engaged either in a focused state of concentrative meditation (averaging 2.7 minutes in length), *or* a relaxed state of "neutral mind" (averaging 1.6 minutes in duration). During these few minutes of concentration meditation, the experts developed widespread increased activation within multiple attentional systems and allied regions. The experts who had longer durations of practice experience showed *lesser* degrees of fMRI signals in their amygdala, medial frontal gyrus, and nucleus accumbens when exposed to distracting sounds.

The most recent fMRI study by Lutz and this Wisconsin team monitored 15 expert Buddhist meditators and 15 novices while they practiced a self-induced form of loving-kindness-compassion meditation.[5] All subjects showed stronger responses to emotional sounds in their anterior insula and anterior cingulate cortex while meditating than during the resting condition. While this particular style of Tibetan meditation also influenced other cortical regions, the experts (10,000 to 50,000 hours of practice) responded to sounds with greater activation of their right temporo-parietal junction (TPJ) and the right posterior superior temporal sulcus (PSTSUL) (see figure 1).

These activations were interpreted as reflecting both the experts' greater capacities to share in another person's emotions and to adopt an intuitive perspective about another person's mental status in general (see table 14). Noteworthy was the experts' greater activation of the right inferior frontal gyrus (iFG). This was consistent with their enhanced sensitivities to unexpected, behaviorally relevant stimuli.

With specific reference to the red regions in figure 3, one observes that these right lateralized functions are in keeping with the emerging hypothesis that long-term meditative training can have a greater influence on the plasticity of the kinds of bottom-up networking that are represented within the lower, ventral subdivision of the attention system (table 4).

It is not a simple matter to design a neuroimaging study of meditation that will satisfy all critics [ZBR:214, 226]. Hölzel and colleagues in Germany recently reported a study of 15 Vipassana meditators, averaging 34 years of age.[6] Their prior meditative experience, while distributed over an interval that averaged almost 8 years, was less than in the two just cited reports based on Tibetan styles. During fMRI monitoring, these German subjects were expected to perform a substantial number of tasks: mental arithmetic, button pressing for correct answers, and button pressing at every first sensation they encountered when they inhaled. The meditators developed increased signals in the anterior cingulate gyrus and dorsal medial prefrontal cortex on both sides, in contrast to controls.

Because the meditation phases were limited to one minute, the meditators did not have sufficient time to reach a deeper meditative state. In addition, the button press–inhaling condition led to their reporting "very diverse subjective experiences." The authors contrasted their results with those in the study by Brefczynski-Lewis et al. (just discussed), in which the more expert meditators had actually shown *less* anterior cingulate activation than did their novice controls. Included among the several interpretations of factors responsible for divergent data is the possibility that when meditators perform complex tasks their internal or external pressures to excel could be reflected in greater anterior cingulate and frontal responses [ZBR:217–218].

Favorable Behavioral Results in Novices of Five Days of Integrated Meditative Training

Tang and colleagues studied the behavioral responses of two groups of undergraduates at a technical university in China.[7] One group of 40 attended a course of "integrative body-mind training (IBMT)." It began with a brief instruction in "mind setting." This approach deemphasized their efforts to control thoughts. Instead, the subjects' alertness was cultivated by listening to instructions on a compact disk that focused on high degrees of awareness of their body and their breathing. Training in a group setting for twenty minutes a day over a five-day period was supplemented by dialogue with a skillful coach. While the 40 controls had the same number of training sessions, their compact disk instructions were limited to the relaxation of body parts.

Subsequent tests indicated that the IBMT subjects showed enhanced positive moods and reduced negative moods. They also had improved significantly on their executive-type responses to conflicting information on the attention network test (see table 5). After undergoing the stress of mental arithmetic, plus one extra session of 20 minutes' training, they also showed significantly lower salivary cortisol levels and higher levels of salivary immunoglobulin A.

These short-term results again suggest that our top-down skills of attentional focusing are relatively easier to acquire. The evidence reinforces the conclusions from the text and table 5 that advanced meditators may slowly be developing more "opening up" meditative styles and engaging in a range of subtle, global, more bottom-up receptive practices.

Commentary

Different research groups are studying distinct forms of meditation, using different performance tasks and dissimilar techniques. The assigned tasks themselves add significant voluntary complexities to how each experiment can be interpreted. The old Chinese phrase *wu-wei* carries a crucial legacy of meaning into Zen meditative practice [ZB:607; ZBR:361]. It implies an advanced *unselfconscious* level of behavior. Behavior has become so efficient that *no sense remains* of "trying too hard," because all action has now become *selfless*.

It would seem worthwhile for investigators to extend their studies toward the more spontaneous, *non*–task-induced changes that develop *after* the initial phase of concentration yields to the more openly receptive phase of each meditative session. Why? For at least two reasons. First, because this would more closely correspond with the way one's experience naturally unfolds on the meditation cushion. And second, because a phase of no-thinking arises sooner or later, and this long moment of non–self-conscious *mental silence in clear awareness* corresponds more closely with the psychological concept of an authentic "baseline." Long sought in neuroimaging research, it can ripen into experiential reality during periods of increasingly silent illumination on the long Path of Zen.

10

Inward Turned Attention: Induced Experiences

> The main limitation of this study was the fact that subjects were asked to remember and relive a mystical experience rather than actually try to achieve one.
>
> M. Beauregard and V. Paquette[1]

Attention is flexible. We can direct it outwardly, to focus on objects. We can also direct attention internally, to explore an abstract concept, to focus on a memory of an actual previous personal experience, or even on some object that we can vividly reimage in "the mind's eye." One practice in Zen is to concentrate attention on an enigmatic statement called a koan. While the content of such a koan is quite obscure, its form can serve as a recurrent focus for the practitioner's undivided attention of the moment [ZB:110–119; ZBR:61–63].

It is traditional in Zen to regard minor "openings" or even "peak experiences" as nothing special. Zen trainees are advised to *let go* of "their" experiences of enlightenment and not to view them as attainments that were "achieved." Yet, the many differing traditions prefer their own ways to meditate, and to interpret the various experiences that occur.

Alternative Ways of Meditating

Within the Catholic contemplative orders, the Carmelites have developed a special interest in mystical experiences. Beauregard and Paquette monitored 15 Carmelite nuns with fMRI during three conditions: "mystical," "control," and baseline. In this study, it is important to note that the "mystical" condition was based on a *retrieved* memory. The nuns were asked to remember, and to *relive* (with their eyes closed), the most intense mystical experience they had ever undergone during their membership in the Carmelite order. Why did the researchers adopt this strategy? Because the nuns had made it clear to them, before the study began, that "God can't be summoned at will."

What other memory had the nuns volunteered to recall? During the control condition, their task was again to remember, and to relive (with eyes closed), that most intense union they had ever felt with another *human* being all during their affiliation with the Carmelite order. During the baseline condition, they entered a state of rest with their eyes closed. Each mystical and control period lasted five minutes. Afterward, the nuns rated how intense had been each of these two newly induced experiences, on a scale of 0 to 5. (They did not so rate their original experience.) A separate psychological rating scale was also employed. It contained 32 items that represented a standard mysticism scale. Qualitative interviews were also conducted. The authors are to be congratulated for including these three measures. Together, the data provide the kinds of subjective and objective documentation essential to interpret the neuroimaging results [ZBR:214–215].

The first-person reports were useful. They confirmed the nature of the relived states (both mystical and control) which the nuns had self-induced from memory. Neither of the retrieved states that were monitored with fMRI precisely reproduced the whole original episode that they had experienced previously. The self-reports also indicated that, during the control condition, they had successfully reexperienced a feeling of "unconditional love" for another person. The nuns rated the average intensity of *both* of these induced subjective experiences at about level 3. On the mysticism scale, responses to three high-scoring descriptive items stood out. They were: "I have had an experience in which something greater than myself seemed to absorb me." "I have experienced profound joy." "I have had an experience which I knew to be sacred."

The results of the study addressed the issue cited in the epigraph: what can we learn from contemplatives who are only *remembering* a previous, intense mystical experience? The fMRI data prove interesting. Let's begin with the control results. In this instance, the nuns' task was to remember an episode involving their *union* with another human being (unconditional human love). At this time, fMRI signals increased in the right and left superior parietal lobule, left caudate nucleus, right inferior orbital cortex, and left anterior cingulate cortex. (These comparisons are all made against the resting baseline data. Statistical formulas among these sites ["Z numbers"] varied over a narrow range, from 3.93 to 3.53, respectively). The superior parietal lobule increases could be associated with the nuns' stated intention of trying to merge the physical Self with another significant person during a period that lasted for five minutes.[2]

In contrast, when the data from the remembered "mystical" condition were compared with this "control" (human love) condition, fMRI signals were greater in the right medial orbitofrontal cortex, the left inferior parietal lobule, the right middle temporal cortex, the left superior parietal lobule, the right medial prefrontal cortex, and the right anterior cingulate cortex. (In this instance, the Z numbers ranged more widely, from 4.91 to 3.34, respectively.)

However, the most significant fMRI signal increases occurred when the remembered "mystical" condition was contrasted with the resting baseline. During these comparisons, the greatest signal increase occurred in the right medial orbitofrontal cortex. Next were increases in the right medial temporal cortex, the left and right inferior parietal lobules, the right superior parietal lobule, and the left caudate nucleus. (Now, the Z numbers ranged from 6.60 to 5.17, respectively.)

In this induced mystical/baseline contrast, the Z-score computed for the nuns' *right middle temporal cortex* was substantially greater (+2.45 more) than it was for this same region during the induced mystical/control contrast (6.24 vs. 3.79). This difference suggests that the right middle temporal cortex may have played a somewhat different role when the subjects remembered their mystical episode than when they remembered their union with another human being. In this respect, we recall that the nuns had estimated that the net, *overall* intensities of their two subjective experiences (mystical and control) had been at approximately the same quantitative level. Given these observations, it is tempting to relate the increased fMRI signals in their right middle temporal cortex with their personal reports either of "something greater than myself which seemed to absorb me," with "profound joy," or with the memory of a "sacred" experience.

In this study, the region of the middle temporal cortex corresponded with BA 21. In figures 1 and 4, note that this middle temporal *gyrus* occupies a lengthy region. It extends just below the superior temporal sulcus and just above the inferior temporal gyrus (BA 20). This region is not to be confused with the middle temporal *area* (area MTA).

During the mystical condition, signals also increased in the left caudate nucleus. This finding might represent some further elaboration of the feeling of love also reported during the control condition [ZBR:255–260]. The nuns' increased signals in the right medial orbitofrontal cortex during both the mystical and control conditions may be correlated with certain kinds of pleasant, satisfying positive associations that some other subjects report at times when this medial orbital region becomes active [ZBR:159–160].

Psalm 23 as an Object of Devotion

Religious sentiments can also be induced during the reading of a familiar text. The Twenty-third Psalm in the Old Testament expresses David's confidence in God's grace. It begins with the familiar line: The Lord is My Shepherd. I shall not want. A well-controlled study monitored six religious teachers of a fundamentalist Evangelical Christian community while they read this psalm, both silently and aloud.[3] All fundamentalist subjects were said to have had a previous "documented conversion experience." Their nonreligious controls were university students. For the purposes of this study, the term "religious experience" referred simply to the experiences that the subjects *induced in themselves* (and sustained during a PET scan) throughout this reading or recitation. PET scans showed that two right prefrontal activations occurred consistently during this particular religious condition: in the dorsal lateral (BA 9), and in the dorsal medial (BA 6) regions.

The authors concluded that the reading of the Twenty-third Psalm under these experimental conditions induced neither an emotional experience nor an arousal-like "happy" state. Instead, it appeared to be more comparable with a deliberate cognitive process. The subjects did rate their feelings (using an affect scale). However, no first-person description is provided that could enable readers to interpret the form and content of the subjects' actual experience in relation to the PET scan data. Lacking first-person reports, several explanations are possible for the right frontal preponderance of activation. One possibility reflects some expectations that the religious teachers themselves placed on their own cognitive/religious/devotional performance during this experiment. For example, if normal subjects try "too hard" on a task, and process "too many top-down instructions," fMRI signals increase in the right lateral frontal region and in the thalamus on both sides [ZBR:396].

Commentary

By definition, top-down attention occurs when a person intends to concentrate on an intense experience and tries to induce it voluntarily. Table 4 has outlined the fundamental distinctions that separate such Self-directed, Self-induced forms of deliberately voluntary attention from the bottom-up, reflexive, openly receptive forms.

As we now turn next to explore the origins of this Self in part II, a lingering question will surface: What kind of world could consciousness open up to, then not only receive but embrace, once attention is liberated from all maladaptive intrusive references to the pejorative Self?

11

First Mondo

> It may very well be that the question is the most basic form of Zen discourse, rather than pronouncements, proclamations, or statements.
>
> D. Wright[1]

Questions are essential in Zen. In Zen, a mondo is one such question asked and replied to. The reply can be far from the answer expected. Zen often uses short questions like "Who?" or "Why?" to probe the depths of existential issues.

While questions are essential in Zen, answers are hard to come by. That's okay, because a questioning mind doesn't *know* yet. The questioning mind remains uncertain. It can stay open for other options. Here, we will adopt the conventional question-and-answer format, using it to summarize and simplify issues discussed in the previous chapters.

You've spent many pages pointing out the functional anatomy of two systems of attention. What's the point?

The point is to realize the basic pointing role of attention. That *is* the point. Our top-down and bottom-up modes of attention serve as the salient vanguard for sensory processing and goal oriented behavior. Moreover, the way these dorsal and ventral systems of attention overlap the networks of our Self-referential and other referential processing have important functional implications for styles of meditation and states of consciousness.

Why is the right side of the brain specialized for attention, whereas the left side is specialized for language?

I don't know. Neurobiologists might hypothesize that some survival advantage was associated with distributing two such vital functions on separate sides. In this way, they (a) wouldn't interfere with each other locally, and (b) wouldn't both be lost during damage to one side, etc.

The bottom line is that our ventral attention system remains watchfully alert. It is quick to respond physiologically to salient stimuli arriving unexpectedly from *anywhere*, on either the right or left side of the distant environment. This attentiveness continues globally even though much of its bottom-up made of processing is represented anatomically in the lower cortical regions of the right cerebral hemisphere.

You've said that you're biased. Which biases would you like your readers to pay more attention to?

I've been impressed by how pivotal a role certain parts of the thalamus played in each alternate state episode that I've experienced. The first was an internal absorption; the second was a taste of kensho. True, each state did shift the foreground of attention in distinctive ways. Yet what each state *subtracted from my Self* was much more impressive than any other functions that it enhanced. In my experience, the long Path of Zen involves a "letting go." This means a deconditioning of the unfruitful aspects of the psyche accompanied by a gradual restructuring of the personality along lower profile, less Self-centered lines. This incremental reprogramming is adaptive. It enables the trainee to become increasingly simplified, stable, and more humane.

Why do stimuli "evoke" gamma waves early, and "induce" them later on?

Evoked is a word that refers to the way the brain's hard-wired, perceptual functions first respond to a stimulus, instantly and automatically. Some gamma wave activities become prominent early in this reflexive response. *Induced* refers to our softer-wired, more conceptual responses. These arise during the later milliseconds, when the brain is drawing on various other resources of its previous experience.

Part II

On the Origins of Self

To study the way of the Buddha is to study your own self.
To study your own self is to forget yourself.
To forget yourself is to have the objective world prevail in you.

Zen Master Dogen (1200–1253)

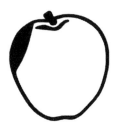

12

You Are the "Person of the Year"

What is the first business of the person who practices philosophy? To get rid of self-conceit.

Epictetus (c. 55–135 C.E.)[1]

One conceit (perhaps still lingering among a few self-anointed Brahmins) is that Boston is the hub of the Universe. Indeed, each person anywhere on the planet is hard-wired to perceive their own Self not just as a mere hub, but as the *whole physiological axis* around which the rest of the world turns [ZB:40–42]. Much of this arises from a simple fact: as soon as sensory impulses enter the brain from that other world, the sites representing our own sovereign physical Self are designed to receive highest priority.

Is each person really *that* important? Readers may doubt that their own physiology confers such a Self-anointed status. Yet, there *you* were—your very own face—on the cover of *Time* magazine. Your face was mirrored in the reflective Mylar of the magazine's final issue for 2006. The message was unmistakable, authoritative: *You* were the "Person of the Year," at the keyboard, in control of the information age.

Time had said so (though countless other candidates were deserving of this honor). By the close of 2006, it seemed obvious: individual persons had thoroughly transformed communication. Consider *Time*'s evidence: Now you can upload your personal video onto your own "easy, edgy" website. It is called YouTube. You can post your personal profile on MySpace, go public on Facebook.[2] You might not agree with so bold a choice, yet *Time* had put its weighty finger on the scales of a major tipping point in the cultural history of our planet.

"The consequences of it all," said *Time*, "are both hard to know and impossible to overestimate." To illustrate these consequences, the magazine then devoted some thirty-odd pages to an array of self-indulgent expressions.[3] In fairness, *Time* acknowledged that "you can waste hours" on such alluring websites, because everyone now could be an instant publisher and create his or her own "amateur hour." If cyberspace limited a person to only one hour of amateurish expression, the trend might not be so troubling. In fact, this new electronic age has outstripped our old Cro-Magnon, hard-wired cerebral capacities. In stealth, unwary "users" have been entrapped into compulsive habit patterns and addictive behaviors reminiscent of those once sponsored by the Japanese pachinko parlors and American slot machines [ZBR:251–255].

Time allotted to Brian Williams, of *NBC Nightly News*, the space on one page to redress the balance. Williams diagnosed, straightway, the dynamic force driving this ominous trend. It was our "celebration of self." He concluded that we had surpassed the excesses of our former "Me Generation." We had now become a self-engaged "User-Generated Generation."

As a physician, I've grown increasingly concerned about habit-forming tendencies that have infiltrated an already ailing society. As a student of Zen, I've seen consumerism invade Buddhism, further complicating the spiritual materialism to which our *I-Me-Mine* is susceptible. Electronic preoccupations consume large segments of our population. We sit in front of screens each day, not through just *one* amateur hour of trivia, but through endless hours that contribute to epidemic obesities, both physical and mental.

It was different in the distant past. When Buddhism entered a country, it usually had centuries to adapt to the prevailing indigenous culture. (Of course, this was all B.C.—*before computers*, before mind gyms, "virtual reality," full-scale consumerism, and habit-forming varieties of electronic expression.) Thus, when Buddhist influences entered China during the first millennium C.E., the early Ch'an meditation practices could evolve in contact with long-established Taoist cultural orientations. One of these was the deep appreciation that people had for the benefits of walking out of their houses into natural outdoor settings. It was a quiet, calming practice to be outside. It elevated one's angle of vision to look up past the hills and mountains into the open sky. It oriented one's attention *externally*, more *selflessly*. It celebrated the world of Nature, as *it* was, not the Self [ZB:644–667]. This ancient practice—paying close attention to each seemingly "ordinary" daily event, observing life as *it* unfolds naturally—continues to be the mindfulness-based activity that inspires a living Zen. It can have important physiological consequences (chapter 23).

No Mirrors

Notice, whenever a mirror beckons, how difficult it is to avoid becoming a candidate for one's own "person-of-the-year" honor? This tendency helps explain why "no mirrors" remains an established custom during meditative retreats at many Zen centers. The covering over of mirrors removes this temptation to indulge in mirror Self-worship, a further reinforcement of the Self-image to which all seem susceptible.

Of course, there's a lighter side to seeing one's own face mirrored on a *Time* magazine cover. Some readers quickly contacted *Time*, applauding this creative approach to its annual cover selection. By the subsequent issue, 110 respondents had already said that the cover was a brilliant move. Others, 106 of them, said that they humbly accepted the award. And 28 delighted souls announced a new intention. They planned to include this new "Person of the Year" award on their own resumé!

13

On the Nature and the Origins of the Self

> The fundamental delusion of humanity is to suppose that I am here (pointing to himself) and you are out there.
>
> Zen Master Hakuun Yasutani (1885–1973)

The plan during the rest of part II is to consider how our personal sense of the "I-Self" arises. After that, we examine how our sense of Self relates to that of the "other" world outside us. This discussion serves as the preamble to part III, where we will inquire: How could such a strong sense of personal identity evolve toward self*less*ness?

One Apple, Two Versions of Reality

In part I, we observed how events unfold when the brain directs attention to any object "out there." Take an apple as the object. In milliseconds, the eye translates that apple's raw photons into crude neuronal impulses. Back in the brain, our "mind's eye" quickly reifies these messages into our own subjective image of that apple. This version is inherently private. Although this synthesized image is based on appearances and personal guesses, we believe it represents "true" reality. We adopt it as "real."

Meanwhile—subconsciously—the brain has been busy reformulating not one, but *two different versions* of that one apple. First priority goes to its Self-centered version. Why do these egocentric circuits automatically assume such sovereign, possessive authority? Because long ago, we constructed our Self to be *the overriding* authority on reality. Simply as a teaching device to emphasize this point, these pages resort to the expedient of spelling this dominant, psychological version with a capital *S*.

You certainly remain free to resist such an interpretation of your own Self-important status. Yet, when I surveyed my old college dictionary recently, it contained over 400 entries for "self." Having started with "self-abandoned," the listings ended with "self-worship," four pages later. (In contrast, the word "other" received no such emphasis, although it did end with "otherworldly," after less than 3 inches of "other" entries.) The sequence of topics in this book might seem designed to follow an order that is the reverse of the way the dictionary lists such words. (For example, though we start here with aspects resembling "Self-worship," our text then moves in a direction toward "Self-abandoned.")

Now, back to the second version of that apple: Why is that version of reality so different? Because brains long ago set up a separate category of circuits. These circuits remain dedicated to the processing of any *external object*, like a fruit. Accordingly, this second version automatically identifies that apple as a separate object, and locates it *out there* in the environment. These "other" objects and things exist as separate entities *outside* of our body. Because we (and our dictionary) tend to value them less as objects than we value our own Self, the word "other" will remain un-capitalized until much later in part III.

Yes, we're returning to an old distinction. It splits subject from object. So ancient is this subject/object dichotomy that we often forget to ask why it exists. Yet, a century ago, the pioneering neurologist Hughlings Jackson (1835–1911) addressed this issue. Jackson employed two useful terms to illustrate the broad interface along which each personal "Self" (within) engages that objective, "other" world (out there). By choosing the phrase "subject consciousness" he was referring to the kind of processing which makes us personally aware of *ourself*. The contrasting term was "object consciousness." It referred to all processing that makes us aware of separate *objects*, as independent entities located in that world outside us.

We've now entered a new century. Why dwell on musty old phrases, words that serve only as substitutes for the tangible brain networks that create Self/other relationships? Because sharp distinctions between subjective and objective are both fundamental and useful. They help to untangle the dual mechanisms that underlie ordinary experience. For example, if you're selected for jury duty, it helps you to use this same subjective/objective distinction to separate the emotionalized impressions by one witness from the accurate perceptions of another witness that are dispassionate representations. It becomes useful to now specify two such distinct categories, because in later chapters their differences will help clarify how meditators can develop an *increasingly selfless mode of nondual experience* on their long path of meditative training.

Our Egocentric Point of View Is Self-Centered, Personal, and Subjective

Once that barrage of photons from an apple out there stimulates our retina, these messages rush straight back to that preeminent central configuration we reserve for our physical Self inside mental space. Indeed, each time we "see things from our standpoint," the midline of our own head and body automatically becomes that long axis back to which the coordinates of these external visual stimuli pointedly refer. We are the physiological terminus for all lines of sight that point back to our body.

This Self-centered mental posture was designed for action. Hard-wired, it was already off to a head start during infancy. Now, as an adult, we find our body leaning forward, hand and arm poised to return the hammerhead to that exact position in space where the nail awaits. During avoidance behaviors we lean back, to escape being hit by a low tree branch.

Whenever we need to focus on the details of each new event—be it a nail or an apple—we narrow the tip of our top-down attention to a sharp point. So, in the first diagram below, let the pointed nose of the subject who looks at an object—an apple—suggest the leading edge of this person's private, head-centered, longitudinal meridian:

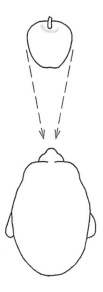

An Allocentric Perspective Is Other-Centered, Impersonal, and, It Seems, Objective

Get ready for some realities that are both unfamiliar and subtle. *Allo-* is a term no-where near as familiar to us as *ego*. (Recall how much the dictionary favors Self entries as opposed to other.) However, allo- means "other" (from the Greek *allos*, other). On these pages, allo- serves to make a crucial distinction. When the visual brain processes an external object allocentrically, it automatically brings into play its second frame of spatial reference. This detached perspective gets off to a much later start, but it can be detected in children between 3 and 5 years of age in the way they play with toys.[1] Why is this object-centered version so *impersonal*, so unsentimental? Because other priorities direct its networks. It is, fundamentally, an *other*-referential perspective.

Its first concern is to *represent the form of some object "out there"* in so categori-cal a manner that it enables the object itself to be identified. When visual stimuli first arrive from such an object, their messages are processed with reference to *their* spatial coordinates. These lines seem to stay converged "out there" in *their* envi-ronment, not to refer back toward us, the viewers. What is the other-referential version of that apple *out there*? It takes the form of an object that (1) exists as an independent entity, (2) already has *its own* intrinsic midline, (3) is a co-occupant along with the other items adjacent to it in the surrounding scenery, and (4) seems innocent of our presence.

Can an object be "seen," yet be independent of your "Self?" Don't expect that you can easily comprehend this counterintuitive concept. It is a foreign, "far-out" notion to think that any object might appear to manifest *its* own "lines of sight." It is like asking us to believe that an apple's midline plane could arise with reference to some vertical pull of gravity from its own distant planet on an orbit "out there," far beyond the pull that attaches us to our own earth.

The next diagram tries to convey visually the flavor of this same curious concept: an apparently independent, object-centered, "apple-centric" situation.[2] The two arrows at the bottom are there to remind us that the viewer's brain is subliminally aware of all three apples out *there*. However, this particular extrinsic version exists in a compartment not yet being referred back to the axis of the viewer's head and body.

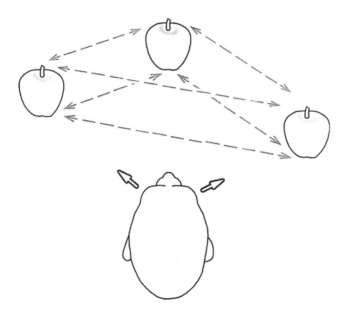

Integrating the Two Frames of Spatial Reference

Of course, we have been speaking very loosely about apples as being coded in "their" terms. Any notion of an "apple-centric" version is an expedient. The intent is merely to suggest how such lines of reference *might seem to begin* out there in an object-based manner. Yes, the processing of this extrinsic version of any object does begin independently. But something else happens. Normally, this second, other-centered version will go on silently to join our first Self-centered frame of spatial reference in a merger as complementary as yin and yang. In this ongoing synaptic alchemy, a mosaic of interactions blends two parallel physiologies into a joint working partnership.

Please remember: We are not informed that these visual transformations exist. They occur *sub*consciously. Ordinary consciousness remains blissfully unaware that our brain has these two separate versions. It knows only the result *after* they have merged seamlessly. This fact explains why we're unable—so long as we remain firmly gripped by the supremacy of our Self-fictions—deliberately to sustain a clear concept of (1) what allocentric perception *alone* might feel like, and (2) how much we are dominated (if not enthralled) by all our Self-referential processing. Don't be discouraged when you find it hard to understand what happens during our two normal versions of visual processing. A casual survey of articles published recently shows that researchers also struggle to find words that describe the differences. Table 6 lists descriptors used that can help us remember why these two versions are so different.

Hyphenated words and curious diagrams on these pages can only point a reader in the general direction of the two strange concepts. Could an *extra*ordinary state of consciousness help clarify this situation? Yes, in one extraordinary flash, kensho strikes off the deepest roots of Self, and suddenly unveils allocentric perception per se. Moreover, attentive readers may already have sensed how subtler degrees of allocentric processing might actually develop practical applications in interpersonal relationships. A recently introduced word, *allophilia*, refers to our becoming open to experience other human beings with the same positive consideration that we usually extend toward our own Self.[3]

Table 6
Examples of Ego/Allo Terminology

Egocentric Processing	Allocentric Processing
Self-centered	Other-centered
Body-centered	Stimulus-centered
Viewer-centered	Object-centered
Self-referential	Other-referential
Body-referential	World-referential
Viewpoint-dependent	Geometric-dependent
Observer-dependent	Observer-independent
Spatial motion–sensitive	Object form–sensitive

Note: In the openly receptive meditative context, other-referential is prefered. Object-centered tends to suggest that a person might still be trying to focus attention on an object.

Some researchers, aware that two networks exist, still have problems disentangling their two separate distinctive functions. Even so, pioneering brain imaging studies have recently identified the functional anatomy of the two pathways at the cortical level, especially early in their course [ZBR:17, 153–154, 167–183, 324–325, 532]. Building on that previous review of the topic, the next sections survey the latest evidence published mostly in the last 2 years. This new research does more than confirm that our intrusive "ego-Self" differs from its "allo-other" counterpart. It invites us to ask: how does any normal brain manage seamlessly to bridge the functional gap between the two networks? A short answer is: the brain is aided by an array of subconscious "*selfothering*" functional connections.

Recent Studies of the Separate Egocentric and Allocentric Streams of Spatial Reference

Neggers and colleagues in the Netherlands studied subjects whose task was to judge how they were processing simple objects in the space in front of them.[4] The subjects' main target was a vertical bar, projected on a screen 2.5 m away. Functional MRI scans monitored the subjects while they viewed this bar in one of two ways. They rendered an egocentric decision when the bar was positioned off to *their* right or left side. Note, in this instance, how the location of the bar was being defined: in relation to the midline of *the subjects' own* head and body. Alternatively, this bar could be positioned in relation to the center of one *other* different, horizontal bar. Note that this second bar lay *behind* the target, in the background. Accordingly, an object-centered, allocentric decision would be involved in this instance.

The fMRI data suggested that normal subjects use two different visuospatial "streams" to process their responses. Moreover, these two streams are represented predominately on their brain's *right* side. (Interesting point: so is attention.)

The Egocentric Stream

Figure 4 shows a long, curving red-and-white dashed line in the back of the brain. It represents the general direction of this *dorsal* processing stream. The fMRI evidence suggested that this Self-centered pathway began posteriorly. First, it traveled *upward* from the occipital lobe, then continued on its posterior path toward a major region of signal activity. This site appeared to be in the right *superior parietal lobule (sPL)*. Consult the legend that explains what figure 4 represents. (see figure 5 also.)

Normally, this superior parietal lobule anchors many covert working images of our physical self—our *soma*—toward the upper end of this dorsal egocentric stream. This superior lobule serves as our main somatosensory association area. Here, we refine our proprioceptive and touch functions [ZBR:148–149]. These messages inform us, subliminally (1) where our own body parts are located with respect to our body image, and (2) what the exact spatial dimensions are of an object nearby that our own body parts (our fingers especially) happen to touch there.

Close at hand, an innate wisdom conveniently locates a major cluster of *attentive resources*. Chapters 5 and 7 emphasized the site of these local, voluntary attentive functions. They are in the *posterior intraparietal sulcus (pIPSUL)*, poised to sharpen the way we focus our top-down, Self-centered physical efforts (table 4) (figures 1, 3, and 4). So, too, is a small region high on top of the superior parietal lobule (msPLB) (figure 2).

That's not all. Resources of many other kinds are available in nearby occipital → parietal regions. They help organize and enliven our sense of visual space. In short, the dorsal watershed all along this same upper trajectory is designed to respond to our personal "*Where is it?*"-type questions. However, the whole dorsal path answers more than this simple three-word question. In fact, its responses are designed to answer the full range of questions that ask: "*Where is it in relation to Me?*" Because our parietal networks employ spatial metrics expressed in absolute terms, they enable us to reach our own arm out accurately to grasp a target, whether it is stationary or moving.

Will our grasp succeed? Will we hit the nail on the head, or only bang it bent? Precise levels of 3-D topographical processing decide the answer. These continue to corepresent, and to track, *where* our own moving body parts are successively placed *in relation to where* the target lies out there in space. The entire action of reaching out into space becomes a supraordinate merger. It integrates our superior parietal lobule into a vast sensorimotor consortium with other regions. The resulting parallel operations translate into an act of *selfothering*. Notice that in this process, selfothering tends to lose much more than one small hyphen between its two components. It also begins to shed that prior capital *S* and any misguided tendencies to look down its nose from some psychologically superior elevated notion of Self [ZBR:201–203].

The Allocentric Stream

In contrast, the Dutch research suggested that this second pathway pursues an initially downward course. Having also begun in the occipital lobe, this ventral stream then runs forward along the *undersurface* of the temporal lobe, then flows into several other temporal lobe regions. In figure 5, the green arrowheaded, dashed *and* dotted line represents the initial *ventral* direction of this allocentric processing stream.

Again, many adjacent tributaries contribute relevant functions all along this lower occipital → temporal watershed. What do they accomplish? In brief, their

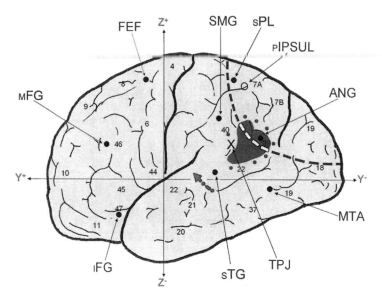

Figure 4 Directions of the two streams in a lateral view of the left hemisphere
The large red area is the *angular gyrus* (ANG) (and it includes the small circles around it). This
represents the smallest of the three major cortical regions in which PET scans reveal high levels of
metabolic activity even during conditions of passive rest. At right, the long, curved, red-and-white
dashed line represents the general dorsal direction of the egocentric stream along the so-called
where? pathway. The short green dashed and dotted line with a large arrowhead suggests the
lateral branch of the lower allocentric stream. It rises up from below toward its representation in
the *superior temporal gyrus* (sTG).

    Starting at the left, in the frontal lobe: iFG, inferior frontal gyrus; mFG, middle frontal
gyrus; FEF, frontal eye field; SMG, supramarginal gyrus; sPL, superior parietal lobule. pIPSUL,
posterior intraparietal sulcus; MTA, middle temporal area; TPJ, temporal-parietal junction. sTG,
superior temporal gyrus.

    The thin, straight, crossing lines suggest the axes of the spatial coordinates. Y+ and Y−
represent the opposite ends of an anteroposterior axis (from the front of the brain to the back).
Z+ and Z− represent the opposite ends of a dorsal-ventral axis (top to bottom). The X and Y lines
represent the kinds of standardized planes that researchers use to localize discrete brain sites in
terms of their 3-D coordinates. The small numbers refer to Brodmann's areas (BA).

    Figures 4 and 5 summarize schematically the nine PET scan reports condensed in the 2001
review by Gusnard and Raichle (chapter 15). These authors emphasize that the regions shown
have a high active metabolism at rest that can be accurately measured with PET scans. Moreover,
they are labile regions that can also become (1) *deactivated* when subjects perform overt tasks
that demand outwardly oriented attention; (2) *more* activated when subjects perform Self-
referential tasks under well-controlled conditions. See plate 2 for the color version of this figure.

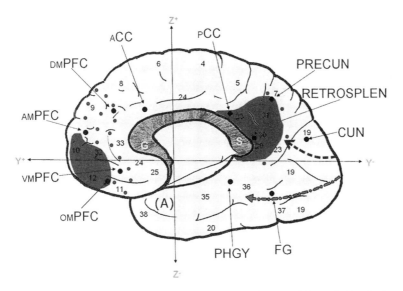

Figure 5   Directions of the two streams in a medial view of the right hemisphere
This view represents the inside surface of the *right* side of the brain. One large red area at the viewer's left (and its halo of small circles) occupies much of the medial prefrontal cortex. Here, normal subjects show high levels of metabolic activity in PET scans even under conditions of passive rest. At right, the red area represents the other major metabolic "hot spot." It lies deep in the parietal region and in front of the occipital lobe. This extensive region includes the *precuneus, retrosplenial cortex*, and the *posterior cingulate cortex*.

The short, curved red dashed line suggests the medial course of the dorsal egocentric stream. Note, below, the longer, green arrowheaded, dashed *and* dotted line. This represents the major initial, ventral direction of the allocentric stream. It begins its medial course on the undersurface of the temporal lobe, along the lower, so-called *what?* pathway.

Starting at the left, in the frontal lobe, are the four subdivisions of the medial prefrontal cortex, namely omPFC, orbital medial prefrontal cortex; vmPFC, ventral medial; amPFC, anterior medial; dmPFC, dorsal medial; aCC, anterior cingulate cortex; pCC, posterior cingulate cortex; PRECUN, precuneus; RETROSPLEN, retrosplenial cortex; CUN, cuneus; FG, fusiform gyrus; PHGY, parahippocampal gyrus. (A), the subcortical location of the amygdala.

The gray curved area in the center is the corpus callosum. G refers to its genu; S refers to its splenium. Fibers crossing over in it enable this right hemisphere to play a predominant role in those merging functions which normally combine both to direct our attention into space and to represent individual objects out there. The lines of the vertical (Z+) and horizontal (Y−) axes are shown intersecting at their zero point, the anterior commissure. See plate 3 for the color version of this figure.

preexisting "templates" help us both to frame *"What* is it?"-type questions and *to interpret* what the identified answers *mean.* If the dorsal, parietal, Self-centered stream is mostly action-oriented, then its ventral, temporal partner is chiefly oriented toward two different goals: identification and interpretation. Its interpretive functions contribute elaborate nuances of meaning. They will become increasingly important when we consider what they infuse into the nature of insight in part IV.

As allocentric messages relay forward, the temporal lobe networks specialized in pattern-recognition functions help reassemble their version of the form and structure of the discrete objects being imaged out there. The temporal lobe can deploy looser metrics when it seeks to decode such messages. When scanning for answers, its looser associations use criteria that are more relative than absolute. Free to explore broad conceptual relationships, the temporal lobe has some flexibility to interpret a range of objects and categories, using optional approaches.

Moreover, regions farther along this lower temporal lobe pathway also enable us normally to infuse subtle atmospheres of values into what was just identified out there [ZBR:247–253]. Possibly assisting in such representations are some "spatial view cells" tucked away over in the hippocampus and parahippocampal gyrus of the medial temporal lobe.[5] These allocentric nerve cells, while primed to represent a location in continuous space "out there," can even infuse *a positive sense of rewards* into such a scene. Certain of these semantic properties, resonating at higher levels of portent and aesthetic appreciation, are the kinds that could be further amplified during a state of kensho.

Ways to Help Integrate These Two Normal Frames of Reference

In this earlier-cited Dutch study by Neggers et al., further fMRI evidence then pointed toward sequences that would involve the prefrontal cortex. Normally, our prefrontal cortex is designed to help search for practical, "intelligent" answers to general questions. For example, it seems to be asking: "What *should I do* about it?" Up here, in the *middle frontal gyrus (MFG)*, fMRI signals increased both during Self-centered tasks *and* during other-oriented tasks (especially during the latter) (see figure 4). The evidence suggested that this middle frontal gyrus (like others nearby in this right dorsolateral frontal region) could normally play an "executive" role. Such a higher-level role could finally help coordinate into one unified, actionable whole the separate message streams and functions implicit in those two earlier ego- and allo- versions that had arisen far back in the parietal and temporal lobes, respectively.

Table 7 summarizes the basic aspects of our Self-referential and other-referential processing pathways. It begins by oversimplifying the way these two

Table 7
The Two Major Processing Streams

	Egocentric Processing Stream	Allocentric Processing Stream
Main theme	Spatial processing in relation to personal Self; inherently more subjective	Object processing in relation to other things in the environment; inherently more objective
Initial course	Occipital → parietal	Occipital → inferior temporal
Major crossroads	Superior occipital region; superior parietal lobule; angular gyrus	Inferior occipital region; fusiform gyrus; parahippo-campal gyrus; superior temporal gyrus
Adjacent interactions	The pathway for localization in space; "*Where* is it *in relation to Me*"	The "*What*" pathway; object identification and semantic interpretation
Metrics	More absolute, and action-oriented	More relative and abstract
Operational aspects	Faster and more accurate	Slower and less accurate
Spontaneous spatial judgments of relative distances	Novel environments tend to be processed with reference to Self-centered criteria	Older familiar environments tend to be reprocessed with reference to other-centered criteria
Nearby local attention resources	Posterior intraparietal sulcus	Superior temporal sulcus
Subsequent frontal lobe integrative activities	Middle frontal and inferior frontal gyrus, R > L	Middle frontal and inferior frontal gyrus, R > L
Thalamic contributions early to each stream	Dorsal tier of pulvinar subnuclei, lateral posterior and lateral dorsal thalamic nuclei	Ventral tier of pulvinar nuclei
Navigation tasks in virtual environments	Parahippocampal gyrus, precuneus, superior parietal lobule	Parahippocampal gyrus, retrosplenial cortex; fusiform gyrus, retrosplenial cortex, parahippocampal gyrus
Directed introspection	Anterior medial prefrontal cortex	
Triadic social contingencies	Dorsal medial prefrontal cortex	
Ordinary level of activity	Self dominates the mental field	Subliminal
Mental field during kensho	Self-processing is deactivated or bypassed	Meaning is amplified to the level of immanence; OTHER becomes overtly manifest

normal spatial processing streams initially diverge when subjects respond to a simple visual stimulus such as a bar. Notice that the table starts by emphasizing how the brain's lateral regions respond over its convex *outer* surface.

Farther down, however, some later descriptions in the table summarize the results of different tasks. As the next chapters will discuss, these other tasks engage the subjects in details of navigation, introspection, or interpersonal relationships. They are interactive tasks, involving higher-order levels of Self-referential processing that had begun at lower levels.[6] Often, these higher levels tap into much more complex resources of intention, emotion, and memory. Note that when the inner and outer surfaces of the brain are now taking on different functions, some higher-order functions are referable more to our brain's *inner* cortical surface.

Commentary

The simple bar experiments highlight the right hemisphere's major role in representing both our ego- and allo-centered frames of spatial reference. Earlier, part I had emphasized how we can also refine the potential of this right side to open up attention in ways that enhance its fast, bottom-up forms of sensory processing. These two right-sided trends—both in attention and in spatial processing—provide an interesting counterpart to the ways in which we represent most of our multiple language skills in the left hemisphere.

The focus of research will now change. The discussion in the next chapter is based on patients who had acute brain lesions. The patients' neurological findings confirm the remarkable fact: the normal brain processes information from the outside world in two very different ways.

14

Selective Deficits of Egocentric or Allocentric Processing in Neurological Patients

> Don't cling to your understanding. Even if you do understand something, you should ask yourself: Is there something I have not fully resolved, or perhaps some higher level of meaning?
>
> Zen Master Dogen (1200–1253)

It was a big controversy. One camp held firm to the belief that only parietal lesions caused visual neglect. The other camp argued that temporal lobe lesions could cause visual neglect. Hisaaki Ota and colleagues in Sendai, Japan devised a simple visual test enabling the contesting theories to be tested in the same patient.[1] It turned out that the two theories could be reconciled because they were not mutually exclusive.

Hillis and colleagues at Johns Hopkins used this test to study how two groups of patients performed after an arterial blockage had acutely compromised their visual functions in two separate brain regions. These underperfused regions of cortex were accompanied by small local subcortical infarcts.[2] In their first report, they selected 15 patients in whom each abnormal region was on the *right* side of the brain.

No patient could attend to a visual target in the normal manner. Why did the two groups have two different kinds of visual problems? Because their brain lesions were in two different places. In one group of 11 patients, only a small part of the right *parietal* lobe was damaged. Had this inferior parietal lobule been normal, it would have processed that opposite, left side of *space* in the conventional *Self*-centered way.

In the other group of four patients, small parts of the right *temporal* lobe were impaired. In the previous chapter, we observed how these temporal regions would normally have functioned. They would have attended to the opposite side of an *object*; they would have gone on to represent and reassemble its form in the usual *other*-centered, allocentric manner. Let's proceed step by step to explain how the visual deficits differ in these two groups of patients. Then it will become clear why the two once-contending views can be reconciled.

The Egocentric Spatial Defect

These patients neglected the visual space (*and all items in it*) off to *their* left side. Again, note what "*their* left" means. "Their left" is a *personal* construct. Its high priorities refer to spatial coordinates that point *back* to the axial midline of their own physical Self. Their "left" means to the left of an imaginary plane that would normally extend far out into space. *Before* their stroke, they had "owned" this left half of space, having in this sense a vested property interest that enabled them to move into it, occupy it, and become attached to it.

To illustrate, suppose we were to ask one such model patient to count the apples in a long row, while looking straight ahead. The eight apples are spread out horizontally in this row, two feet apart, in front of the patient. Four of these apples are in a line off to the patient's right side; the remaining four are similarly located off to the left side.

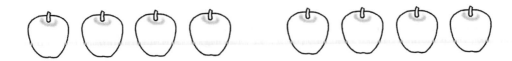

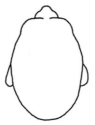

The patient counts the apples, yet reports seeing only "four." Which four are seen? Only those four off to the patient's *right* side. None of the four apples on the *left* side—1, 2, 3, and 4—are seen. They are there, but they are neglected. *Unattended to.* This is what the patient sees:

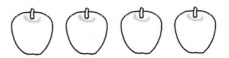

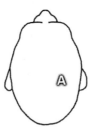

Which part of the right inferior parietal cortex was impaired in this select group of neurology patients? It was the *right angular gyrus*, designated above by the letter *A*.

- *The parietal lesion causing this egocentric defect.* How could dysfunction of this small part of the occipital → parietal stream stop egocentric processing? Normally, this right angular gyrus is one of several Self-referential sites. Jointly, they help us both to pay attention to space *and* to put it into practical use based on our very own, intimately *remembered* prior experience.[3] Bearing in mind these overlapping functions, let's return to figure 4. It shows how strategic is the location of this angular gyrus (ANG). It straddles the normal route taken by messages passing up and down along the posterior parietal egocentric pathway. Note that discrete damage to the cortical surface here could delete those local intrinsic cortical functions that help activate their other connected parts in a larger network. Furthermore, a slightly deeper extension of the lesion could also disconnect some passing *subcortical* fiber connections which normally enable visual impulses to relay up toward the superior parietal lobule (sPL).

The Allocentric Spatial Defect

This second group of patients had a different visual deficit. Their visual problem expressed the abnormal way they processed the stimuli from *individual objects*. These patients neglected that half of any discrete *object—anywhere in outside space, left or right*—which was opposite the site of their brain dysfunction.

For example, suppose we were to ask such a model patient to look straight ahead at a different long row of apples, also spaced 2 feet apart. Now the "apple task" is slightly different. Only apples 3 and 7 are intact in this whole row of eight apples. All other apples have a dark rotten area on one side. Note how the two sets of dark areas differ in the diagram below. In those apples numbered 1, 4, 5, and 8, the blemished area covers almost half of "*the apple's right side.*" In contrast, apples 2 and 6 have that dark rotten area on "*the apple's left side.*" (Please try briefly to adopt an "apple's point of view." You might even consider standing on the other side, *behind* the row, now facing the patient, even "becoming an apple," if that approach could allow you to appreciate why such unusual wording might be used to convey such an object-centered notion.)

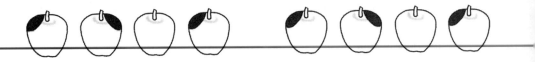

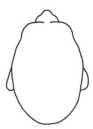

The visual task diagrammed above seems straightforward. The task for this model patient is to count only the six apples that are *spoiled*. The patient understands the task.

Yet the patient reports seeing only two spoiled apples. Apples 1, 4, 5, and 8 are overlooked. Below, four symbols (X) indicate each apple that is missed. Notice that these four apples are the only ones in which the rotten area is on the *"apple's right side."* They are neglected. *Un*attended to. The diagram below shows the scene from the standpoint of this model patient who sees only two spoiled apples.

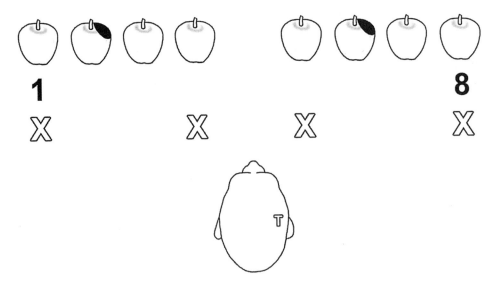

Apples 5 and 8 are crucial to your diagnosis. Why? Because the patient who also neglects apples 5 and 8 clearly has a defect restricted to the opposite side of an *object*. This object-centered, opposite visual defect applies to a discrete *object that is anywhere* in outside space, right or left. This defect is not confined to the opposite half of the whole spatial world off to the left, as had occurred in the prior example of the model patient who had an angular gyrus lesion in the parietal lobe.

- *The temporal lesion causing this allocentric defect.* This second group of patients had one or two damaged regions in their right temporal cortex (T) that were compromised by poor circulation: the *fusiform gyrus* and the *superior temporal gyrus*. Returning first to figure 5, one sees how ventral is the location of this fusiform gyrus (FG). It occupies the junction between the inferior temporal lobe and the occipital lobe. Hidden on the brain's undersurface, this fusiform region occupies a strategic crossroad. It lies directly on the path of the green arrow that represents the lower visual stream of object-centered, other-referential processing.

Returning next to figure 4, a short green arrow is seen overlying part of the superior temporal gyrus (STG). Part of this long, plump gyrus is included in the upper course of the allocentric pathway. Notice how each branch that this "other-centric" stream pursues through the temporal lobe is relatively far removed from the Self-centered *dorsal* stream as this latter stream rises through the angular gyrus of the posterior parietal lobe.

Why, when parts of their right temporal lobes were compromised, did the second group of patients neglect that *half* of any discrete *object* opposite the site of their brain damage? For the same reason that the model patient overlooked apples 1, 4, 5, and 8. Once again, when the right temporal lobe is damaged locally (as indicated by T), the defect does not interfere with vision in only one half of *all* external space. Instead, the damaged right temporal lobe cannot attend to and transform into patterned messages the particular visual stimuli that radiate from any object's "right" side, no matter where that object is located.

The latest study from this same research group reports on the right-sided spatial defects that are caused by *left*-sided lesions, and confirms their earlier observations.[4] It also extends them in a manner suggesting that our right hemisphere is the more Self-relational, and the left hemisphere is more other-relational, at least with respect to the way they each enter into spatial attention processing. Table 8 summarizes these differences.

So What?

You may wonder: Of what benefit is it to my normal brain to pay attention in this complex manner? Contemporary theories are oversimplifications. But perhaps to

Table 8
Hemispheric Differences in Self/Other Processing

	Right Hemisphere	Left Hemisphere
Kind and degree of specialization	For more viewer-centered, global forms of spatial attention processing For a more general role in egocentric processing	For language, and for more local, other-relational forms of spatial attention processing For a more general role in allocentric processing
Contralateral neglect that is self-centered	Caused by more dorsal damage that includes the *right* inferior parietal lobule	Caused by more dorsal damage that includes the *left* inferior parietal lobule
Contralateral neglect that is object-centered	Caused by more ventral damage that includes the right inferior temporo-occipital region	Caused by more ventral damage that includes the left inferior temporo-occipital region

From J. Kleinman, M. Newhart, C. Davis, et al. Right hemispatial neglect: Frequency and characterization following acute left hemisphere stroke. *Brain and Cognition* 2007; 64:50–59.

a primitive creature eons ago, it afforded some survival advantage if one ventral perceptual compartment was specialized quickly to identify a reasonably objective facsimile of a dire threat to life, while the rest of its rudimentary brain was scrambling to escape and vocalize its alarm to others. (Even later, in a hominid era, invoking the image of a sabertooth tiger as a threatening object might help illustrate a potential advantage.)

In summary, up to this point, the results have emphasized the two broad streams of cortical sites that go on to be linked physiologically. Thus far, some ego- and allocentric networks appear to be represented in modules more on the brain's convex outer surface, sometimes more on the *right* side. So, not incidentally, were most of the bottom-up attention networks discussed in part I.

Contemporary meditators may wonder: What practical significance does this recent brain research have for me? The next brain-imaging studies to be discussed follow a different experimental design. The researchers were seeking a baseline. Now, they finally chose to consider what the normal brain was doing during quiet, passive resting conditions. The results are fascinating.

15

The Brain's Active Metabolism during Resting Conditions

> What is most difficult is to be perfectly at rest, not activating the conceptual faculty.
> Master Yuan-Wu (1063–1135)

It is difficult to let go into perfect rest, hard not to activate the conceptual faculty. As the twenty-first century dawned, Gusnard and Raichle published a series of landmark articles on this Self/other interface.[1] They began with a seeming paradox in the data collected from many positron emission tomography (PET) scans. Even though the subjects had been resting, certain parts of their brains still showed especially high levels of metabolic activity. Figures 4 and 5 have summarized the main findings.

Where were the two most metabolically active regions? To recap the PET scan evidence, they were *not* on that outer cortical surface with which we have just become familiar. Instead, both sites occupied the inside surface, *next to the midline*. Figure 5 has shown that, in front, one very large medial region covered the *medial prefrontal cortex* (MPFC). The second highly active region was deeply centered farther back. Its vast expanse included the *precuneus* (PRECUN), the *retrosplenial cortex* (RETROSPLEN), and the *posterior cingulate* cortex (PCC). A third, smaller region was that same angular gyrus (ANG), discussed above in its egocentric context. It was located on the outer surface of the posterior parietal cortex, shown in figure 4.

So the question is: Why are these fronto-parietal regions so highly active metabolically? They stay active even when normal subjects—seemingly at rest—are approaching conditions reasonably close to those of meditators who are settling down into a passive relaxed state. Maybe there is a simple answer. Perhaps it is because *some multitasking operations are still ongoing in these regions*, driving them automatically.

What kinds of activities? These pages propose that the ongoing activities in at least two major categories of Self-relational functions could be:

- Helping us consolidate the circumstantial details of our lifelong personal history;
- Keeping our personal files partially accessible to be opened selectively and actualized for immediate use during each present moment.

What does that first category mean? It means that *each of us has been actively maintaining a covert journal*. We tend to overlook how many private entries we have consolidated here, in these capacious networks of polymodal associations. Their matrix of 3-D space and time enables us to register every event and location that we wished to stamp with our own time frame and wanted to claim with our own nametag. *These are the places where we built, stored, owned, and continue to update the semifictional realities of our own life story.* (If you doubt how much each person is Self-driven to construct the narrative of his or her own life story, check out some I-generated entries on YouTube and MySpace.)

"Monkey Mind"

Clearly, each of our personal life stories implies a brain that keeps updating its own ongoing journal. We keep on file vast amounts of subconscious, incidental, autobiographical, and highly detailed data which are but thinly disguised when they surface in dreams.[2] Yet, if each elaborate entry is to be an event we can index in "our" own time, it must do more than refer simultaneously to "our" personal, Self-centered physical space. It must simultaneously record this event *in terms of many other relevant circumstantial details that document the way various objects are placed in the scenery of the world outside at the same instant.* Of course, our Self-referential nouns and pronouns will play the major active role in such entries, but adjectives and adverbs will still be included in this Self-other journal.

The downside is obvious. Swirling into our turbulent streams of consciousness are accumulations of mental debris. This discursive, mind-wandering phenomenon—"monkey mind"—is familiar to all meditators. Stirred up by habit energies and emotions from subconscious limbic levels, these trivial thoughts contaminate our meditation. Few such memory traces and imaginary plans turn out to be of practical immediate survival value. Still, everyday we make new journal entries.

That said, the next reports illustrate how our second category of covert multitasking operations can still perform an essential practical service. How? By helping spatial memory files to remain sufficiently open. Somehow, this remarkable random accessibility allows discrete memory traces of various ages to be tapped into selectively and used for *immediate* selfothering purposes. Some memory traces were obviously laid down long ago; others could have entered working memory only moments earlier. Each index is scanned, and the relevant trace is selected automatically. The next sections illustrate that such brisk, highly selective, open accessibility has practical applications.

Navigating the Streets of a Long-Familiar City

Rosenbaum and colleagues selected normal subjects who had become experts at navigating through their native streets of downtown Toronto.[3] Then they challenged their subjects to solve "virtual" mental tasks that were based on these same familiar streets. The subjects had to access some of their older spatially street-smart navigational skills in order to pass such tests of spatial working memory. At these times, fMRI signals increased in their right *parahippocampal gyrus* (PHGY) (figure 5). In contrast, signals increased in the *precuneus* (PRECUN) and *superior parietal lobule* (sPL) when the subjects imagined themselves being Self-engaged in other positions that could imply more egocentric kinds of processing.

Signals also increased in the *retrosplenial cortex* (RETROSPLEN) when the subjects' task was to assign *a given directional heading* to a place in space. This task also involved their retrieving old familiar landmark information, memories they had acquired long before, laid down during relatively more allocentric frames of reference. Sometimes, the researchers created a new, artificial roadblock. Now their subjects, forced to detour, needed to combine both immediate and remote spatial memories into complementary selfothering interactions. During such novel executive decisions, their dorsal lateral prefrontal regions now came into play, including the *middle frontal gyrus* (MFG) cited in earlier chapters (figure 4).

Making Spatial Judgments in Recently Encoded 3-D "Virtual" Environments

Frings and colleagues in Freiburg, Germany, used simple cube-shaped objects to generate fresh "virtual" environments.[4] The subjects' fMRI signals increased in the *precuneus*, bilaterally, when their initial task was to encode novel arrangements of these objects into new memories with the aid of chiefly allocentric criteria.

Subsequently, the subjects had to retrieve these fresh, 3-D spatial memories in order to solve an object recognition task. Then, precuneus signals increased a second time. During the very earliest (searching) phase of this delayed retrieval, signals also increased simultaneously in the region around the *inferior frontal gyrus* (IFG). This evidence suggested that their frontal lobe had now become an active participant in this deliberate search.

In a separate study, subjects needed to rely on external landmarks in a park-like virtual environment as their basis for making allocentric 3-D spatial judgments.[5] fMRI signals increased in their *fusiform gyrus* (FG), *retrosplenial cortex* (RETROSPLEN), and *parahippocampal gyrus* (PHGY) on both sides (figure 5).

Using Verbal Descriptions to Induce either Egocentric or Allocentric Coding

Zaehle and colleagues in Switzerland chose to *verbally* describe spatial information to their subjects.[6] In this way, they sought to exclude the effect that direct, external visual stimulation would have on the results. fMRI monitoring followed the 16 subjects while they processed this auditory information and transformed it into visual-mental imagery. Precuneus activations were more strongly involved during egocentric than during allocentric spatial coding. Allocentric coding recruited both the hippocampal formation and the ventral visual stream bilaterally, as well as the right inferior and superior parietal lobule.

In general, the evidence surveyed suggests that the precuneus plays more of a Self-referential role [ZBR:205–206] (part VII). In contrast, the retrosplenial cortex functions more in an other-referential context. When we require a quick selfothering merger of functions, notice how useful it becomes to have these two regions positioned right next to each other. In these pages, both the retrosplenial cortex and its close neighbors are envisioned as contributing to the normal journal-like functions that we use to consolidate entire scenes into narrative memories of discrete events in our past. On one occasion when I was meditating, a random sequence of free-running snapshots occurred that may have represented a surge in these metabolically active medial circuits [ZB:390–391] (chapter 20).

Self/Other Changes in Medial Regions during Normal Development

The medial prefrontal cortex is relatively more active when both children (age 10 years) and adults (age 26 years) respond to short phrases that describe their own Self as opposed to some highly familiar other person (e.g., Harry Potter).[7] In contrast, the medial posterior *parietal* cortex shows relatively more fMRI signals when the topic refers to other social information, not to Self-knowledge exclusively.

However, children continue to activate their medial prefrontal cortex during Self-relational processing much more than do adults. Moreover, back in their medial parietal regions, children chiefly engage their anterior precuneus and posterior cingulate gyrus. In contrast, adults chiefly engage the region farther back in the posterior precuneus.

How Does Our Self Learn Normally Both to Introspect and to Relate to Other Persons? Medial and Other Frontal Lobe Contributions

Fortunately, as children, we become socialized. We learn how to relate with greater empathy to other living persons "out there" than we do to our mechanical toys and other objects. The inner surface of the frontal lobe contributes to these maturing adult interpersonal skills.[8] Here, once our "social cognition" skills become more subjective, interactive, and abstract, they tend to be represented farther forward near the frontal pole.

The way one of these medial clusters of Self-oriented fMRI sites functions may be of interest to introspective meditators who also have to keep reminding themselves to meditate. The sites are located in and around the *anterior* part of the *medial prefrontal cortex* (AMPFC) (figure 5). Signals increase here when the task for normal subjects is to shift into an introspective mode to answer private "Who am I?" types of questions. These tasks are designed to test their abilities to select which words best characterize their own basic personality traits, or to specify which emotional state their Self is in at a given moment. Nearby anterior medial regions become active when the subjects' task is to encode their own freely chosen, voluntary intentions. These are the willful goals that they plan to maintain during an interval of time.[9]

Close comparisons also provide intriguing data, both literally and figuratively, in this medial prefrontal cortex. For example, some Self-oriented introspective sites also lie near other-relational "close-affinity" sites. These latter regions turn out to be activated most when we are called upon to judge certain other persons with whom we feel an especially close personal relationship.[10]

In contrast, sites farther away tend to be activated when our task is to evaluate strangers at a distance, and to judge their potential behaviors. These sites, more distant themselves, lie higher up near the *dorsal medial prefrontal cortex* (DMPFC). This dorsal region also enters into higher-level, more convoluted mental interactions. These higher functions can focus attention on decoding *three*-way social contingencies rather than our two-way relationships.[11] For example: How might you and a second person interrelate with some object, under two very different conditions? Suppose in one, the object is an ice cream cone, while in the other, it is an axe.

fMRI signals increase in the medial prefrontal cortex when we restrict our Self-evaluations to more cognitive, descriptive factual levels.[12] However, signals increase in the ventral anterior cingulate region once we're called upon to evaluate our Self using *emotionally* valenced descriptions. We assume that normal people will put a positive "spin" on their own better qualities. As La Rochefoucald phrased it back in the seventeenth century, "Self-love is the greatest of all flatterers." However, after some patients damage their orbitofrontal region, they go on to develop expansive Self-assured delusions, exaggerating these flattering notions about their own social skills to unrealistically lofty heights.

Deactivations during Attentional Shifts toward Externalized Goals

Thus far, our discussion has cited high resting activities and briefly increased brain activities. It is time to correct this imbalance. *Deactivations are of at least equal importance all along the Path of Zen* [ZBR:195–199].

- How can one define genuine *deactivations*? Gusnard and Raichle emphasized how important it was first to define an equilibrium state of normal "baseline" *activity*.[13] Once this level is approximated, then brief increases can more readily be seen to represent *activations*, and brief decreases can be more accurately defined as deactivations.

- When do deactivations occur? PET scan studies show that deactivations are most easily defined when we shift our attentional resources toward the processing of immediate, externalized goals. These *deactivations are reactive, caused by this quick shift in attentional processing*.

- Where do the deactivations occur? They occur both in the anterior medial regions of the prefrontal cortex, and in the posterior parietal cortex. Note that while they chiefly involve the medial parietal regions, lateral regions like the angular gyrus are also deactivated.

- How are these deactivations to be interpreted? As a normal, brief, reorganization of Self-referential networks *triggered by tasks that compel attention to immediate external goals.*

- How are these deactivations relevant to the meditative path? They point to comparable normal mechanisms poised instantly to decrease our notions of Self during a quick shift toward external attention and/or intended movement [ZBR:201–203]. They point also to a testable hypothesis: namely, that if *genuine* no-thought intervals are reached during an effective level of deep meditation that arrives at *total rest*, these silent intervals could show even lower metabolic activities than occur during the prior so-called baseline resting conditions when one's ordinary mind-wandering mental phenomena tend to prevail. Finally, they point to two major themes soon to be developed: a) mechanisms comparable to those causing our normal reactive deactivation could shift the brain in the direction toward selflessness; (b) long term meditative training could cultivate and amplify these capacities to shift toward selfless insight-wisdom.

16
Internal "Mirrors" Facing Outward

In humans and monkeys, the mirror neuron system transforms seen actions into our inner representation of these actions.

Gazzola and colleagues[1]

Over a decade ago, serendipity graced a physiology experiment: researchers just happened to be in the room to witness the firing of what soon came to be called "mirror neurons" [ZBR:267–269, 348–350]. These motor nerve cells were in the most anterior and inferior part of this monkey's *premotor* cortex. What caused them to discharge? They fired not only when this monkey broke open a peanut shell. They fired not only when this monkey chanced to passively observe a lucky researcher who just happened to be breaking a peanut shell. Mirror neurons also discharged when the monkey merely heard the *sound* of a peanut shell being broken. So, though the monkey might have appeared totally passive, certain of its motor and sensory nerve cells seemed joined into receptive circuits poised to perform a kind of mimicry.

Since then, it has become clear that monkeys have whole systems of sensori-motor cells ready to monitor relevant behavior. Do human brains have comparable nerve cell systems? Is this how we feel empathy, anticipate what the other person has "in mind," learn by example to "mirror" other person's social behaviors, tennis serve, or golf swing?

As the research field expanded, its elastic complexities required a more speculative vocabulary. "Embodied simulation" was a recent addition.[2] "Embodied" began as a useful word. It suggested the direct way one human being might develop an internalized "experiential understanding" of the other person. A noteworthy qualification remains: in themselves, mirror nerve cells serve to match each observer in only a relatively "compressed fashion" with what he or she observes. In themselves, each mirror matching system is *neutral*. Its local circuitry is as cool and unsentimental as any glass mirror on the wall that reflects the combing of one's hair. It relies on many *other* intervening sets of memory-based functions. These interpret what some other person might be intending and project what might be the outcome of some external event. Indeed, the artificial acts of an industrial robot also provide a human brain with a bare stimulus source sufficient to develop such human "intuition."[3]

In human subjects, first to be described was the visual mirror system, followed by the auditory mirror system.[4] fMRI signals respond in comparable brain areas, both when one person acts in a way that produces a sound, and when a second person makes this same sound. In each instance, the auditory stimulus causes increased signals in a circuit that links the temporoparietal and premotor regions on the left side.

An interesting observation is that this left hemispheric premotor circuit tends to be more activated among normal persons who score higher on an empathy scale.[5] In contrast, other research suggests that patients who have autism are deficient in the functions of their mirror neuron system, a finding that has significant medical and social implications.[6] Future claims that one or another style of meditation is more efficacious might be based on how the subjects' empathy is being tested for, and on how conservatively their parallel neuroimaging studies are being interpreted (chapters 45 and 46).

Subtle Aspects of One's Physical and Psychic Self

When "mirror" is used in the neurosciences and in Zen, it can become a term so slippery and elastic that it needs to be interpreted with care [ZB:48, 593]. This is especially true if we accept the principle that only in a rigidly "compressed" manner do a given observer's mirror nerve cell functions per se match what they witness.

How will *mirror* be defined? This question bears on some issues raised during a previous discussion of different varieties of oneness and unity [ZBR:333–357]. It was the second category of oneness (category II) that presented the clearest paradox.[7] It represented a state that was rendered internally empty of Self. Yet the mental field also included a sense of some outward, quasi-physical representations of such a "Self." Indeed, the Zen-trained subject who was serving as an example had used the following words to describe this second variety of oneness: "the universe was me and I was it. I looked up at the sky and that experience was exactly like looking at a mirror" [ZBR:345]. In this instance, we can only wonder if some *somatic* elements of "quasi-mirror-like" functions were being enhanced, and if they represented the kinds of projections of a residual Self that were then being displaced externally.

It was proposed in the previous chapter that we engage the mostly midline cortex of the frontal and parietal lobes in two major categories of functions. What could help to bridge the conceptual gap between the basic simulations of our relatively small core of mirror neurons and these larger networking activities that we employ during our normal Self/other referential processing? Perhaps what we use to close this gap might correspond with the soft self-portrait lens of our flexible, creative imagination. How could normal "leaps" of this imagination help to integrate these two systems? The links could connect the inside of the cortex with the outside of the cortex, its medial side with its lateral side. For example, farther back one set of connections might link the precuneus with the inferior parietal lobule. In front, another set might link the medial prefrontal cortex with the inferior frontal gyrus.[8]

Embodiment?

"Embodiment" began as another useful word that went on to acquire confusing implications. Leggenhager and colleagues define *embodiment* as "the sense of being localized within one's physical body."[9] Their studies emphasize that one such embodiment, thus defined, could be coded at the temporoparietal junction (TPJ).

The 20 young women studied by Devue and colleagues showed *decreased* fMRI signals in their right anterior insula at times when they visually recognized their own bodies. Decreases also occurred in the right anterior cingulate while they were recognizing their colleagues' bodies.[10] When embodiment is defined experimentally as "body ownership," it has also been associated with *increased* PET scan activity in the right posterior insula and the right frontal operculum.[11] When we generate mental imagery, a more inferior occipital region, the extrastriate body area (EBA), might also contribute, at least to the degree that it responds selectively to the external appearance of human bodies and body parts[12] (see table 9).

Subcortical Contributions to Self/Other Distinctions

The conscious mind may be compared to a fountain playing in the sun and falling back into the great subterranean pool of the subconsciousness from which it arises.

Sigmund Freud (1856–1939)

As far is Buddhism is concerned, the main thing is the crushing of the ego; and one is to go about it with all one's forces—irrespective of higher or lower.

Nanrei Kobori-Roshi (1918–1992)[1]

Freud championed the view that most of our mind is hidden from view.[2] He gave some very Zen advice to would-be psychoanalysts. He counseled them to keep open their own unconscious processes, to maintain a measure of "calm, quiet attentiveness—of evenly hovering attention," to remain receptive to, but non-judgmental about, what their patients were saying. I encourage my psychiatrist colleagues to learn how to meditate, and to have a small room in which their patients can meditate before they are seen in follow-up interviews.

Kobori-Roshi came from a different tradition, yet he developed a similar perspective about the workings of the mind. His statement above is taken from an interview, in the first part of which he emphasized how much our high-level sophisticated thoughts were constructed on a foundation of dualism. This deep-seated dualism is the basis for our always separating "this" from "that," inside from outside, Self from other. The result turns our discriminating intellect into "a convenient but treacherous instrument." In this context, how does he describe the Buddhist approach? It is one that will free *both* levels of the mind, "higher" and "lower," from the maladaptive influence of the egocentric Self.

How can you examine what's going on in your mind? When only one thin cognitive thought stream glistens high in the sunlight of consciousness, mental events are more easily identified. Much harder to discern are the outlines of what goes on down in the deep, murky pool of the subconscious at lower levels. Here, things hide we'd rather forget. Meditation trains such an "evenly hovering attention." Growing more selfless, it becomes more objective about what it chooses to witness, less disturbed by what it finds.

Subcortical Considerations

If research illuminated only the higher cortical levels uppermost in our mind, it would miss the crucial events that relay during the early milliseconds. These are the sequences, surveyed in part I, that determine how we will separate inside from outside, *this* Self "in here" from *that* "other world out there." In these closing pages of part II, we continue to emphasize our lower-level pathways. This discussion of the infrastructure of Zen will continue throughout part III.

- An early visual coding of the subject/object distinction begins in the relay between the *superior colliculus* (SC) and the *pulvinar* (PUL). (See the bottom of figure 6.) This lightning-fast subcortical step begins in the roof of the midbrain. It starts as early as 6 milliseconds, long before the more elaborate ego- and allocentric refinements unfold in cortex that are suggested in figures 4 and 5.

- During this early phase, the thalamus serves as a kind of Grand Central Station deep in the center of the brain. Its large *pulvinar* plays an active role, helping to "switch" our attentional resources appropriately from one potential "track" to another. Once the pulvinar confers its perceptual salience on an incoming visual, auditory, or touch stimulus, the medial temporal lobe and other cortical sites are alerted. Instantly, they pay more personal attention to *where* this stimulus is coming from, and *what* it is most likely to be.[3]

- Suppose that the incoming sensory messages are from an apple. Soon after they relay into a monkey's medial temporal lobe, one out of eight nerve cells curled up in its hippocampus will register the *place where* that apple is positioned in space. Ten percent of these "place cells" use Self-centered coordinates. This means that they help the monkey *personalize* this exterior spot. Now this place exists *in relation to* the position of the monkey's own head and body. Most other cells (69%) respond allocentrically. This means that they're tuned with reference just to *that* particular apple as an object out there in space [ZB:186].

- However, when human patients have bilateral hippocampal damage, they cannot imagine any such new coherent Self/other experience.[4] Why not? Because their mental images no longer have the receptacle of space within which they can construct all the circumstantial details of an event into an integrated, selfother version. Lacking the requisite spatial context, their images are fragmented, incoherent.

Commentary

Normally, we represent our action-oriented cortical functions in dorsal modules all along the parietal pathway. These networks quickly decode whatever Self-centered spatial discriminations we need most for the task. The more nuanced aspects of allocentric processing relay all along the lower watershed. They may take a little more time to evolve. Parts of the lower visual path are longer, and some impulses can meander as they stream through the temporal lobe. How can the normal brain integrate its parietal version of spatial processing with its temporal version—its *"where"* with its *"what?"* How can it prioritize the delicate attentional balance between two so very different systems, the one so Self-centered, its partner so other-centered? Chapter 7 introduced the frontal lobe as providing one of the options for such integrations at the cortical level (figure 3) (part VII).

But there are others. The brain has three basic mechanisms to excite, or to inhibit, a distant site. First—and foremost for our purposes in this chapter—it can use its *frontal → thalamic* projections. These top-down frontal lobe interactions with the thalamus (including its pulvinar, lateral posterior, and reticular nucleus) help channel which kinds and amounts of salient information flow along each separate stream.[5] Second, it can use other *cortical → subcortical* connections. Third, it can use its direct *transcortical* connections to supplement these effects.

The discussions in parts I and II have now reviewed how the brain attends both to *that* other world out there and to *this* personal Self inside. A few questions raised during such a cavalier survey are the kinds that might serve to stimulate further investigations. Beyond that, could any such provisional "map-making" attempts serve the needs of travelers who contemplate setting off on a long spiritual journey? Maybe, at least if the discussions may also suggest a plausible biological basis that might help sustain some meditators in their aspirations to become *less* Self-centered.

With these considerations in mind, we turn next to examine in part III some physiological resources that meditators might be drawing upon when they walk this long rigorous Path toward selflessness. As my teacher, Myokyo-ni, often observed, not until meditators happen to lose "the delusion of I" will they "suddenly see clearly."[6] And with this first authentic "awakening," their subcortical transformations of consciousness really begin. Now, meditators become motivated to start advanced Zen practice [ZBR:394–396].

18

Second Mondo

Nothing is easier than self-deceit. What you wish for, you also believe to be true.
Demosthenes (384–322 B.C.E.)

Why is the Self capitalized in these pages?

In the past, I've followed the standard literary conventions: spell the personal self with a small *s*, and reserve capital letters for the "Universal Self," the "Ultimate Reality." Always in this diminutive spelling of "self" is there the full acknowledgement that each human being is but an infinitesimal, transient aggregate of the original stardust in a cosmos too vast to be imagined.

Yet, this small *s* also vastly understates the root cause of our everyday problems. In fact, overconditioned Self-centered responses are the real cause of our psychological predicament. Most psychological problems become inturned, Self-inflicted. So, the point in capitalizing the Self here is simply to call attention to how obviously we've overinflated it. (Any Ultimate Big Picture could hardly be concerned if such trivial attempts with wordplay might seem briefly to give humans equal billing.)

Why do so many wild thoughts interrupt my attempts to meditate?

There's no reason to be surprised by your normal so-called monkey mind. It illustrates the free-running associations of your lifelong personal journal. You maintain this narrative in the metabolically active, so-called resting networks of your mostly medial, frontoparietal regions. It takes active metabolic work to consolidate all these detailed memory scenarios. They not only keep your life story accessibly on file, but also lay busy plans for your future. Moreover, when the *subconsciously* driven habit energies of your emotional state keep agitating the limbic nuclei in your thalamus they go on to activate these regions of cortex. A program of regular meditative practice enables you to witness each discursive subjectivity calmly—without becoming attached to it—and to examine each emotional wave more objectively—without being hijacked by it.

Are you suggesting that our parietal lobe cortical networks are more oriented toward Self, whereas our temporal lobe networks are more oriented toward "other?"

Yes, that's the general idea, and the message of those apples.

Isn't that an oversimplification?

Yes. Because pivotal events occur at the thalamic level as part of each reaction to a quick shift of attention. Simultaneously, when these deep thalamic mechanisms enhance other-referential processing, they also decrease Self-referential processing. (Deferred until later sections is this discussion of the thalamus and some integrative roles performed by fronto-temporal connections).

What is a "reactive" deactivation; and why is it important?

The two words refer to the deactivation that occurs as part of the normal reaction to attentive processing. It will be proposed that the selflessness of kensho reflects a sudden, major increase in the amplitude of this normal response. The result could be an unusually enhanced reciprocal *de*activation of those regions in which the Self had been chiefly represented.

Why is the concept of other-referential processing so difficult to grasp, and to retain?

It is difficult because Self-centered processing dominates our experience. In addition, only recently has a critical mass of information begun to clarify how cortical and subcortical processes combine in different brain regions to generate consciousness. Moreover, only recently have we appreciated all of the implications to Zen of the normal physiological mechanisms of attention. When sudden shifts into attention deactivate the networks of the Self, consciousness can become transformed toward an other-referential state. This selfless state is discussed next in part III.

Part III

Toward Selflessness

There is nothing true about Buddhism except for the manifestation of no-Self.

Joshu Sasaki-Roshi (1907–)

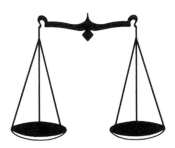

Seeing Selflessly in a New Dimension

It is not that something different is seen, but that one sees differently. It is as though the spatial act of seeing were changed by a new dimension.

Carl Jung (1875–1961)

Non-I, *Anatta*, is not an academic subject of discussion, but an immediate, vivid experience which rends the veil of delusion so that the eyes suddenly see clearly.

Irmgard Schloegl (Myokyo-ni)

The research just surveyed prepares us to understand how our brain *normally* pays attention, constructs a personal Self, and links these subjective constructs into the detailed circumstances of actual events at one particular time and place. The previous chapter closed by introducing some subcortical levels that help integrate our basic sense of Self. Part III proposes a more formal explanation for how this sense of Self can disappear. The ancient Pali term for this state of non-I is *anatta*. Zen traditions call this new dimension of consciousness a state of "no-self."

Explanations for this state of selflessness now resume, starting with pivotal events down in the thalamus. The purpose of figure 6 and its caption is to provide an illustrated discussion of how our thalamic pathways normally interact with the cortex in ways that set the stage for a state of no-self to develop.

The Pulvinar

In humans, the pulvinar becomes very large, so large that it now occupies about one quarter of the volume of our thalamus. It preserves its ancient "hotline" connections from the superior and inferior colliculi in the upper brainstem. Whenever these primal circuits detect some threatening visual or auditory stimulus, they instantly relay signals on to the amygdala—subconsciously. These sophisticated survival circuits mediate many phenomena of blindsight (and its likely auditory counterpart, "deaf-hearing") [ZB:240–244].

Why has the primate pulvinar become so bulky when compared to its size in lower animals? Because as hominids evolved into a highly socialized species, the pulvinar coevolved with our expanding cortex, becoming its *pivotal association nucleus*. In this key bidirectional role, it confers *salience*. This vital automatic process enables us to separate the key stimulus of potential interest in the foreground, hold on to it, and transform it into a subject worthy of further, meaningful, attentive interest.

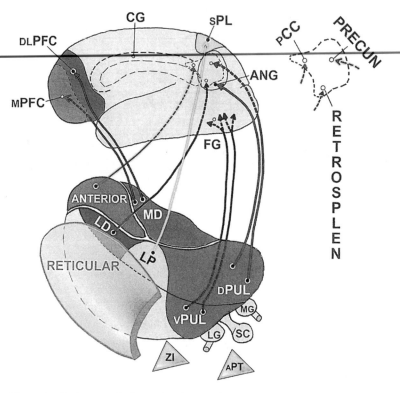

Figure 6   Thalamocortical contributions to the dorsal egocentric and ventral allocentric streams
This composite view shows the normal pathways leading from the thalamus up to the cortex. For convenience in viewing, only left-sided structures are shown. These connections rise up from the left thalamus to supply both the outside and inside of the left hemisphere. Pathways from the dorsal tier of nuclei predominate. Thus, at bottom right, one path leads from the *dorsal pulvinar* (DPUL) to the angular gyrus (ANG) on the *outer* cortical surface. A second path from this dorsal pulvinar leads up to the *precuneus* (PRECUN). Dashed lines indicate that this path projects to the *medial* parietal surface. Other projections from the *lateral posterior* (LP) nucleus supply the *superior parietal lobule* (sPL). These help to anchor each person's subliminal sensate impression of existing as a physically articulated Self-image.

In front, the *medial dorsal* (MD) thalamic nucleus projects to the prefrontal cortex, both to its outer, dorsolateral (DLPFC) and to its medial (MPFC) surfaces. The deep medial area in the back of the brain is shown enlarged at the top right. Here, two other adjacent dorsal nuclei of the limbic thalamus project to this medial surface (dashed lines). Thus, the *anterior nucleus* projects to the *posterior cingulate cortex* (PCC), and the *lateral dorsal nucleus* (LD) projects to the *retrosplenial cortex* (RETROSPLEN).

Note that relatively fewer pathways from the thalamus are shown serving the allocentric processing stream. However, messages from the *ventral pulvinar* (vPUL) are shown passing first through the region of the *fusiform gyrus* (FG) on the undersurface of the temporal lobe. These continue on their way forward through the other-referential pathways in the rest of the temporal lobe and on toward the superior temporal gyrus. (*continued on page 89*)

The pulvinar does more than assign *immediate sensory relevance* to all varieties of complex incoming signals. Instantly, it relays these priorities up to influence the responses of higher cortical levels over much of the back of our brain, and even as far forward as the orbital cortex [ZBR:168, 175–176]. The pulvinar also enters into specialized functional connections with the angular gyrus. These become especially enhanced when we focus spatial attention.[1] This normal liaison between the pulvinar and the angular gyrus will become an important avenue for enhancing their joint functions. Moreover, it explains why the reticular cap that inhibits the pulvinar also deactivates the angular gyrus. Separate projections from the pulvinar to the amygdala and to the cingulate cortex further emphasize how vital an influence its signals play in shaping the habitual emotional processing of our limbic system.[2]

Two Main Divisions of Subnuclei in the Pulvinar

Primate studies provide important clues about how the pulvinar assigns its coding priorities. The pulvinar divides many of its normal functions between two main groups of subnuclei.[3] The attentive reader will soon notice a point of crucial importance. This natural grouping into *two tiers*—dorsal and ventral—is relevant to other major themes in this book. Indeed, it resembles many similar functional divisions of the cortex for attention that were discussed in part I. It is especially intriguing with respect to the Self/other representations discussed in part II, and therefore to our understanding of how selfless insight occurs.

The Dorsal Group of Subnuclei in the Pulvinar

Two arrows in figure 6 illustrate how separate paths enable the more dorsal group (dPUL) to interact both with the angular gyrus *and* with a part of the precuneus, respectively. Moreover, the discussion in chapter 16 hinted that some normal "leaps" of imagination might be facilitated by a triad of interconnections capable of linking associations from the posterior thalamus with both lateral *and* medial cortical sites. Note that these pathways linking the dorsal pulvinar with both the outside and inside of our parietal cortex can help integrate the

Three important inhibitory nuclei are shown, artificially detached, at the bottom. They are the *reticular nucleus*, the *zona incerta* (ZI), and the *anterior pretectal nucleus* (aPT). Two relay nuclei of the thalamus are also shown at the bottom right. The *lateral geniculate nucleus* (LG) relays visual data to the occipital cortex. The *medial geniculate nucleus* (MG) relays auditory information to the auditory cortex. The *superior colliculus* (SC) in the midbrain relays its reflexive visual and related polymodal messages quickly through both the dorsal and ventral pulvinar to the cortex. Its counterpart, the inferior colliculus, plays a similar auditory role. See plate 4 for the color version of this figure.

network of conventional egocentric functions distributed along the dorsal occipital → parietal path.

A separate thalamic nucleus in this same dorsal tier has been singled out to play a special role. This fact illustrates the general bias of the dorsal nuclei toward Self-referential leanings. Why is this *lateral posterior nucleus* (LP) distinctive in its physiological orientation? Because it interacts with the major somatosensory association region underlying our physical sense of Self, the whole *superior parietal lobule* (sPL) (a site shown also in figure 4). This LP nucleus also interacts with parts of the *precuneus* (a site also shown in figure 2).

Why are these normal dorsal thalamic ↔ cortical interactions so important? Because they help incorporate the higher-order functions of our Self-centered soma into the various 3-D topographical mergers involved in representing an ongoing external event. How could such joint efforts transform other-centered space? In a sense, they could enable us to "imagine" extending our body out into the matrix of our environment, envision ways to embed our physical image inside this shared space, and truly "embody it" [ZBR:148–152)]. In short, they enable us to act in the outside world.

The Ventral Group of Subnuclei in the Pulvinar

The pulvinar's ventral group of subnuclei (vPUL) assign salience to the messages that are processed *allocentrically*, enabling them to play a role in other-referential functions. Figure 6 suggests that this version of object-centered information could then relay forward throughout the lower occipital → temporal pathway.[4] Recent primate studies indicate that the most lateral nucleus of the inferior pulvinar connects with this ventral other-referential stream.[5]

These last three sentences make explicit the earlier suggestions in parts I and II: The lower, ventral, occipital → temporal stream processes other-referential messages, injecting its portent of salience into the way we normally process object-centered types of information.

The Limbic Nuclei of the Dorsal Thalamus

A distinctive group of thalamic nuclei is also arrayed along this same dorsal tier of the thalamus. They line up just in front of the pulvinar and lateral posterior nucleus [ZBR:168]. Their limbic connections make them especially important [ZBR:171–175]. Of course, a variety of impulses from the limbic system rise up to influence the emotional responses of parts of our cortex—for better or worse. But many of these impulses will undergo processing in these so-called limbic nuclei of the dorsal thalamus. Which parts of the cortex are the next targets for such strong limbic influences that relay up from our dorsal thalamus?

Chapter 15 introduced them. Figure 5 highlighted them in orange. Indeed, the PET scan data condensed in figure 5 ranks these medial cortical targets of the limbic thalamus as having the highest ongoing resting metabolic activities in the whole human brain. It is no coincidence that these large cortical "hot spots" are connected with the three "limbic" nuclei of the dorsal thalamus, nor that the angular gyrus (orange areas in figure 4) is a special target of the dorsal pulvinar.

To-and-fro oscillations normally reverberate among the various circuits in this bidirectional cortical-subcortical partnership:

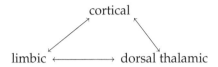

What are the dysfunctional consequences of these connections? They are substantial. Agitating such a turbulent coalition are the cognitive dissonances, emotional valences, and hard-wired instinctual drives that lend dynamic qualities to our *psychic* Self. We acquired overinflated notions of Selfhood when we were infants, and further embedded their emotional constructs in a lifetime of journal entries. So deeply conditioned are our longings and loathings that now, in adult life, their resonances shape our covert attitudes and their misdirected energies distort our interpersonal behaviors. (And, as meditators soon learn, these same energies help to drive the "monkey mind" into random discursive thoughts.)

The arrows in figure 6 specify the particular pathways that link the three limbic nuclei of the dorsal thalamus with their highly active counterpart regions in the higher cortex. The limbic nuclei include:

1. The large *medial dorsal thalamic nucleus (MD)*. It engages in interactions with all regions of the prefrontal cortex (PFC).

2. The *anterior thalamic nucleus*. Its links are shown here with the posterior cingulate cortex (PCC) and with some adjacent portions of the retrosplenial cortex (RETROSPLEN), yet it also supplies the whole anterior extent of the long cingulate gyrus. Notably, it contains many head direction nerve cells, as does its neighbor.

3. The *lateral dorsal nucleus* (LD). Its functions also contribute to enhance the high metabolic activities of the medial and posterior cortex.

Various lines of evidence suggest that the resulting thalamocortical interactions help us generate and store countless Self-relational (and allied circumstantial) memories. Represented at mostly subconscious levels, these narratives remain tightly attached to our psyche. Therefore, without our knowledge, they easily bias our versions of reality, and mislead us into counterproductive thoughts and attitudes. Closely attached to our soma are still other memories that we con- ~~solidate unknowingly. They could motivate us to "head" in impulsive, impractical~~ directions [ZBR:172–173].

Well, so what? It's easy to acknowledge that we have a Self, and to be flat-tered into believing that its assets greatly outweigh its liabilities. So what good is a map that shows some of its anatomical and physiological correlates? Does this map show how such an omniSelf could *shed* its biased Self-centering, cut off those liabilities caused by its overconditioned limbic system, become more self*less*? Not yet.

What is missing? Selflessness requires another explanation. It needs a system that can *subtract* or *bypass* the networks that link this dorsal pulvinar and limbic thalamus with their counterparts up in the cortex [ZB:614, 653–659]. Selflessness requires a major source of *deactivation*, a way to dampen the ordinary oscillations that reverberate between thalamus and cortex [ZBR:174–175].

Potential Inhibitory Sources in the Subcortex

Additional, subcortical mechanisms now reenter our discussion, helping to spec-ify how certain frontoparietal target regions can be deactivated (chapter 15). Ch'an Master Huang-po once said there was a "Gateless Gate to the Stillness Be-yond All Activity" [ZB:367]. In this regard, three groups of γ-aminobutyric acid (GABA) nerve cells now play a pivotal role. They can serve as a "gate" in the thalamus. The largest by far is the *reticular nucleus of the thalamus.* Its insulating blanket of inhibitory neurons envelops *all* nuclei of the thalamus, selectively.[6] It prevents their nerve cells from overfiring (and it shields them from becoming "overheated," in a sense).[7] Cast in a similar role are two smaller nuclei shown at the bottom of figure 6. Their lesser GABA pathways also ascend to inhibit the thalamus. One nucleus is the *zona incerta* (ZI). The other is the *anterior pretectal nucleus* (APT). Each of the three inhibitory nuclei can exert a *potent, selective influ-ence* that negates the functions of the higher-order thalamic nuclei cited above [ZBR:176–179].

These GABA nuclei are small, thin, inconspicuous. Can they act decisively to change the way larger cortical ↔ thalamic networks synchronize their firing pat-terns? Yes. Their inhibitory functions can shift the critical frequency rates of the oscillations that normally shimmer back and forth between the thalamus and the cortex. Inphase oscillations can unify and enhance the shared functions of the two levels; out-of-phase oscillations become disorganized, ineffectual.

In short, GABA *nerve cells can shift our usual physiological bias.* Its usual bias has been to keep our two frames of Self/other reference always tilted toward expressing our most Self-centered functions. But suppose a shift were to occur acutely that stopped this former bias. Now, our internal compass could abandon its standard polarized, Self-referential tendencies. Now, instead of an attitude that points all messages *inwardly*, into a Self-centered awareness, the new mental field could open out into a seemingly new dimension of OTHER-consciousness. Why does perception now seem to register so clearly and directly inside this novel state of consciousness? Because it has been emptied of all prior maladaptive limbic associations linked to the old, overconditioned *I-Me-Mine* [ZBR:22, 333–334].

On the other hand, some reports of kensho leave the impression that a residual quasi-physical representation of the self-image is projected out into an enveloping "Oneness" of external space [ZBR:342–345]. What might explain such a paradox? Perhaps, when dorsal Self-centered processing is suspended, the spared ventral pathways in the thalamus permit elementary somatosensory messages from the head and body still to be represented by ongoing functions from the ventral posterior nucleus [ZB:263–264; ZBR:456].

Implications of Changing the Physiological Balance between Self and Other

This discussion points to deactivations that decrease the functions of three limbic and two other specific nuclei, all in the dorsal thalamus. These deactivations could cause a significant decrease in the maladaptive influences of the Self.[8] What kind of *residual* effects could *repeated*, major sudden shifts into selflessness have on one's personality? Ideally, a person who underwent repeated states of awakening could evolve into a sage who was free from unfruitful overconditionings, unattached to Self-centered conceits, unburdened by habitual indulgences and heartaching resentments [ZB:579–584; ZBR:240–250, 394–396].

For ordinary long-term meditators, such shifts away from their overly subjective Self toward other-referential processing can also evolve slowly, incrementally. When little insights arise, they can help the meditator prune back the *I-Me-Mine* before it regrows toward its original size. As part of a general working hypothesis, shifts of various degrees and durations in the direction toward other-centered processing have two corollary implications.

1. They could help explain why long-term meditators often discover that their greater degrees of self*less*ness coincide with the impression that their mental state is becoming increasingly clear, and that they have grown more mindfully aware of ongoing events.

2. They sponsor testable hypotheses, helping ultimately to clarify the physiological basis for the major transformations of consciousness during advanced states of awakening [ZB:491–533; ZBR:337–338, 369–371]. Such proposals have been relatively straightforward:

- During such extraordinary states, called kensho or satori in Zen, the whole mental field shifts instantly into allocentric processing.
- This *OTHER-referential* processing becomes the sole mode of undiluted comprehension.
- During such novel states, shorn both of Self and of personal time, penetrating insights probe deep into existential issues.
- The accompanying affirmative changes have a potential to revise the patterns of impulse flow in ways that transform the person's subsequent behavioral traits [ZB:653–659].
- The late moonlight phase of kensho can be envisioned as a delayed inhibitory wave of reactive deactivation. It serves to confirm that the earlier sequences represented an imbalance of activation within temporal lobe allocentric pathways [ZBR:418, 425–432].

Commentary

Are such states so mysterious? Ancient Zen traditions downplay kensho-satori as "nothing special." Moreover, brain research in recent decades, including reports discussed in these pages, can be interpreted to suggest that normal, inherent biological mechanisms are plausible candidates for many mental phenomena that arise during the superficial absorptions and the deeper alternate states of consciousness. Why then, should the advanced states remain so puzzling?

They certainly puzzle the witness. Consider some reasons:

- There is no simple precedent for any deep state of insight-wisdom that suddenly wipes out every biased entry you've handwritten in your lifelong journal, leaving only an anonymous mirror to behold a whole new dimension of transformed objective consciousness.
- When this OTHER perspective flashes in to reify the entire mental foreground, it comprehends a simple fact. This new level of understanding was previously inconceivable: This, JUST THIS, is the way all things REALLY are, in themselves!
- Then, as the pace of flashing insights slows, a realization of Oneness dawns: The ordinary world of phenomena (one's prior impression of relative reality), and THIS fresh, underlying absolute, objective (noumenal) world are *One and the Same!*

Research in this new century has barely begun to explore the normal, commonplace allocentric origins underlying states so extraordinary that they dissolve not only the witnesses' sense of Self but enable all personal time to evaporate into ETERNITY. Subsequent generations of neuroscientists may begin to appreciate why the ancient sutra records that a man called Siddhartha once said:

"The end of the conceit 'I am'—that is the truly greatest happiness of all."[9]

20

On the Long Path toward Selflessness

Your subjective ideas are deeply rooted, and hard to pull out all at once. So I employ temporary expedients to take away your coarse perceptions.

Master Yang-shan (807–883)[1]

The Path of Zen leads toward selflessness incrementally. This long Path emphasizes the Self-imposed discipline of regular meditation (*zazen*) and the daily life practice of mindful introspection in the workaday world (*shugyo*). It also develops one's capacities to endure the rigors of repeated meditative retreats (*sesshin*). Zazen exercises each trainee's determination to make—and *keep*—a firm, ongoing commitment: to dedicate a block of time for silent meditation every day. This habitual decision—to withdraw in solitude from the hyperactive 24/7 world—demonstrates a key principle: There's no need to be constantly "*doing* things."

Levels of calm, no-thought, perceptual clarity develop when one adheres to a regular schedule of morning meditation. This morning setting helps foster subtle, intuitive realizations. Thoreau understood that "All memorable events … transpire in morning time and in a morning atmosphere," and he supported this claim by referring to the ancient saying from the Vedas that "All intelligences awake with the morning" [ZB:621].

Retreats are essential to carry the benefits of daily meditation to yet another level. Rigorous retreats develop one's capacities to adapt and to persist despite inevitable physical and mental discomfort. Retreats are highly educational. They lead you to an intimate appreciation of how much you are indeed the source of your own anguish, resistance, and boredom.

Many transient physiological surges warp one's perceptions along the meditative path [ZB:457–460]. They too are educational. How are we to interpret these "quickenings?" One way is simply to view them as the functions of normal networks that have become briefly overactive. The previous chapter serves as a reminder: Overactivations are followed by *de*activations, at levels both cortical and subcortical. Whenever a physiological imbalance prompts causes excitatory functions to surge into consciousness, a secondary surge of reactive inhibitory responses stands ready to contain them.

The Feel of Two Hands

Quickenings occur not only while one is seated on the meditation cushion. I once experienced a memorable quickening ten minutes *after* my morning meditation [ZB:399–404]. The episode was triggered by the simple act of drying my face with a towel. Though the incident lasted only 5 or 10 seconds, it greatly amplified my sensation of tactile awareness in both hands, R > L. This physiological surge appeared to have engaged *selective* regions of my cortex in dynamic combinations with their deeper thalamic counterparts. With reference now to the red-and-white dashed line in figure 4, it is plausible that this overactivity of touch perception had involved a local branch of the dorsal egocentric pathway as it streams through the anterior parietal lobe.[2]

Bytes of Memory

A separate episode of quickening occurred (also after meditating) one evening in the zendo. It was a fastforward mode of mental scanning that leaped beyond the sentences by Hakuin that I was actually chanting at that moment [ZB:395–397]. This surge had easy access to my memory of this familiar chant, and anticipated big bytes of its next lines. It then expressed these lines in a rush of "heard-thoughts" that were being projected out into the space directly in front of me. So agile was this process that it operated equally well during a fast-reverse mode. An episode of hyperfluent language processing appeared to have taken over some normal functions of the left inferior frontal region. The thalamic counterpart to this frontal region is the medial dorsal thalamic nucleus (MD) (figure 6). One speculation is that some transient increase in dopamine processing had overcome its usual local GABA inhibitory constraints.

Chanting and Imagining

When normal subjects are monitored by MEG while they are either singing or humming a popular song, they develop increased alpha and beta activities bilaterally in their premotor, sensorimotor, and superior parietal areas.[3] On other occasions, even though they are still only imagining this song, beta oscillations (15 to 30 cps) occur in these same regions. Moreover, only during this same kind of imagining mode do they also develop high-frequency gamma oscillations (60 to 200 cps) in Broca's area (BA 44). This gamma activity appears to represent a silent interior rehearsal, one that serves as a preliminary step for their actual, subsequent singing.

The Hippocampal Formation: Implications of a Division of Labor

The parahippocampal gyrus rolls up into the hippocampal formation near the front of each medial temporal lobe (figures 2, 5). Important point: Both egocentric and allocentric local circuits reside close together down here in the hippocampus [ZB:180–189; ZBR:99–108]. The evidence suggests that some hippocampal circuits can enter into the early tagging and indexing of Self-centered memory functions, whereas others can contribute similarly to allocentric functions. It becomes of interest to consider how the different ego-/allo- modules in the two networks might have participated during two other episodes that were previously described.

The first episode was a brief quickening. It occurred during the final sitting in the zendo around 9:00 P.M. [ZB:390–391]. Abruptly, a succession of static images projected themselves into vision just *below* the center of gaze. Each was a snapshot, a framed memory of an actual event, involving recognizable people and places. Each individual scene lasted for a fraction of a second. Each such image was selected from widely separate decades, fell into no clear sequence, and had no obvious unifying theme. It was as though I were flipping at random through a personal album of old, faded color prints, during an interval that lasted perhaps a total of 10 to 15 seconds.

Parts I through III have suggested how such scenes might have originated. They could have represented personal Self/other journal entries retrieved within a network that linked the hippocampus with medial parietal and frontal regions and with the inferior parietal lobule. Posterior regions in this network seemed to have gained access to the entries in this visual journal, flipped through its scenes, then retrieved *and* recognized the gist of random samples drawn from its pages. These old scenes were colored only faintly, an observation in keeping with the mostly egocentric dorsal stream orientation of this medial network. This dorsal stream lacks the heightened color sensitivities that would be conferred by the fusiform gyrus (FG), a ventral-stream region located on the undersurface of the temporo-occipital junction (figure 5).

A Taste of Kensho

The second experience was a much more complex surge of overactivity. It occurred in London on a Sunday morning. I was looking up into the sky from a train platform, while traveling to the second day of a retreat [ZBR:407–432]. Initially, such a kensho experience might seem to present a paradox. When a person's sense of Self dissolves, *if* the hippocampus were the sole gateway into every kind of memory, and *if* this one route into memory flowed *only* within a single dorsal egocentric stream—and *if* that one stream were now all bypassed—then why should one's memory functions continue to record the immediate and ongoing memorable details of the selfless state of kensho?

The apparent paradox can be resolved. We can postulate that other hippocampal and parahippocampal circuits still continued to index ongoing events and interact within the remaining allocentric pathway. Such a selective sparing of place cell functions on the allocentric pathway can account for the fact the details of kensho are preserved in the sequences of one's ongoing visual memory.[4]

A similar proposal could help account for the way an entire perceptual scene becomes indelible during major insights of other kinds. After Charles Darwin's insight into natural selection, he wrote: "I can remember the very spot on the road whilst in my carriage, when to my joy, the solution occurred to me."[5]

An Experience of Internal Absorption

One evening, while meditating in Kyoto, a major hyperattentive surge entered an aroused and successively heightened mode of one-pointed attention [ZB:470–518]. It hallucinated a color-saturated leaf as it spread within attentional and memory networks represented more on the right side of the brain. The evidence suggested that both the right and left sides of the reticular nucleus of the thalamus could have reacted, secondarily, in response to the earlier phases that had activated both attentive systems. GABA nerve cells in this reticular nucleus appeared to play a major inhibitory role in blocking sensory transmission in the back of the thalamus. This blockade could have occurred at the level of the *lowermost* sensory relay nuclei (figure 6). Norepinephrine and serotonin systems could also have shared in an accompanying stress response and contributed to the scope and depth of this unusual state of consciousness.

Commentary

Zen traditions regard a variety of such episodes as nothing special [ZB:373–387]. From the neuroscience point of view, we do not need to regard them as esoteric. They simply represent three quickenings and two extraordinary states. Each happened to be expressed in sequences involving different regions and levels of the brain.[6]

21

Neuroimaging during Tasks That Shift the Brain from Self-Referential into Other-Referential Forms of Attention

> Inclusion of a control condition referable to a physiological baseline puts one in the best position to correctly understand imaging data.
>
> Marcus Raichle and Mark Mintun[1]

In their 2006 review article, Raichle and Mintun reemphasize the need to determine the true resting "baseline" functions of key networks in the human brain. They also call attention to the remarkable ways certain networks shift—*up or down*—from this resting baseline. Each direction of functional shift is of central importance.

The article begins with the data cited earlier, in chapters 13 and 19. Recall that these PET scan data showed that two of the brain's largest metabolic "hot spots" occupy regions along the *midline* of our frontal and parietal cortex (figure 5). Indeed, these medial regions stay highly active even when the person's brain might seem to have settled down toward a relatively quiet state of baseline, "resting" equilibrium. Why is it useful to keep returning to this concept of resting equilibrium?

Because even if such a resting condition provides only a tentative baseline, it still enables one to observe how the brain can shift its activities—*up or down*—in several intriguing ways. Note for example, that some of the resting hot spots become even "hotter" when they become further activated. Precisely when does this activation occur? *It occurs when our attention turns internally and shifts into Self-referential (egocentric) tasks.* No surprises here. Such tasks do seem to be Self-oriented, Self-centered. But this alone can't prove that our "Self" components are the sole, exclusive agencies that function in such spots. Nor does it mean that our "Self" is housed only in such cortical spots.

Why not? Because, as part I discusses, any such introspective, goal-directed tasks also involve an inevitable *inturning* of attention. Therefore, let's not regard hot spots as occupying just some narrow niche where we store only the Self content of our personal database. What else do the high metabolism and the limbic connections of these regions indicate? These two clues point to a context that is much larger, almost "holographic." Hot spots are foci of activity in a huge network. They represent *how and where and when this person had once attended to events in the past, had registered and elaborated on such detailed information, then kept it indexed and instantly accessible.* Why would anyone do this? *In case he or she ever needed to retrieve it.*

More About Deactivations

Remember how the early PET scan data also showed something surprising (chapter 15)? Something else happens when we turn our attention *outward* toward various ordinary *external* goals.[2] Now those same frontoparietal regions—the ones that were previously hot spots at rest—get slightly "cooler." Therefore, the act of directing attention *outward* toward the environment partially *de*activates these same mostly midline regions. Note: Partially means only *a small fraction*, not the whole. The distinction introduces a sense of proportion that has practical implications.[3]

Why, even when we seem to be at "rest," do these particular frontoparietal, mostly midline modules already bustle with so much activity? Part II already suggested one reason why these regions work so hard: it requires constant effort to straddle a Self/other fence. It takes work to maintain, integrate, and keep accessible the reams of detailed data we have stored in these *two* huge domains. We forget that our actual "global" experience is fundamentally a *blend*, one that combines data from *two* frames of reference. Why does such a *two*-sided enterprise seem to run counter to our usual, comforting impression? Because we've long been firmly attached to one notion: that our *I-Me-Mine* controls the axial center of every action. Indeed, its supremely Self-fulfilling priorities seem fully to dictate the course and dominate the memories of every event. We've simply not been made aware that there is another object-centered, form-sensitive style of other-referential processing. It's always been there, but we've been deceived (table 6).

A simple experiment illustrates how the absolute supremacy of one version of vision dominates another. Select a distant spot. Reach out with your right arm and point your index finger at it, so that this spot seems directly in line with your nose and your fingertip. First close your left eye. Then open it. Next, close your right eye. Note the jump. For most people, the right eye is their "master eye." Its version dominates when we align our head, eyes, and arm in space. The nondominant left eye still has its own field, and still contributes to 3-D vision. However, its own version is overruled in the ordinary act of eyes-open pointing.

Usually, we have little reason to question such biased working impressions. Normally, our personal Self (like our "master" eye) automatically assumes sovereignty over its private domain. This dominant Self has a long history. We've reified it in thought and action, documented it in time and in space. Yet, in actual fact, we've also *co*registered huge quantities of other historical and geographical details *subconsciously*. These items are referable to the scenery of that rather messy world outside. They remain as invisible as the submerged bulk of an iceberg, suspended mostly out of sight and out of mind. Consider how much is involved in this huge, complex *subconscious* operation:

- We maintain not only a journal that records older Self-centered entries and loosely integrates them with corresponding external circumstantial details.
- We also register and attend to brand *new* events—and meld *them* too—along both sides of the Self/other boundary![4]

Relationships at the Interface between Self and Other

To appreciate the huge dimensions of this subconscious Self/other task, it helps to consider a clinical analogy. It relates to the techniques health professionals use when they are called upon to judge a patient's mental competence. A premise underlies this determination: human memory hinges on recalling multiple prior associations. Indeed, because each patient's personality develops in such a larger multirelational context, the consultants tend to begin with a list of elementary questions. The key words might seem to have only a literary ring, for they start by asking the standard adverbial questions: "who-what-where-when-why?" In fact, the answers will help assess the connections among the association cortex of all four lobes.

Thus, when neurologists and psychiatrists begin to determine a patient's intellectual competence, they pose tasks that search for evidence not just on one side of the patient's Self/other boundary. Their lines of questioning are essentially *relational*: can the patient blend together the *two sets* of facts—Self/other—*in both space and time?* Does he know more than *who* he really is? Does she also know, say, *what* the current president's name is? *Where* she is now, and *where* she lives? Moreover, does he know *when* it is (the correct time, date, and year), and also understand the reasons *why* he is being seen?

We have noticed that neuroimaging researchers also tend to be task-driven individuals. When they're on a quest for the sources of human Self-identity, it seems only natural for them to assign tasks for their subjects to solve. As a result, most early PET scan studies were task-driven. Researchers usually required their subjects to make mental shifts. These were either externalized (toward other) or internalized (toward Self). Therefore, the chief findings, just summarized, were that the hot spots deactivated during external shifts of attention and activated during Self-centered introspections. Nowadays, specialized fMRI techniques are most often used. The sections reviewed next continue to regard this actively emerging field as work still in progress.

Recent fMRI Imaging Correlates of an Ongoing Self-Referential Orientation during Assigned Tasks

After the previous review of this topic went to press [ZBR:193–199], fMRI researchers worldwide continued to confirm and extend the original PET scan findings. Again, the recent data point not only to a few spots where a so-called Self per se might be located. Instead, the fMRI findings suggest that (1) networks and modules are widely distributed and consistent more with an "omniself"; (2) *some* Self-referential functions are *co*registered *in relation* to "other" frames of reference, within a much broader context; and (3) some multimodal Self/other associations are now sharing coordinates in a dynamic process that codes for space and time along a scale of values. A brief survey of these recent fMRI findings begins with the frontoparietal network, most of which is *medial* in location.

- It maintains a very substantial, dynamic, online activity when the eyes are closed at rest. This ongoing, tonic activity also occurs during passive open-eyed tasks when the subject enters into simple, ordinary low-level functions of visual observation. Meditators may find some reassurance in the latest reports. It turns out that certain normal people who show more baseline fMRI signals in their medial regions at rest are also predisposed to report more mind-wandering thoughts that are like "daydreaming." Their thought streams arise both when they are placed in a passive resting condition and when they become bored by overpracticing routine tasks.[5]

- Thereafter, the prefrontal regions of this medial network can be recruited into additional, active, higher-order Self-referential functions that engage the psyche in more complex executive and autobiographical operations. Farther back, both the medial parietal and the inferior parietal lobule components can enter into other subtle higher-order elaborations. If, in a sense, these functions help to "embody" aspects of our physical Self-image in the scenery they do so by consulting a wide variety of visuospatial functions that are *also* other-referential in nature.

- *Particular increases occur.* One small percent of this resting network's substantial "baseline" activities can increase briefly (phasically). When? When we superimpose a particular additional task that involves interoceptive, *Self*-referential kinds of internal attentive processing. Clearly, this slight increase in fMRI signals is a partial phenomenon. Sometimes its shifts are so subtle they can be appreciated only when the researchers clearly establish a resting control period, one that has allowed their subjects to settle down quietly for many minutes.

- *Particular decreases occur.* This resting network's "baseline" activities also respond quickly with brief (phasic) *decreases*. When do these *de*activations occur? In response to tasks of a different kind. These tasks evoke externally directed attentive processing, the kinds that remain exteroceptive and *other*-referential. Again, these deactivations are also relatively slight. They too are often revealed only when the research design has provided an adequate resting baseline. An important point: greater decreases occur when the tasks are more difficult, demand more mental effort, *and require more attentional resources.*

- Yet this mostly medial frontoparietal network doesn't respond quickly only by such obviously task-*driven* increases or decreases. The fast resolving powers of fMRI now reveal something crucial that PET scans had missed. *Even at rest, fMRI signals also undergo a slow, spontaneous fluctuation. This normal variability of fMRI signals is of a very remarkable kind.* When do these slow fluctuations occur? The answer bears repetition: Spontaneously, even during rest.

The spontaneous fluctuations recur several times a minute, much more slowly than do the peaks of the old, familiar EEG waveforms. We turn to their important implications in the next chapter.

Commentary

During meditation, what sustained interval could come closer to representing a "real" psychophysiological baseline? Surely, one candidate remains those longer intervals when more proficient meditators let go and sustain moments of genuine "no-thought" clarity and bare awareness. This combination occurs increasingly during the more advanced levels of meditative training. At this writing, no reports have yet focused exclusively on *just this* interval during prolonged open receptive meditation. It is a curious omission, for the whole phenomenon deserves a comprehensive investigation. When even a shallow period of no-thought supervenes during this writer's usual state of (eyes partly open) meditation, the scope of the whole external environment expands, becomes experienced through a heightened and globally clarified awareness, only part of which is attributable to the spontaneous elevation of the eyelids.

22

Slow Fluctuations, Revealing How Networks Shift Spontaneously

> Union gives strength.
>
> Aesop (sixth century B.C.E.)

Brain regions grow stronger when they cooperate. "Nerve cells that fire together, wire together." How do they join forces? All the answers aren't yet in. Indeed, Michael Fox and colleagues at Washington University in St. Louis reported in 2005 that parts of the Self-centered network are connected more at some times, but less at others.[1] They detected these recurrent variations in "functional connectivity" in the *resting* brain. Their data, documented impressively in color, showed that our brain constantly undergoes *slow spontaneous* shifts in signals—up and down, at rest—when *no* tasks were added.

Even more intriguing: when spontaneous shifts occurred in the Self-referential network, simultaneous shifts often took place in the *opposite* direction in the other-referential network. It happened almost like a seesaw: When Self went up, other went down. When other went up, Self went down. Are you a meditator, wondering how you might decrease the influence of the Self? Here it is, happening spontaneously!

In this 2005 report, ten normal adults served as subjects. fMRI monitored whatever transpired in each subject's mental field during one of "three different rest conditions." Note how this passive "rest" was being defined. It was a condition of very *minimal* mental effort, comparable in many respects to an elementary form of meditation. For example, each subject was then passively engaged either in (1) simple, soft visual fixation on a crosshair; (2) resting, with eyes closed; or (3) resting in dim lighting, with the eyes open, but not fixed on a particular object.

No subjects were actually engaged in formal meditation, and their minds often wandered. However, these preliminary data showed that some intrinsic to-and-fro undercurrents were underlying the flow patterns of our normal streams of consciousness and unconsciousness. Most intriguing to the theme of this book was the possibility that if we could clarify the mechanisms for both the overt fMRI responses and these covert fluctuations it might help us understand how the brain could shift into extraordinary states during long-term formal meditative training.

Notably, to begin with, the baseline fMRI signals were similar during each of these three passive "rest conditions" cited above. However, once sufficient time was allowed to elapse to detect the slow, spontaneous fluctuations, the two opposing networks again tended to shift their fMRI signals in an up-or-down reciprocal manner. Suppose, for example, that resting signals happened to *decrease* in the Self-referential network. Simultaneously, signals often *increased* in the other-referential attention network.

The Other-Referential Network

Let's now be specific about which modules constitute this other-referential network. They showed (by virtue of each slow, spontaneous increase in signals) that they were then interconnected with the others in this same category. They included

- the intraparietal sulcus (IPS) and the supramarginal gyrus (SMG) of the inferior parietal lobule;
- the frontal lobe in its orbital, frontal eye field (FEF), and supplementary motor area regions;
- the frontal lobe in its dorsolateral portions;
- the posterior temporal lobe in its lower lateral portion (the so-called middle temporal [MT] portion (BA 19/37);
- the region of the insula and adjacent frontal operculum.

When we examine this first article by Fox et al.,[1] we see that its figure 3 deploys "hotter" colors to illustrate these *spontaneously increased* fMRI signal intensities. The use of such red and yellow colors highlights the enhanced "functional connectivities" that briefly strengthen the links among this constellation of *lateral* regions just listed above. "Hotter" connections mean that when these particular sites join together, not only do they share their stronger activities but they also tend to co-vary them *at the same time and in the same direction*.

It is no accident that this pattern of hot colors tends to overlap with much of the same *lateral* cortical attention network discussed in chapter 7. We've seen how the overt responses of that lateral network activate during *externally goal-directed attention and working memory* (and seen a comparable representation of that attention network illustrated, asymmetrically, in figure 3 of this book).

Now, what about the different kind of slow, spontaneous shifts, the ones that recur in the mostly *medial* regions of the frontoparietal network? These regions fluctuate, simultaneously, in the *opposite* direction, showing shifts that *decrease* their fMRI signals. The fMRI data show that this network overlaps with the *Self-referential* regions.

The Self-Referential Network

This network includes:

- That very large cluster of sites back in the posterior medial region. As discussed in chapter 13 (and illustrated in figures 4 and 5), this region consists of the posterior cingulate cortex (PCC), the precuneus (PRECUN), and the retrosplenial cortex (RETROSPLEN).
- Much of the medial prefrontal cortex (PFC; both BA 32 and 10).
- The angular gyrus (ANG) of the inferior parietal lobule (BA 39).
- The superior frontal (BA 8) and inferior temporal cortex (BA 20/21).

Accordingly, we find that the same figure 3 of Fox et al. used "cooler" colors to illustrate these linked regions that had all shifted, simultaneously, toward *decreased* signals. These cooler green and blue colors represented connections that were *decreased* in modules throughout the Self-referential network.

Now observe carefully. When we turn back the pages to examine figure 1 in the article by Fox et al. we must immediately switch our own mental sets. Several times. Because their figure 1 illustrates the set of changes that had taken place many seconds later, *after* the resting subject had undergone a slow, spontaneous *fluctuation*. This subject is still simply looking out passively, as before, toward the same crosshair. Yet, now we discover what happens when the brain undergoes a *slow, spontaneous* shift in a *reciprocal* manner. Each patterned set of colors in their figures 1 and 3 is seen to have *shifted places*. Hotter colors occupy the regions of the former cooler colors, and vice versa.

No new task was involved. No directed thought process, no intention. The two Self/other networks had shifted spontaneously. Normal, intrinsic, slow cyclic fluctuations during this resting state had reversed the two sets of color-coded images in diametrically opposite directions. Simultaneously, the hotter regions in one network became cooler, and the cooler regions in the other network became hotter. A coherent, reciprocal, seesaw-like process had taken place. (A comparable shift might exchange the colors of the attention network in figure 3 in these pages with the orange colors of the egocentric stream in figures 4 and 5, respectively.)

How often did the two networks continue to change slowly, back and forth, spontaneously? It is tempting to search for a gross, first-order approximation of the ego/allo cycle. The timeline at the bottom of their figure 1 indicates how many fluctuations occurred during a five-minute interval in one human subject. This person's two sets of color-coded patterns appear to go through reciprocal cycles: peaks in one cycle tend to coincide with valleys in the other. Their figure 1 suggests that a slow, switching process tends to recur three times a minute.

Confirmation of such a reciprocal cyclic tendency is evident in Peter Fransson's report.[2] There, figure 6 illustrates the slow fMRI fluctuations in a different subject who was also studied during rest. This person's signals fluctuated spontaneously between a Self-referential (introspective) mode and what Fransson called an "extrospectively oriented mode." The two sets of signals appear to alternate directions four times a minute. Notably, when Fransson's subjects shifted into such an external (extrospective) mode, the data in figure 6 indicated that the active regions corresponded with *both* the top-down and bottom-up systems of multimodal attention discussed in part I.

Questions and Commentary

- What are these slow, *reciprocal* fluctuations? Are they an index of genuine neuronal activity in the brain? Or only artifacts? To pick up raw fMRI signals requires sensitive imaging techniques that can detect low levels of blood oxygen. But some of these blood oxygen level–dependent (BOLD) signals can be mimicked both by the rhythm of cardiac contractions, and by changes in carbon dioxide levels secondary to variations in respiration.[3] However, significant signals still survive after the raw data are corrected appropriately. What do these corrected results reveal? Similar robust, reliable patterns of distinct brain networks, each one of which is functionally coherent.[4] These fluctuating changes correspond with real networks (this discussion continues in part VII).

- How many separate networks each show evidence of their coherent functional connections when subjects are resting passively? Not just the two major Self/other networks discussed thus far. By 2006, De Luca and colleagues at Oxford University had identified *five different coherent patterns*.[5] Each pattern was composed of a distinct cluster of subregions. All subregions clustered in any one network shared in its distinctive, independent intrinsic "idling" mode at rest.[6] In 2006, Vincent and colleagues at Washington University in St. Louis confirmed that the hippocampus can share its memory-based connections with the other sites in their already-identified consortium of robust, spontaneously active mostly medial resting-state regions (These regions continue, as before, to link into the lateral cortex of the inferior parietal lobule on both sides)[7] (figure 4).

- What would any resting brain gain by engaging slowly, only several times a minute, in such reciprocal "tilting?" Do such covert, intrinsic fluctuations somehow prepare our brain briefly to shift back and forth between its Self-centered, interior orientations (shifts that we don't consciously recognize), and its other innate perspectives that represent externalized modes of attention? Could these silent other-related inclinations represent a kind of exercise, as it were, that prepares them to become more overtly influential, lending greater amplitudes to their reciprocal shifts? While certain spontaneous fluctuations seem also to carry silent, *preoperational potentials* that incline us toward such overreactive functions, present evidence has yet to prove that the mental coherence of a potential cognitive counterpart is poised to enter human consciousness to the same degree. Further answers to these key questions await research during which skilled subjects, at rest, can begin to specify precisely the mental form and content of deeper eddies in their streams of consciousness. While highly skilled mediators could provide some essential first-person reports, they would need further specialized training before they could become expert witnesses capable of making the requisite subtle discriminations[8] [ZBR:3, 48–50].

- In the interim, what's the point in discussing recurrent, spontaneous shifts if they do not seem to register as distinct cognitive changes in our ordinary landscape of consciousness? Their value lies beyond the fact that they show our brain has intrinsic, dynamic capacities to "shift gears." We knew that already. More intriguing are the normal mechanisms that could cause such a distinctive pattern of changes to develop. Consider the facts: Simultaneously, these mechanisms not only are periodically activating one kind of processing. They are also *deactivating* a very different kind of processing in many other modules. In one sweeping shift, vast cortical networks are being reorganized in a reciprocal, seesaw-like manner. *This spontaneous inverse change is transforming physiological connections on both sides of the brain.*

- What is the standard explanation for an intrinsic operation that instantly changes *both* sides of the cortex simultaneously? A switching process that operates from a deeper *sub*cortical level. Chapter 19 discusses why the thalamus is an obvious candidate. The basic mechanisms have many implications for how we understand the shifts toward selfless insight that are discussed throughout parts III and IV.

- Fast corticothalamic oscillations could superimpose a top-down modulating influence on any final throwing of a deeper switch [ZBR:167–175]. For example, the glutamate released by descending cortical fibers quickly excites GABA neurons down in the reticular nucleus of the thalamus. However, glutamate also acts on these GABA nerve cells' slower *metabotropic* receptors. This causes, subsequently, a long-lasting *decrease* in the synchronized inhibitory firing of the reticular nucleus. On the other hand, electrical coupling among reticular nerve cells enhances their inhibitory functions.[9] Similar to-and-fro physiological shifts in the net balances among various other firing rates could overlay the slower intrinsic neurochemical and metabolic mechanisms that generate the fluctuating cycles of functional connectivity and show up as slow rhythmical changes in fMRI signals.

- Are other messages implied in the rhythmical aspects of reciprocal shifts? Thus far, we have discussed several categories and levels of shifting functions. Some immediate responses are more Self-directed internally. Others are evoked by the attention required to accomplish goal-directed explicit exogenous tasks. Still others occur slowly, spontaneously. A deep "central pacemaker" is one plausible explanation for a bilateral slow rhythm, but the thalamus is not the only candidate. The evidence that spontaneous, inverse, fluctuations tend to recur at very slow rates— perhaps only three or four times *a minute*—raises other possibilities. Maybe slow cycles reflect rhythmical activities interconnecting the thalamus with more primitive circuits still farther down, say in the hypothalamus and the brainstem. The next research steps seem obvious: use multiple electrodes to record the firing of nerve cells in primates directly; monitor the electrophysiological and neurochemical correlates of the fMRI fluctuations all over both hemispheres *and* the brainstem during the states of waking, slow wave sleep, REM sleep, and anesthesia.[10]

- To date, light sleep has been studied with fMRI in human subjects, despite the noisy fMRI environment.[11] Slow signal fluctuations did increase in amplitude in the visual cortex during sleep, and they persisted in the other intrinsic network regions as well. Deep anesthesia in monkeys did not stop the spontaneous, coherent fMRI signal fluctuations.[12] These preliminary studies suggest that the biological role of slow fluctuations reflects some fundamental ongoing metabolic patterns of reorganization, the neurochemical and electrophysiological origins of which are not yet clear.

- What *is* clear is that the reciprocal nature of these intrinsic fluctuations confirms the changing patterns of the PET scan responses in similar coherent networks. Major shifts of greater amplitude could be envisioned to underlie the reciprocal phenomena in kensho (see figure 7).

23

The Balance of Opposing Functions: Age-Old Perspectives and the Destabilizing Effect of Triggers

> Nothing so promotes the growth of consciousness as the inner confrontation of opposites.
>
> Carl Jung (1875–1961)

Opposing forces temper a person's character. Carl Jung believed that we went on to mature psychologically after the age of 35 only to the degree that we had confronted and resolved "the problem of opposites" [ZB:660–663]. This is what happened to Siddhartha. One set of opposites is fundamental, to Zen, to the purpose of this book, and to neurobiology in general. It is the pairing of inside with outside. Each time we explore the nature of Self/other relationships, we confront this crucial pairing.

The opposing aspects of inside/outside confront us with far more problems (and opportunities) than we realize. Many chapters in this book specify physiological processes that are normally in opposition. We might label such opposing processes as activation or deactivation. Sometimes we also call them excitation or inhibition. The important point remains: when opposites contend and sculpture our normal biological functions, they often combine forces in practical ways to arrive at a harmonious *balance*.

The terms *egocentric* and *allocentric* also imply opposites (table 4). It is in our best interest that the two network models complement each other, not unlike the ways opposites are paired in the ancient Taoist belief system. It was a fundamental Taoist belief that each of Nature's seemingly contrasting phenomena (such opposites as night and day, hot and cold) were constantly alternating spontaneously and effortlessly. Yet while yin and yang were clearly opposite in sign, they shared *coequal* status in a larger creative partnership, jointly shaping One Universal grand design. The seeds of early Ch'an Buddhism would be planted in this indigenous Taoist cultural soil.

Today, let some serious challenge strike, perhaps while driving on the highway, at the office, or in the home. We must respond instantly. In this immediate moment, what is relevant? Not every old overconditioned network. Only the nitty-gritty, a tiny fraction of our whole mental array. Instantly, attention must shed attachments that had accessed irrelevant contentious, valenced memories. This means bypassing virtually all conflicting circuits that had been preoccupied with trying to insert our old autobiographical Self-in-the-world. Jung foresaw the benefits: once our opposites stop their internal discord, we become free to rechannel their energies efficiently along more harmonious lines.

Are such soft, outdated conceptual models applicable to any simple-minded working hypotheses being proposed in these pages? A few speculations here might become of heuristic use, stimulating later investigations designed to clarify how opposing mechanisms interact along the spiritual path.

Three caveats:

- The mindful, introspective path toward insight might seem to offer one's intellect a gentle way to start pruning off some pejorative branches of the Self [ZB:125–129, 141–145]. Fortunately, our capacity for Self-reflection is innate. Yet, the Self exerts a subversive influence during any naïve internal probing attempts. No short-term, shallow attempts to willfully achieve "selflessness"—however well-intentioned—suffice to cut through the extensive, deep root systems of the *I-Me-Mine* complex. During a retreat, receptive meditation allows us to cultivate our natural attribute of reflection with increasing degrees of objectivity.

- Multidisciplinary research in this field requires subjects who can skillfully conduct an exacting, timed, detailed personal inventory—an ongoing chronicle of consciousness. Their first-person reports must be intimately correlated with an array of neuroimaging and psychophysiological techniques.[1] The goals are threefold. To clarify how the basic physiological parameters of various responses arise; whether they coevolve during, and correlate with, certain psychophysiological events on the meditative path; how they then go on jointly to reshape and transform its outcome [ZB:338–347].

- Such a major research agenda implies serial, repeated, genuinely longitudinal studies of many experienced meditators, a group that represents the normal range of differing temperaments. It means monitoring their fast *and* slow rhythms—at rest, awake, during slow wave sleep, during REM sleep. It means studying meditators not only at moments when their attention is oriented toward simpler external visual, auditory, and tactile cues. It means monitoring them while they wrestle with social dilemmas that present tough conceptual, ethical, and intuitive problems. A tall order. Note how difficult it still is for researchers to prove which fast EEG rhythms called "brain waves" correlate with particular mental functions, three quarters of a century after Hans Berger first introduced the term, "electroencephalography."

Among the speculations about the states of absorption that might be tested, supported, or refuted in the future are these:

- Could some *external* absorptions represent overactivities that surge within the top-down, externally oriented ("other") attentional networks (as shown in figure 3)?

- Is *internal* absorption more likely initially to be associated with a surge of over-activities involving some arousal of bottom-up functions within the ventral association network? [ZBR:319–320]. Of potential interest in this regard was the early appearance of the red leaf referable to the witness's right fusiform gyrus and the impression that his gaze was being held involuntarily, fixed straight-ahead.

Meanwhile, our emerging concepts might tend gradually to soften the impact of a seemingly hard-nosed old Zen teaching. During many past centuries, Zen masters have followed a useful tradition. The masters have tried to check their trainees' understandable enthusiasm with this caveat: the brief awakenings of kensho and satori are "nothing special." And of course, their trainees have resisted. How could anything ordinary shift a person into such extraordinary states? Yet, such a traditional line of interpretation might find reinforcement somewhat as follows:

- Aren't the latest neuroimaging findings lending support, albeit qualified, to the old masters' stance? After all, these data suggest that normal brains—under the most *ordinary* of resting conditions—are undergoing reciprocal ego/allo shifts, perhaps on cycles as often as three to four times a minute.[2] Indeed, the normal brain's repertoire includes covert mechanisms already so well organized that they can routinely deactivate its intrinsic Self-centered orientations and tilt its other-referential network's connectivities in a more allocentric direction.

- Perhaps under our ordinary conditions of rest, we normally keep a very tight rein on the amplitudes and durations of such intrinsic network fluctuations.[3] As a result, only minor "tiltings" in the resting fMRI scans remain as token hints, suggesting that rare—and much greater—shifts in amplitude might potentially transform our external attentive processing by completely dropping out its Self-referential mode.

- Viewed from this simplified perspective, the phenomena of kensho might then seem to begin as a kind of brief imbalance. Perhaps the normal mechanisms of the person's ordinary shifting responses could become briefly "overextended," as it were. Such an enhanced shift could represent a major change in the amplitudes, cyclic frequency, duration, and patterning of that person's Self/other networks. The result would reflect a deep change in innate physiological mechanisms.

- At such a major tipping point, which phenomena of the moment could emerge? The anonymous witness to this extraordinary state of consciousness could awaken into a wide-open field of clear consciousness. Why would such a fresh, unifying, allocentric perspective seem to represent a dramatic, otherworldly departure from the norm? Because it had bypassed all the old biased conditioning responsible for that person's former Self/other sense of duality.

Equipoise

The normal neuroimaging research reviewed thus far points to pivotal shifts. Some responses to stimuli begin in milliseconds. Others evolve only several times a minute. The shifts enable functions within one large network to be selectively accessed and enhanced, whereas other functions in an opposing network are diminished simultaneously. Indeed, our Self-referential and other-referential networks are the two crucial "opposites" sharing such a similar seesaw relationship, yet on different scales of time.

Analogies exist with the way an old-fashioned balance scale operates. Consider the familiar symbolic image of Justice. As she holds up such a balance, why is Justice blindfolded? So that she can weigh *objectively* the individual merits of competing claims. Societies worldwide recognize the underlying principle: Eliminate subjective biases, weigh objectively the realities of a given situation, then render a balanced judgment. Such a scale might appear stable when equally heavy loads weigh down each of its two opposing pans. But breathe on it, and it freely undergoes little fluctuations. It remains in a delicate state of dynamic balance, poised to go up or down.

In the brain, the term *equipoise* can suggest similar natural, physiological capacities for balance. Yet, brain systems retain similar potentials for tipping their functions instantly—indeed, sometimes with substantial released force—in opposite directions. Our neural excitatory mechanisms are so leveraged, and so coordinated with their inhibitory counterparts, that when regions linked into one network swing into activation, their opposite functions in another network can tilt toward corresponding degrees of *de*activation. Symmetrical modules in the opposite hemisphere can be yoked to support and strengthen each other, yet remain free to contribute their own innate responses—some excitatory, some inhibitory—when they are recruited into the constellation of a different network [ZBR:546, chapter 96, note 13].

What Role Does a Triggering Stimulus Play in Upsetting the Balance?

If you watch bird watchers in action, you see them deploying a variety of top-down and bottom-up attentional skills. Pursuing multiple attentive roles as searchers, seekers, and listeners, bird watchers remain open on heightened alert for a new sensory experience. Distant bird calls pierce consciousness. Zen bird watchers, aware that Ikkyu was enlightened by the sound of a crow's caw, appreciate the potency of such an auditory stimulus.

Zen literature often cites the ways an unexpected sensory stimulus is the catalyst that triggers kensho and satori [ZB:452–457, 591–592, 615–617] (see also chapter 39). On such occasions, a sharp, penetrating sound in the world outside excites an instant overreaction. Attentive networks have several options when they overrespond to such an alerting stimulus (chapter 4). Perhaps they happened then to be in an allocentric phase, one already tilted to orient out *toward it*. Or, if in an egocentric phase, their bias was to refer this stimulus *back* to personal coordinates. Or maybe they were in a more top-down or a bottom-up attentive mode. In each case, once a trigger sets off an extraordinary degree of excitation, impulses spread throughout the reticular activating system and its extensions, setting off brisk mixtures of complex activating (and deactivating) discharges [ZBR:303–306, 351–356].

Moreover, at this moment, the slower fluctuations within the brain's *intrinsic* circuits also become potentially important, because they provide additional ways for inhibitory circuits to be enhanced as they shift forward to contain excessive excitation. Slow endogenous rhythms are already poised to shift major networks in the brain—several times a minute—into varying degrees of reciprocal opposing functions. Suppose the two sets of activations and deactivations—the one immediate and exogenous, the other more innate and endogenous—each happen to rise, and to fall so that they reach their polar extremes simultaneously. Now, with high peaks soaring out of deep valleys, all prior Self-centered functions could briefly drop out of that person's mental field. No longer a partial deactivation, no longer a small silent fluctuation, such a major shift could represent total freedom from the old dominant version of a Self-centered consciousness.

Syzygy

The National Weather Service uses the term *syzygy* to describe such a rare conjunction. In this instance, the gravitational forces of the sun, the moon, and Earth line up to cause extraordinary high tides on Earth [ZB:346–347, 592]. Can a similar conjunction of events serve as a metaphor for the physiological tidal wave that could wash away Self-centeredness? An explicit hypothesis, testable in the distant future, is that the timing inherent in the periodicity of a person's intrinsic fluctuations could contribute to the syzygy of that vulnerable instant. Figure 7 ventures such an interpretation in a preliminary form: an external trigger coinciding with an internal configuration sufficient to precipitate the state of kensho.

An Upper Visual Field Advantage Favoring the Impact of Triggering Stimuli

Kensho's fresh, anonymous version of the environment is clear and directly other-referential. Often enough to be interesting, similar "peak experiences" tend to happen in *natural outdoor* settings, not indoors. It is no accident that many such

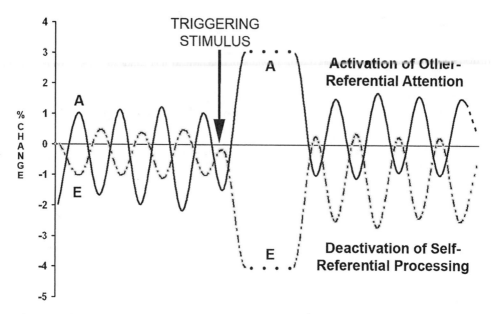

Figure 7   The dual effect of a triggering stimulus: a hypothesis for the precipitation of kensho
At left, the continuous wavy line represents the usual slow spontaneous fluctuations of our intrinsic stream of *other*-referential (allocentric) attention (A). Note how this up and down course bears a see-saw, reciprocal relationship with the course of the second, interrupted line. That dashed and dotted line represents the slow fluctuations of connectivity within our intrinsic stream of *Self*-referential (egocentric) processing (E).

Suppose a triggering stimulus (↓) now captures the attention of a meditator who had been engaged in a long prior program of attentive meditative training. This trigger prompts an immediate physiological overreaction. Two neuronal responses unfold simultaneously: (1) a major *deactivation* stops Self-referential processing (E). This dissolves all prior constructs of the *I-Me-Mine*. This interval is vacant of Self. It leaves the impression of emptiness, and it lacks all sense of time; (2) a major *activation* enhances attentive processing within the ventral, other-referential network (A). This leaves the impression of "suchness." All things are experienced as THEY really are.

In the immediate afterglow, allocentric processing still appears substantially enhanced, whereas self-centered processing is shown reduced to a lower level. This leaves the impression of a much lower profile i-me-mine.

natural settings engage the brain in what is literally an elevated mode of receptive attention [ZB:664–667]. It was when I happened to look *up*—into a bit of distant, open sky—that a taste of kensho arrived [ZB:537, ZBR:305–306]. Perhaps some physiological bias at that instant might have been referable to the elevated point of view registering in the sky in my upper visual fields. These other-centered upper fields are subserved more by the lower visual stream as it flows on through the temporal lobe.

The arrows in figure 5 show that the ego/allo processing paths diverge once they leave the occipital lobe. In fact, the anatomical destinies determining their different processing efficiencies had begun milliseconds before. Two clinical correlates are implicit first in the way the lens of the eye inverts the raw visual image of an apple, and next in the divergent course that these retinal fibers pursue as they then transmit messages from the eye toward the back of the brain. Furthermore, as medical students, we also learned that

- our upper visual fields are represented in the lower part of the visual cortex. This lies nearest to the temporal lobe. In contrast,
- our lower visual fields are represented in the upper part of the occipital cortex. This lies closest to the parietal lobe.

These two different representations are relevant to Zen and the brain. Sdoia and colleagues presented a discrete visual task to either the upper, or the lower, visual fields of normal subjects. The tests called upon them *selectively* to process each stimulus using either their allocentric or egocentric frame of reference.[4] The subjects responded to each stimulus by pressing on a button with either index finger. Their reaction times showed that the efficiency of their upper and lower fields of vision were distinctly different.

Faster processing speeds showed that their *upper* visual fields were more efficient when the subjects made other-referential spatial judgments. These greater allocentric capacities could have been an advantage for remote ancestors, the ones who survived by detecting a threatening stimulus early while it was still far off in the distant scenery near the horizon. In contrast, the subjects' Self-centered spatial judgments were performed much faster in their *lower* visual fields. These attributes help us look down while eating food, try to strike a nail with a hammer, or perform the visuomotor transformations involved in pressing a button. On balance, evolution seems to have designed intelligently.

"Spiritual awakening" is a phrase sometimes used as an alternative for enlightenment. The visual research just cited suggests that a potential physiological basis could exist for a legend about Siddhartha's awakening. It is that his final transformation into the Buddha—the Enlightened One—began when, after meditating all night under the Bodhi tree, he looked up before daybreak and glimpsed the bright "star" in the sky *above the horizon* [ZB:621].

Ancient astronomers knew this wandering planet (Venus) by several names. To the Greeks, she was "the bringer of dawn." A silk painting discovered in the Buddhist caves at Dunhuang on the old Silk Road portrays her as a white goddess holding a stringed musical instrument. The rooster portion of her crown suggests the early hour at which she shines in the eastern sky.[5]

The sentence in Psalm 121, "I will lift up mine eyes unto the hills, from whence cometh my help,"[6] is but one of several age-old Judeo-Christian expressions that might lend itself also to hint at a physiological bias oriented toward our upper visual fields. A more recent phrasing makes the point in an explicit manner. It is by Shabkar (1781–1851), an enlighted sage in the Tibetan tradition.[7]

> I raised my head, looking up,
> And saw the cloudless sky.
> I thought of absolute space, free from limits,
> ... Then experienced a freedom
> Without center, without end.

It is noteworthy that during the Tibetan technique called sky practice or sky gazing, the adept meditator cultivates a stable form of receptive, intensified "open presence" awareness. This practice involves (deliberately) keeping the eyes open and directed somewhat upward toward empty, cloudless space, while still maintaining an empty mind open to realize the unity of space and awareness.[8]

An intriguing exhibit in the Seattle Art Museum is of further interest, with regard to the direction in which a monk might be gazing during kensho. It is a polychrome statue entitled *Monk at the Moment of Enlightenment*. It dates to the Yuan Dynasty, in late thirteenth to fourteenth century China. This statue depicts a Buddhist monk looking up and to his left.[9] It remains possible that earlier religious iconography might have had some cultural influence on the artist who created such an unusual statue. The Nestorian Christians had traveled the Silk Road to establish a mission near Ch'ang-an (Xian) during the seventh to tenth centuries,[10] and the Archbishop of Peking in 1307 was the Franciscan, John of Montecorvino.

Different brain regions undergo activation when we are indoors than those that are activated when we are outdoors. When subjects are monitored with fMRI while they gaze at various images, indoor scenes activate the posterior parahippocampal region, including the parahippocampal place area.[11] The retrosplenial cortex, in contrast, shows no such activation, although it activates preferentially to full scenes rather than faces.

One general hypothetical scheme would emphasize a substantial role for the neuromodulator dopamine in a variety of religious activities (including beliefs, experiences, and practices).[12] It draws general support from the suggestions that dopamine systems could be directed more toward functions in space at a distance from the person, and from the evidence reviewed later in part VI that dopamine's faster responses influence the inclinations of the nucleus accumbens, whereas many of its other modulating functions develop more slowly.[13]

Seeing through "No-Self" and Beyond

The Zen phrase "No-Self" is a term that needs to be interpreted with care. No-Self (Skt: *anatta*) does not mean that the person stops witnessing. It does not mean that kensho's open mental field beholds "nothing" at all in some "empty" world outside. It means that witnessing happens with none of the old intrusive, Self-conscious *I-Me-Mine* standing in the way. It means that no former veils of Self obscure or distort everything in that outside environment. Once these old concepts drop off, the anonymous observer is finally graced by the glimpse of an unimaginally "objective vision." This fresh reality sees clearly *into* the eternal perfection of "all things as THEY really are."

Coming out of this state of oneness, the person finally grasps the error inherent in the old Self/other mode of dual perception. The new understanding is based on direct, impersonal, other-centered, authoritative experience. Why is such an insight qualified to be called insight-*wisdom*? One of several reasons is that it finally comprehends that all of the person's earlier Self/other constructs had been centered from the inside, looking out (chapter 41).

Arriving in the diminuendo of kensho is another realization that appreciates its ineffable nature. The inexpressibility of such an extraordinary state flies through the gaps in any net of mere words that one might try to cast in its direction. That said, could any form of communication help readers edge a little closer to what its essence is? Kobori-Roshi once suggested that poetry could serve this function.

And so this chapter closes with two spare lines of poetry by Seido Ray Ronci, a Rinzai monk and contemporary Zen poet.[14] The words hint at how much is usually obscured by our veils of Self and lies in the all-inclusive beyond.

How much I long to see through the man who sees through the moment.
I sit.

Third Mondo

> Anatomy is to physiology as geography is to history; it describes the theatre of events.
>
> Jean Fernel (1497–1558)[1]

How would you summarize the PET and fMRI data thus far?

It shows that during a normal passive resting condition, certain of our medial frontoparietal and angular gyrus networks have several options. They can (1) maintain their already high degrees of tonic resting activity, (2) respond quickly with brief dynamic shifts—up or down—toward added tasks, each direction depending on whether they orient the point of our attentive processing either inward or outward. Meanwhile, the same networks are also undergoing *spontaneous*, intrinsic, coherent, cyclic fluctuations. These covert fluctuations develop on a much slower time scale. However, their up or down shifts resemble some of the same reciprocal shifts toward activations and deactivations that occur during the immediate responses to obvious stimuli and tasks.

So what?

Intrinsic mechanisms connect our different cortical regions into well-defined separate networks. Each network is poised to serve our needs for specialized functions. At rest, certain mostly medial frontoparietal networks maintain unusually high metabolic rates and functional activities. When these same regions become further activated, they service our normal, more Self-centered functions.

However, this egocentric network also shares in a diametrically different, crucial tendency: It is *de*activated not only during our ordinary top-down attentional and external goal-directed responses but also when a brisk sensory stimulus event captures our attention and activates its other-relational counterpart. A similar seesaw reciprocity is inherent not only in such normal shifts but also in the slow, spontaneous, intrinsic fluctuations.

Why is this Self-referential deactivation important?

It is important for three reasons. The first is that it offers a plausible explanation for why a sudden sensory stimulus that captures attention might help precipitate a state of kensho.

The second is a corollary reason. It offers a potential rationale for meditators to practice strengthening their bottom-up and top-down powers of attention. Theoretically, the regular meditative practices of attention might both augment the reactive amplitude and prolong the duration of such a deactivation response.

The third reason is that it is a complex operation to yoke both cerebral hemispheres into such a major reciprocal Self/other shift. To cause one cortical network to increase its functions while those of its opposite counterpart are decreasing speaks for mechanisms organized at a deeper, *sub*cortical level by some *centralized* switching agency.

So?

Such a sudden shift—away from egocentric processing into allocentric processing—is characteristic of the state of kensho. These lines of evidence suggest how a brief, major imbalance of normal pivotal mechanisms could underlie kensho's selfless seeing into "all OTHER things as *they* really are." The slower metabolic and immediate physiological origins of a shift that organizes both hemispheres can each be determined at deeper, axial levels in the thalamus and brainstem.

Then why draw a demarcation line between the dorsal and ventral nuclei of the thalamus?

Because this is a pivotal anatomical boundary. It defines the theater of plausible physiological events. Arrayed here, in one dorsal tier are five thalamic nuclei highly relevant to our normal sense of Self. All their physiological contributions to the Self could be blocked at one time by a shift in the inhibitory cap of the reticular nucleus. Such an interpretation of thalamocortical relationships provides a testable, working, GABA inhibitory hypothesis for why a person's sense of Self dissolves suddenly in kensho. It also suggests one of several levels where our Self-centered biases could drop off incrementally in the course of long-term meditative training.

Which five nuclei in the dorsal thalamus are most relevant to Self-centeredness?

The dorsal pulvinar, the lateral posterior nucleus, plus the three important limbic nuclei: the lateral dorsal, anterior thalamic, and medial dorsal nuclei.

With which parts of the cortex do they normally interact?

With the same mostly medial frontal and parietal regions that have the highest resting metabolism in PET scans. These normal connections can help account for many of our Self-driven, discursive, mind-wandering activities.

What could be some functional consequences of inhibiting these normal interactions with the overlying cortex?

A field of consciousness liberated at higher somatic and psychic levels from its old, Self-referential burdens of limbic system overconditioning.

Is there another name for this state?

Anatta, No-Self, Non-I.

Then what still remains in conscious experience during the state of kensho?

Consciousness opens up to experience an unveiled version of its underlying allocentric processing. *Allocentric* is a general term that describes our usual covert, other-referential version of sensory processing.

What regions in the back of the brain normally enter into this relatively unappreciated category of other-referential processing?

The ventral pulvinar and other ventral thalamic nuclei of the sensory thalamus, in collaboration with their cortical partners. This larger configuration includes the normal overlapping representations of networks in the ventral attention system (table 4) and the ventral processing stream (table 7).

Then why does the perception during kensho seem so astonishing: a "spatial act of seeing, changed by a new dimension?"

This perception is unveiled. No intrusive, Self-referent subjectivities are interposed. Kensho's perception is sel*fless*, nondual, direct. A mode of other-referential processing is attending to all things as THEY really are, not as they had previously been seen, heard, and conceptualized by the *I-Me-Mine*. This leaves the impression that the reality of all things is being experienced objectively.

Is kensho then a whole "new way of looking at the world?"

It might seem so, at first. However, we have always been engaged in a normal, hidden mode of allocentric, other-centered processing. We just haven't been fully aware of it as an isolated phenomenon. This covert mode of object-centered perception has been overshadowed by our prior Self-centered overconditioning. A helpful analogy is the way one master eye dominates our ordinary visual perception.

As a practical matter, are there implications for meditators in the way some temporal lobe functions share an upper visual field processing efficiency?

This processing advantage raises the possibility that some receptive meditation practices might become more efficient at a stage after thoughts drop off when we allow bare, open awareness to drift toward levels *above* the horizontal. My current morning indoor practice begins with the usual soft focus on a spot low on the wall. Later on, I'll *let go and let my eyes drift upward*. One message for meditators is to consider "raising your sights." You often do this anyway when you are relaxing outdoors in natural surroundings [ZB:664–667].

Suppose that genuine selflessness gradually became someone's major ongoing character trait. Suppose that the rare sage who had arrived at this extraordinary stage might actually be manifesting some of the greater degrees of other-referential processing being proposed. Could existing visual and auditory techniques be refined to determine if this sage did manifest an associated upper field processing advantage—both relative and absolute?

This is a far-out, but currently plausible, working hypothesis. During the rare exceptional stage of an ongoing enlightenment, trait changes toward selflessness and other-referential processing might correlate with corresponding measurable patterns of brain plasticity. These changes develop at cortical and subcortical levels. They could reshape the discriminations, attitudes, and behavioral functions of the genuine sage person.

How does the explanation proposed for kensho differ from that for internal absorption?

In internal absorption, the GABA cap of the reticular nucleus inhibits sensory transmission through the most ventral sensory *relay* nuclei far down in the back of the thalamus. This blocks the sensory input through the two geniculate nuclei, resulting in both the "sound of absolute silence" and an ambient form of visual perception that is "blacker than black." Such a blockade stops representations of the physical Self at a relatively low level. However, only a partial anonymity occurs, because the Self of the psyche remains spared.

Why do these pages pile more layers of neuroscience concepts on top of the alien cultural notions about Zen that we've imported from the Far East?

Sorry about that. The latest neuroscience publications are quickly overtaking the vast Buddhist literature of the past two millennia. I've tried to select basic facts from each domain, then synthesize a fresh perspective. This approach, like that of Zen, intends to cut to the key issues. The ultimate hope is to enable the Path to become less mysterious, more practical, and easier to follow. Meanwhile, let go of the top-heavy layers of concepts from either culture, return to the cushion, and to your natural home in the outdoors.

Part IV

On the Nature of Insight

There are moments in our lives when we seem to see beyond the usual, become clairvoyant. We reach then into reality. Such are the moments of our greatest happiness, of our greatest wisdom. At such moments, there is a song going on within us to which we listen ... it is the desire to express these songs from within that motivates all masters of art.

Robert Henri (1865–1929)

Intuitions about Insight

> Certain contents issue from a psyche that is more complete than consciousness. They often contain a superior analysis or insight or knowledge which consciousness has not been able to produce. We have a suitable word for such occurrences—intuition.
>
> Carl Jung (1875–1961)

Henri and Jung introduce us to several issues in the next two parts. Among them: (1) What is the nature of insight? (2) Do the phenomena of an ordinary insight differ from those that strike during a so-called peak experience? In particular, does ordinary insight differ from the brief state of "enlightenment" called kensho in Zen? (3) Can recent research into our ordinary kinds of insight clarify how triggers precipitate these "awakened" states of insight-wisdom? (4) Can recent brain research clarify how kensho's flashing sequences of insight-wisdom evolve? (5) What does a visual artist like Robert Henri mean when he speaks of "songs from within" during moments of "greatest wisdom"?

I first became curious about the nature of insight back in 1967. I had been invited to talk about some discoveries our team had made in laboratory research. I chose instead to focus on the often haphazard ways the creative process had evolved during the course of this bench research. By 1978, this topic had expanded into a book that reviewed the psychological aspects of creativity. In the interim, I had become distantly aware that *insight* was the cornerstone of Zen enlightenment. I did not really understand what that might mean, because my Zen practice had only just begun in 1974. Still, as a neurologist, I could see that we knew very little about the physiological basis for any kind of insight.

The decades since then have witnessed a flourishing literature that describes the (sometimes) overlapping topics of creativity[1] and of ordinary insight.[2] And, as research continued to explode in the neurosciences, it became possible to venture preliminary working hypotheses about how the flash of insight-wisdom might arrive in Zen.[3–6] Even so, researchers rarely used neuroimaging techniques to explore the physiological basis of ordinary insight. Indeed, some scholars still debate the issue: Is insight a "special process?" Or is it "nothing special?" Zen might respond by nodding "yes" to both questions.

It seems prudent to begin with some dictionary definitions:

- *Cognition*: Our process of knowing in the broadest sense. Rational thought processes are not the sole cause of our knowing.

- *Intuition*: Our generic faculty of direct knowing. Intuition usually refers to ordinary levels of intuitive understanding, our hunches that proceed quickly without obvious rational thought processes.

- *Insight*: The sudden act of seeing clearly and comprehensively—without intervening thought—into problem situations or into our own inner nature. This is a more refined level of intuition.

Other definitions become useful in a Zen context:

- *Insight-wisdom*: The profound, insightful comprehension of the existential essence of all things.
- *Kensho* (J.): A brief, extraordinary alternate state of consciousness during which one sees deeply into the existential essence of things. In Zen Buddhism, kensho (and the next deeper state, termed *satori*) represent only the beginning of true spiritual training.
- *Prajna* (Skt.): The flashing process of enlightenment that confers insight-wisdom.

Inside Insight

Ordinary insights are common. These pages view them (1) as expressing the part of general intelligence that we devote to resolving more intractable problems, and (2) as refinements along the broad continuum of creative intuition. To illustrate, stop reading for a moment, look up, and try to recall a seismic insight you've had about something or someone. You may remember that it arrived

- suddenly;
- spontaneously, with no apparent effort on your part;
- wordlessly, with no intervening thoughts;
- surprisingly;
- offering a clear, correct novel resolution of a hard problem which the rest of your conscious intellect had failed to solve (or perhaps had never acknowledged).

Restructuring the Problem

We can also define *insight* as the sudden, major reconstruction of the earlier problem, one that realizes a novel solution. This definition is useful because it helps to disengage and reorient our attention. It points back a few steps to our earlier hang-ups, not onward toward the more impressive solution. These former mental blocks were the kinds of "functional fixedness" that had kept us stuck in a mental rut. The obvious way out of such a logjam is first to *restructure* the original problem, then develop a fresh, creative approach. How can we accomplish this?

When no routine solutions exist for a hard problem, most scholars believe that we then enlist "special" kinds of selective processing to create a breakthrough discovery.[7] Three such major, special processes are identifiable:

- *Encoding*: New features are envisioned, details that were not obvious before.
- *Combination*: Existing facts now bind together in a new coherent fashion.
- *Comparison*: Past information finally becomes relevant, aided by fresh analogies and metaphors.

Restructuring during Incubation

Restructuring can proceed incrementally, at subconscious levels, for a very long time. *Incubation* is a good term for this process, because it reminds us how patiently and how carefully the hen must attend to the eggs before they are ready to hatch. Incubation serves as a loose metaphor for Zen training, though the Zen approach has a timeline of years, not days [ZB:457].

Incubation goes on during waking and sleeping hours alike. In one earlier study of the effects of sleep, the subjects faced a difficult ongoing task. It was to analyze eight-digit long strings of variable numbers in order to discover which hidden, underlying, general abstract rule governed their sequence. Subjects who went to sleep *after* they had worked on this numbers task were twice as likely later to gain a novel insight into this covert "rule."[8] Yet, long before this fresh insight flashed into their consciousness, these successful subjects were manifesting *slow* reaction times in a particular manner. Analysis of this subtle evidence suggested what the future problem solvers had long been incubating, subconsciously: it was the weak representation of this seemingly hidden "rule."

Sleep can help consolidate memories, and rest periods can enable memories of earlier task procedures to be replayed spontaneously [ZBR:103–104]. Recent research by Ellenbogen and colleagues illustrates how a night's sleep acts. It seems to shield the ordinary memories we use for remembering various facts (facts mediated by the hippocampal system) from being interfered with when competing facts arrive subsequently.[9]

Sleep also heightens our capacity to develop helpful inferences about relationships hidden among recently acquired facts. These enhanced capacities enable us to dip into our so-called relational memory, and to extract from its files only those relevant entries that can be bound into a coherent cluster. Prior sleep improved (by 93%) the subjects' relational memory skills (as defined in this manner) for drawing such distant covert inferences. In contrast, a much lesser improvement (only 69%) was associated with the control interval (merely being awake for 12 hours). However, the subjects who slept were not convinced that their memory had rendered correct judgments to a degree commensurate with how much they had actually improved.[10] This evidence suggests they benefited from sleep with the aid of mechanisms operating at subconscious, intuitive levels of processing.

Insights often arrive during the interval of reverie, between the last REM episode and the morning awakening.[11] The sleep studies just reviewed suggest why this is an optimal interval. It is one in which our incubated Self-relational data can fall into fresh creative configurations with various kinds of other-relational data. To the degree that regular meditation enables some meditators "to sleep better" and/or to tap into sleep's subconscious benefits, some of the improved performances assumed to be associated with that day's meditation may in fact have been determined during sleep many hours before [ZB:311–324; ZBR:237–239].

Preliminary Warmth

Leading up to some ordinary kinds of insight, a solution seems almost at hand. Seekers may feel as though they are getting "warm." The phrase "high warmth," describes this "getting close" phenomenon.[12]

The preliminary feeling that "I'm getting warm" seems to originate closer to one's prior conventional knowledge of facts and/or experience. Often, such an ordinary insight is relatively smaller (in size and complexity) when it is the kind that develops incrementally, through subtle gradations of warmth. It turns out that the first process, that of selective encoding, is the one frequently involved during such preliminary "feelings of knowing."[13]

In other instances of ordinary insight, the second and third processes of combination and/or comparison gather sufficient momentum to coalesce. Now the solution arrives in a flash. Notably, during the immediate prelude to such a sudden resolution, warmth is absent (or seems very low), and the solution often seems more substantial.

The "Aha!" Phenomenon

When an insight strikes, a kind of mental light bulb seems to turn on. This analogy evolved after Thomas Edison invented the light bulb, and the phrase is often associated with insights of various sizes. Some people prefer a different expression, one that describes their feeling of release after they abruptly solve a tough puzzle. They associate it with an interior feeling akin to an "Aha!" Two kinds of realization blend into this emotional impression:

- The new solution represents the problem in a way that differs—surprisingly and substantially—from how they had first conceptualized it.

- The novel solution strikes abruptly, flows effortlessly, and completes itself instantly.[14]

During ordinary insights, Ippolito and Tweney observe that the "Aha!" feeling might also include "a corresponding increase in self-esteem; nature has just patted us on the back."[15] In marked contrast, the flash of insight-wisdom during kensho is totally self*less* in nature, both in form and content. It lacks all feelings of prior, partial knowing that may enter during the course of ordinary insight. Its vast existential dimension extends far beyond the limited scope of any ordinary kind of factual knowledge.

The "Eureka!" Moment

Archimedes (c. 287–212 B.C.E) had a legendary insight. It arrived about three centuries after Siddhartha's awakening under the Bodhi (pipal) tree. Much later, in the first century B.C.E., the Roman writer Vitruvius cited the story that Archimedes had uttered the phrase, "Eureka!"[16] Archimedes himself left no written account of this incident, leading deconstructionists to question the accuracy of this legendary tale. Various calculations suggest that Archimedes was perhaps only about 22 years old when he could have had this insight. His youth is not the problem. Indeed, Isaac Newton (1642–1727) may have been only in his early twenties when the falling apple triggered his brilliant insight into the principle of gravity. (Apples can serve as food for thought in a variety of ways.)

Few scholars dispute that Archimedes *would* have realized—insightfully— that the volume of water his body displaced from a bathtub could accurately measure his own immersed volume. At issue is not whether Archimedes could have experienced such a sudden flash of insight or become excited enough to cry out. Rather, the question is: were the methods then used for measuring a small volume of displaced water sufficiently accurate to prove how much cheap silver the smith had melted into the gold wreath in order to cheat Hiero, the local tyrant? Be that as it may, the "Eureka!" legend survives to this day, capturing the crowning delight inspired by a major flash of insight.

26

A Lotus Puzzle

In Zen, a koan is an enigmatic unsolvable statement. The following puzzle is different. It is the kind of riddle that researchers might ask their subjects to solve.[1] Think of it as an example intended to convey the nature of ordinary insight.

Suppose you plant one lotus plant in your small pond on the first day of spring. Assume that it multiplies as it grows, such that every seven days the total leaf area of all plants will have doubled in size. By the end of 12 weeks, your pond is entirely covered. How many weeks did it take for the pond to be *half*-covered?

After you incubate the question for a length of time, the solution may come to you in a flash. If so, pause and inquire: how impersonally did your answer arrive? Often, one's impression is not so much "*I* found it!" (e.g., "Good for *Me*!"). But more like: "*It* suddenly came!" (and "*i*" had relatively little input into the way "*It*" arrived.)

Note also how simply and conclusively the solution arrives.

27

Our Normal Quest for Meaning

A monk asked, What is the essential meaning of Buddhism? Master Mazu Daoyi responded, What is the meaning of this moment?[1]

The Meaning of Meaning

Back in eighth-century China, Ch'an Master Mazu went straight to the point. In any era, what do we mean by the word *meaning*? (And how many thousandths of a second does a "moment" contain?) Meaning refers to that particular idea which something calls forth in our mind. Suppose we look at an object in a new scene, read a printed word, hear a word spoken. Having transformed these stimuli into impulses, it takes us only a few more milliseconds to decode what each item or event *means* (chapters 4, 5, and 6) [ZB:521–529].

Even though we examine these sequences in slow motion, the silent interrogation flows quickly. It seeks to *know*: Which incoming messages cluster into this configuration that becomes meaningful? Does the result translate into something good or bad? Strong or weak? Active or passive? Our brain takes but a few hundred milliseconds to "connect the dots." How could any 3 pound lump of tissue recognize all these stimuli and interpret what they mean, in a half-second or less?

Much more goes on automatically than even Freud wished to credit to the unconscious. True, reams of data stored in "relational memory" must first be accessed, tapped into, and drawn together inside some kind of "semantic space." Only then does the gist of this temporary cluster of partial meanings start to leap into its final shape as a coherent idea. Yet, consciousness is still not fully convinced that this closure is genuine. Two more things must happen: (1) the correct "keystone" of fact drops into its yawning arch of associations, completing the requisite architectural logic; and (2) hints of truth-authenticity-reality, lurking in deep recesses of personal memory, flesh out this factual result.

This chapter and those that follow in part IV set ambitious goals for understanding what "meaning" means. Their pages explore three working hypotheses: first, that interactions between the temporal and frontal lobes participate substantially in the impression that we have reached a meaningful closure; second, that contributions from both temporal lobes, right > left, enter often into our more meaningful impressions of reality; third, that extraordinary experiences of enhanced reality develop only during certain moments of closure. At these rare times, the heightened amplitudes of reciprocal responses combine to (a) enhance the processing functions along allocentric pathways, and (b) infuse novel depths of meaning into the pattern recognition templates nearby in the temporal lobe.

Meaning Drops Out, Selectively, in Certain Neurological Conditions

When 35-year-old Sigmund Freud ventured into this complex arena, he was still a promising neurologist. The field of neurology was still in its infancy. It lacked a diagnostic term to describe a select group of his patients in whom localized brain damage had caused a discrete *loss* of knowledge. Freud viewed their distinctive loss as an a-gnosis, and coined the word *agnosia*.

Nowadays, neurologists diagnose *pure* visual or auditory agnosia only under restricted circumstances, usually in patients in whom a stroke has damaged small parts of the temporal lobe.[2] An isolated loss of *visual* meaning (visual agnosia) develops when such discrete damage is confined to the undersurface of the temporal lobe (e.g., BA 37, 19). (See figure 5, at the site near FG.) In contrast, they develop an isolated *auditory* agnosia when a small lesion damages their superior temporal lobe convexity higher up (BA 22), near the primary auditory cortex. (See figure 4, near the site STG.)

Note that back in part II, the arrows in both figures—the one near this fusiform gyrus, the other in the superior temporal gyrus—were originally intended to show which paths impulses follow during *object-centered (allocentric) processing*. Now, in part IV, the same arrows and the same temporal gyri will help develop explanations for some of the heightened sense of meaningful "reality" that infuses kensho. Relevant to the mechanisms now being proposed is this same intriguing convergence in the temporal lobe: the normal overlap between our major auditory and visual functions that confer *meaning* and those regions that sponsor our *other-referential processing*. So the two green arrows in figures 4 and 5 will now help make explicit a plausible hypothesis: in kensho, some temporal lobe functions that normally help interpret the visual and auditory meaning of events could be recruited to infuse fresh impressions of resonant meaning into the adjacent functions of other-centered processing, now unveiled.

Consider this clinical example. A patient is alert and able clearly to see a set of keys that you are holding up. What is lacking? The patient's capacity to *recognize* (by sight) what they *are*. The ability to *know* what they are used for. Yet, the word for key isn't completely lost, nor is its meaning. This same patient will readily identify the keys (by sound) when you jingle them, and will easily recognize them (by touch and proprioception) when you place them deftly in the patient's hand. What's lacking is *visual meaning*.

So, in visual agnosia, *seeing is okay*, only visual meaning drops out. Meaning drops out because visual events in the present are cut off from all visual memory links that the person had gained during past experience. Why must the underlying damage be so discretely placed? Because it must strip only the sense of *meaning* from an object. Therefore, it must spare the earlier occipital → temporal pathways, the ones that enable the patient to *see* keys in the first place. Those early visual impulses begin far back in the primary visual cortex of the occipital lobe (BA 17). From there, they first flow forward through the visual association regions (BA 18, 19). Their course then takes them on into the pattern recognition templates of the temporal lobe (figures 4, 5). In keeping with how much the normal temporal lobe contributes to meaning, neurologists now use the term "semantic dementia" to categorize the kinds of mental symptoms patients have when their temporal lobe degenerates.

Recent Studies in Visual Agnosia and in the Imitation of Meaningful Acts

When we consciously recollect the visual attributes of familiar things, our right fusiform gyrus makes a major contribution. Vandenbulcke and colleagues studied one 58-year-old woman who sustained a right fusiform gyrus infarct (FG in figure 5). Afterward, she could no longer understand the visual attributes of living creatures or nonliving entities.[3] Her visual-perceptual, linguistic, and naming abilities were spared. She could still engage in actions that involved semantic categorization. However, she could not *consciously* recollect the normal shape and parts of familiar objects. In short, she had lost her ability to organize and envision a "mental image" of objects at the level of her "mind's eye." When normal control subjects attached meaning to visual concepts that they had represented in the form of *pictures*, not words, fMRI signals showed that they all activated this same right fusiform gyrus region.

Rumiati and colleagues asked other normal subjects to imitate actions of two very different types. Some actions were familiar and meaningful. Others were novel yet meaningless.[4] PET scans showed that the meaningful actions increased cerebral blood flow in the left inferior temporal gyrus. In contrast, most of the meaningless movements increased blood flow farther back in the right parieto-occipital junction. This study showed that our semantic interpretation of meaning is linked to the way it activates the ventral visual stream. In contrast, when an action is only imitated—without regard to the meaningfulness of its interpretation—the dorsal visual stream contributes to the requisite visuospatial transformations (tables 4 and 7).

Temporal Lobe Specializations for What Some Things Mean at a Distance

Does anything else about the wiring diagram of the temporal lobe help explain why small lesions here cause such an isolated loss of meaning? These discrete agnosias reflect an anatomical fact: our temporal lobe is designed to serve functions fundamentally different from those of the other three lobes [ZBR:152–157].

It is true that evolutionary pressures sculptured many temporal lobe circuits to specialize in decoding the audiovisual messages conveyed by patterns of language. However, other temporal lobe networks retain their primal, distant early warning (DEW) orientations. These are wary circuits. They still stand watch. They listen. They remain poised to recognize and warn us about what kinds of other things lurk way out there, at relatively *long distances* from our body. Auditory and visual messages are relayed quickly from the brainstem colliculi and the pulvinar to alert these other-referential temporal lobe circuits. Instantly, they interpret what such other unexpected things *might* mean, long before they advance close enough to do us harm (chapters 14, 23). Allocentric processing evolved in a far-sighted manner.

Temporal Lobe Affirmations of Meaning; Déjà Vu

In these respects, the functions of multiple temporal lobe portfolios help us bridge a crucial gap. Why is this gap, when reduced to words, both conceptual and physiological? Because on one side is what an object or event might "mean" *out there* (say to some extraterrestrial-like witness in the most general, matter-of-fact, and objective terms). While on the other side is what this same object or event *really means* to Me (because I've translated it into the Self-centered terms of My own subjective, internalized, memory-based experiences that made it "*Mine.*") The medial temporal lobe might begin to develop some hints related to such bridging, self-othering functions [ZBR:241–242]. In fact, we've observed that many place cells in the hippocampus are tuned to respond to object-centered spatial coordinates. In contrast, their close neighbors are coded to use Self-centered, head-body coordinates as their frame of spatial reference (chapter 20) [ZBR:101].

The normal phenomena of déjà vu help illustrate how the temporal lobe plays a leading role in our affirmations of meaning [ZBR:153–154, 372–373]. Déjà vu seems instantly to sense the gist of an external event. In all truthiness, it concludes: "Sure, I've already *seen* this same scenery before. *I've* scanned the present scene, reviewed the index of *my* journals that had recorded *my* relevant past, evaluated both of these time domains, felt their now-then familiar tug, and finally condensed *my* yes/no options into *one* affirmative response." Temporal lobe interpretations are never that simple, yet their algorithms flow much faster than that sentence.

Several points about déjà vu are worth noting. One is the lightning-fast processing speed with which the medial temporal lobe consults its index and then inventories the relevant memory sites where our old journal entries had been stored (chapter 15). Other major points relate to how much déjà vu accomplishes. In a flash, the brain affirms that two events—widely separated in *time*—share meaningful links that refer them back to one *place* and one *person*. Circumstantial details of time, place, and person cluster into one coherent triad. Yet, during this whole episode of déjà vu, no distinct epistemological thought sequences appear on one's mental horizon. All elementary decision-making goes on at levels of "no-thought" logic. Each such closure rushes to its own impression of truth, certainty, and authenticity. Right hippocampal fMRI signals respond more when an object occupies a familiar location. In contrast, the left hippocampus is more engaged when its comparator functions address novel associations.[5]

What happens when we engage in more complex levels of meaningful (semantic) decoding? Recent fMRI studies of visual humor show that the lateral regions of the temporal convexity contribute when we decode visual meanings.[6] For example, both the superior temporal sulcus (L, R) and the middle temporal gyrus (R) respond with increasing activation to "funny" cartoons in which the humor is visual *or* language-based. Moreover, the left inferior and middle temporal gyri and the left inferior temporal sulcus all contribute when we base our interpretation of the humor in a cartoon on judgments involving interactions between *both* vision and language.

So, when does meaning emerge? In the temporal lobe, various lines of evidence converge, suggesting that meaning arises not from any one single spot. Rather meaning becomes an associative function. It "happens" when multiple regions enter into harmonious, coherent unifying interactions.

Doesn't the Parietal Lobe Also Attend to Meaning?

Yes, but in its own ways, in both its superior and inferior lobules [ZBR:148–152]. In general, the parietal lobe remains much more attentive to our own physical Self-referential processing. Its wiring patterns seem designed to personalize events for actions in space that arise much closer to our own bodies. Egocentric processing is near-sighted. When its percepts evolve in the parietal lobe, we identify them so intimately with our *physical* Self for two reasons. Each reason is related to the anatomical location of particular sensory receptors and their subsequent neuronal pathways.

- The first are the touch receptors on the skin. The parietal lobe is designed to process the touch stimuli entering from tangible objects *close* to us. We can reach toward and actually feel these nearby items. Grasp an apple in the dark, sight unseen. Sensitive touch receptors on the surface of your skin help you recognize the distinctive, smooth memory-based feel of this apple skin.
- The second receptors are those conveying deeper sensations. These signal the ways the muscles, tendons, and joints are moving inside your fingers. As you cup your hand around the apple, these *proprio*ceptive messages inform the opposite parietal lobe of the position of each of your fingers. In pitch-black darkness, this position sense helps you recognize that apple by its round shape.

Multiple Contributions to Spatial Meaning

But suppose you see a snarling Doberman pinscher crouched in front of you only 5 feet away. This could get nasty. Yet, this time you're fortunate. Parietal-temporal-occipital regions not only decode the dog's position. Your 3-D spatial skills and figure/ground decisions now show that an intervening high chain fence lies between you and the dog [ZBR:152–153]. Otherwise, had this Doberman actually been right *behind* you and ready to bite, the signals from your pulvinar and limbic system to the central gray in your midbrain would have caused you to be intensely frightened[7] [ZB:232–235].

28
Studies of Meaningful Coherence in Visual Images

> No problem can be solved from the same consciousness that created it—we must learn to see the world anew.
>
> Albert Einstein (1879–1955)

If you're a researcher, how can you detect the instant when your subjects see their world anew? How do you know when a totally fresh meaning transfigures what they see? Shihui Han and colleagues at Peking University reasoned as follows: First, let's select the few essential visual images from a short movie.[1] Then, let's assemble these isolated film clips in their original, meaningful order. Finally, we will use fMRI to monitor our subjects while they're trying to discover the coherent plot that unfolds in this logical sequence of abbreviated images.

To illustrate what the subjects saw, here is one example of the few film clips they selected to show such a coherent sequence: a student first entering a class-room, then sitting behind a desk, raising a hand, and finally asking a question. As a control, the researchers used these same film clips, but arranged them in a random way that had no coherent narrative links.

Their subjects were twelve normal adults. Their assigned task was to watch sets of coherent epochs that were interspersed with sets of disjointed epochs. Each of the two different kinds of epochs contained 60 selected *static* visual images. Each image was displayed for 1 second. A blank screen, lasting for 10 seconds, served as the baseline control period before each epoch. After the subjects had finished, they reported which sets of epochs had evolved in a coherent order.

Three *right*-sided regions showed increased fMRI signals during these coherent visual epochs (when contrasted with the random order, meaningless epochs):

- The right middle temporal cortex (BA 21)
- The right posterior superior temporal cortex (BA 42)
- The right inferior postcentral gyrus (BA 1, 2, 3)

The authors suggested that two interacting explanations could account for these right-sided activations: (1) Our right hemisphere regions respond preferentially during tasks of *visuospatial* problem solving (as discussed earlier in part I). (2) Our posterior visual association cortex also interprets various actions. It confers meanings on visual events when they seem to be in motions that are either explicit, inferred, or imagined.[2–5]

Table 9 summarizes a sample of these recent reports. They suggest that we normally arrive at various meaningful inferences when networks in the posterior temporal-parietal-occipital region begin to decode the figure/ground relationships of visual events. Note that when this visual association cortex and the pulvinar combine to resolve the crucial figure/ground distinction, the figure of salient interest leaps out as distinct from the incidental scenery in the background (chapters 17, 19). Attention points the way.

We tap into a variety of networks to explain and predict what another person intends to do [ZBR:348–349]. Key modules include the medial prefrontal cortex and the right temporoparietal junction (TPJ). The right TPJ and the precuneus help process all inferences about prior intent. The left TPJ becomes activated when the intention is to engage in social communication.[6]

Meaningful Visual Coherence during Humorous Sight Gags

Zen is enlivened by a deeply embedded comic spirit [ZB:415–418]. Readers who have appreciated Gary Larson's humor in "The Far Side" or the classic cartoon

Table 9
Decoding Functions That Correlate with Particular Processing Regions

Decoding Function	Cortical Processing Region
Processing specific actions during a visual task	Posterior middle temporal gyrus and superior temporal gyrus
Processing specific actions during a linguistic (word-based) task[2]	Areas anterior and dorsal to the two gyri above
General processes of semantic matching involving an action, word, object, or picture	Posterior prefrontal cortex (L > R) and fusiform gyrus (L > R)
Interpreting intent to a living action, based on how its trajectory relates to the larger environmental context[3]	Posterior superior temporal sulcus (R)
Responding to pictures of human bodies	Extrastriate body area (EBA)
Responding to objects including faces	Fusiform face area (FFA)
Responding to particular places	Parahippocampal place area (PPA)
Early visual responses to certain objects[4]	Lateral occipital complex (LOC)
Attributing (while reading) transient thoughts or feelings to another person that are implicit in a short text[5]	Temporoparietal junction (TPJ) (R > L), and posterior cingulate region

humor of the old *New Yorker* can understand why researchers select particular cartoons to study humorous responses.

First, their subjects have to get the joke. The best visual cartoons have no caption. They need no wordy explanation. (The Charles Addams cartoon showing ski tracks that mysteriously straddle a tree comes to mind.) In order for any joke to work, an intuitive flash must occur. It strikes the essentials, discerns incongruities, and enables old barriers to collapse. In these three respects, the instant when one grasps the essence of a cartoon becomes vaguely reminiscent of the way one sees into a whole new reality during the flash of kensho[7] [ZB:413–418; ZBR:154, 165–167].

Tastes for humor vary greatly. Dog owners might delight in books like *Zen Dog*, with its 51 photographs of dogs and Zen sayings.[8] But not every person who volunteered for the humor study conducted by Watson and colleagues could get the sight gags they chose.[9] During the preliminary tryout, one out of every five candidates did not survive the cut. The remaining 16 subjects were monitored with fMRI while they looked at cartoons drawn with simple lines. Only half of these cartoons were intended to be obviously funny. In the funny category, half were pure sight gags; the language used in the captions beneath the other half also contributed to their interpretation.

The visually funny cartoons increased fMRI signals throughout a large mosaic of regions. Most visually responsive areas were in the posterior association cortex. They included the right precuneus, the superior temporal sulcus (in its posterior segment; R, L), and the middle frontal gyrus (R, L; BA 9/46) among many others. Both the purely visual and the language-based funny cartoons also increased signals in the midbrain (L), amygdala (L, R), and hippocampus (L). Unfunny cartoons and language-based controls provided the appropriate contrasts.

The subjects also specified (by pressing a button) *how* funny they found both types of cartoons. Two regions in particular now showed intriguing increases in fMRI signals:

- The frontal operculum/insula (L, R)
- The left anterior cingulate gyrus (BA 24)

What Do Big Nerve Cells Contribute to Human Brain Functions?

Why did the authors emphasize the signals in these two regions? Because large, spindle-shaped nerve cells reside deep in layer 5 of both this anterior cingulate gyrus and the frontal operculum-insular cortex [ZBR:82–85]. Now called von Economo neurons, these distinctive cells were first reported only in humans and great apes. The fact that they were not found in lesser primates points to nerve cells that have evolved only recently, say in the last 15 million years of evolution.[10]

These are big nerve cells. Often enough, "big is beautiful" in terms of neuronal functions. The neurons' size and other histological properties suggest that large axons enable them quickly to transmit simple signals elsewhere. Have von Economo nerve cells given humans a special evolutionary advantage? The authors' current speculations draw on recent reports that particular emotional responses *coactivate* these same two frontal/insular and anterior cingulate regions.

These emotional responses are the kinds associated with *uncertain* expectations and with interpersonal relationships. If this is true, then what relevance does the authors' joke-decoding data have to the nature and mechanisms of human insight? It suggests the interesting possibility that von Economo neurons might contribute to such intuitive sequences as those *helping us quickly assess and resolve complex problems*. Previous chapters have emphasized that a restructuring of the original problem is one essential step in insight. Similarly, in order to get a joke, one must quickly detect any mismatch and instantly come up with a fresh interpretation. Accordingly, in a book about Zen, one far-out question might be: how much of one's meditative training could engage von Economo neurons and be contributing to the brisk efficiency of Zen behavioral and intuitive functions (ZB:668–676)? Recent data on the cingulo-opercular network (summarized later in chapter 55, table 16) suggest the possibility that such cells might also participate in prolonging the interval of an extraordinary state of consciousness.

Seely and colleagues in San Francisco found recently that seven patients who died with certain forms of frontotemporal dementia showed a selective loss of von Economo nerve cells.[11] The cell counts in FTD were 74% less than in controls (R > L). It might be useful to study a broad psychometric profile of various patients who are still in the *early* stages of a dementia. Then, if the hypothesis of Watson and colleagues is correct, a subset of tests based on visual cartoons might detect a selective *early* loss of the intensity of humor in certain patients who had frontotemporal dementia. An early, selective loss might stand out disproportionately until it was submerged in a sea of the other mental deficits.

Is the Impression of "Meaningful Reality" in Kensho a Kind of Superficial, Esoteric "Add-On?"

When we continue to search for the mechanisms underlying extraordinary insights in a state like kensho, our questioning must probe issues that are deeper and more complex than those involved in tasks of ordinary insight. For example, private cultural resistances may stand in the way [ZBR:447–457]. Moreover, it can be too easy to remain satisfied with superficial results. In this regard, the absorptions prove notoriously misleading. No Zen master would accept that their overvalued, blissful episodes, glossy with esoteric interpretations, are equivalent to authentic insights (chapter 48) [ZB:373, 589–592].

One important difference is that, during kensho, "all things are seen as THEY really are." This fresh impression of suchness lends memorable degrees of depth and scope that transfigure the experience [ZB:542–544, 549–553]. During the author's taste of kensho, the major portent of such objectivity extended far beyond the elementary sense of meaning that enters when one's ordinary semantic associations undergo a superficial closure. In this awed experiant, no impulse arose to utter either "Aha!" or "Eureka!" Later, such qualities of reality would lead me to wonder: what ingredients confirm the impression of reality, both during our ordinary moments and extraordinary states?

However, any quest to explain the enhanced "meaningful reality" of an extraordinary state of consciousness per se would seem premature if it were only a quick search narrowly restricted to a few cortical gyri that might generate some esoteric "added-on" value (likened by some to a "God-spot") [ZB:613–621; ZBR:417–503]. Why? Let us begin with one explanation so obvious that it might escape notice, were it not for the aspects of preattention already discussed in chapter 8.

The Early, Immediate, Implicit Role of Preattention in Meaning

One fact is implicit in the automaticity underlying each focused act of attention: *this target event, this object of attention, already has some salient meaning for me, at this instant.* Indeed, I'd waste no time on it unless it was *potentially meaningful.*

Let's review briefly what converges into our perceptions within the first tenth of a second as we glimpse a fruit-like object out there in the environment. Instantly, at *subcortical* levels, preattentive systems scan our instincts, life experiences, and memories for safe, useful options. Orienting toward one particular configuration, their pointed salient impales that target on its pre-sharpened tip. The rest of the brain now has the leisure of further milliseconds of recurrent and reflective processing to decode what this target really *is* and to analyze what it *means* (see tables 1 and 15).

These four sentences summarize how quickly we've *already* projected a substantial gist of the elementary categories of meaning into those early milliseconds. Their influence begins long before that object's original wavelengths could become translated into impulses conveying our linguistic label for "apple" (chapter 4).

What is Zen? Taking a millisecond perspective, we might view it as an ancient, ongoing, wordless celebration of our earliest resources of comprehension [ZB:648–653]. These earlier synapses operate subconsciously. They work silently on behalf of our native virtues, innocent of most top-down directions. Much of the current literature has yet to isolate these vanguard properties of instant attention per se in a manner that distinguishes their immediate focal or global functions from other mechanisms during the rest of our mental processing. These later distributed functions play their own vital overlapping roles. We use them in our more refined perceptions, memory processing, interpretation, language, insightful restructuring, etc.

In confirmation, studies of gamma EEG oscillations suggest that when our brain reacts to an object, its gamma wave activities undergo at least two general categories of responses.[12] Thus, in the first 100-ms phase of "evoked" gamma activities, the brain combines both its initial automatic response of selective pre-attention, and its preliminary coarse visual representation of the particular stimuli that are already arriving from such an object [ZBR:44–47]. High-frequency gamma oscillations (90 to 250 cps) correlate with the matching processes involved in short-term working memory tasks that can begin just after this first 100-ms phase.[13] Thereafter, the second phase of "induced" gamma oscillations peaks at around 200 to 250 ms (chapter 4; table 2). These later gamma waves are associated with the cognitive steps that integrate these immediate visual representations in terms of our own prior personal experience (table 9).

Let us now briefly disengage our focus of attention from gamma activities so that we can redirect it to analyze the object that we believe is a real apple. Let every reasonable association link confirm that this fruit we focus on out there seems in truth to be an *actual* apple. Under ordinary circumstances, we never stop to contemplate the hair-splitting scientific reality: all such impressions depend on a human interpretation of wavelength energies radiating from an object; this makes its independent existence a mere contingency. Instead, to us, we not only believe we're seeing a *real* fruit, we feel comfortable in our ability to identify it as an apple and so label it with a word that seems truly meaningful. Do we keep injecting some personal layers of comfort into our opinions about "real truth?" Then, how much does this truthiness contribute to our believing that an object is genuine and meaningful? These issues become the next topic for discussion.

29

Dynamic Aspects of Truth

Truth *happens* to an idea. It *becomes* true, is *made* true by events. Its verity *is* in fact an event, a process: a process namely of its verifying itself, its veri-fication.

William James (1842–1910)

We cannot escape the conclusions that our earlier notions of reality are no longer applicable.

Werner Heisenberg (1901–1976)

Truths happen. Over time, truths evolve. Before hominids arrived, this planet knew no word for truth. Much later, during years that humans arbitrarily labeled the "twentieth" century, we came smack up against Heisenberg's uncertainty principle. One lesson from atomic physics was that many things we had believed true about the "real" material universe were no longer true.

This chapter returns to address the issue raised in the preface: how do we generate personal truths? How does each brain create its own "truthy" sense of tentative "truths," private truths unverifiable by any scientific methods that might dare to challenge their coherence and devalue their validity? It follows from William James's observation that what *happens* to ring true at first is subject to later change. Sunday's "truthiness" might become Monday's Self-deception.

Meanings Evolve as They Become Multimodal and Associative

During childhood, we gradually realized there was more to an object than a mere name. Apples came in different colors, had a pleasant taste, a smell, a texture. These early descriptors referred to the initial sensory avenues of perception in the back of our brain. Other kinds of abstract knowledge evolved in later years. We learned how an apple grew—from blossoms on trees—into a fruit, which ripened rather slowly. A maturing cognition bound each new facet of information into one larger package of coherent associations, strengthening our positive concept of what a real apple was.

At present, our temporal lobe's pattern recognition systems instantly recognize an apple. Gnosis *knows* it, knows how it differs from a wax facsimile, understands all that's meant when it hears the word spoken. Recent studies suggest two more reasons why the superior temporal sulcus is an important interface in this processing.

- Many semantic messages first traverse the *posterior part of the superior temporal sulcus* as they flow forward toward the temporal pole.[1] Figure 1 shows this sulcus (pSTSUL). Beginning here, along its valley walls is a preliminary, coarse-grain, cross-modal, *presemantic* organization of perceptual features. Then, for finer-grain levels of analysis, the resulting messages stream forward toward the anterior temporal regions. Here, in the perirhinal cortex, objects already known develop the more intimate tug of being newly recognized as such.[2] Further integrations decide in which familiar semantic category they belong.

  The hungrier you are, the more you need to know *where* food is located in space. (Is this apple still up there ripening on a branch? Lying half-rotten on the ground?) Therefore, the meaning that gets attached to each such location of the fruit soon requires interactive consultations with the parietal and frontal lobes.

- Some of these other semantic messages also pass through the superior temporal sulcus on the upward path that connects the inferior temporo-occipital region with the inferior parietal lobule [ZBR:433].

Yes, but Is This Really, Truly an Apple?

Unfortunately, our biases distort perception. They cause us to remember false information. Mere impressions of "truthiness" can be false, not only at a visceral level. In this respect, it is important to appreciate that frontal lobe intelligence is not infallible. fMRI studies suggest that both true *and* false recollections arise when our prefrontal cortex engages in further semantic elaborations.[3]

However, as meaning evolves, the *medial* temporal lobe can play a more objective role. Its left posterior region contributes to our remembering most accurately (more "truly") whether *in fact* we had, or had not, actually processed a given event once before (the déjà/jamais vu decision). As anticipated by that old adage "seeing is believing," an even earlier level of less biased objectivity arises far back in our primary visual cortex. This visual region helps construct the "truest" memory formations.

These several lines of evidence suggest an important take-home message: the more directly we integrate our earliest perceptual messages—the simpler ones that first register *seeing* and *hearing*—with our medial temporal lobe memory functions, the more likely we are to record details accurately and remember an event in ways that consciousness might regard as valid, at least tentatively. Otherwise, greater degrees of uncertainty arise, and will persist.

The world is like a Rorschach ink blot test. We insert the imaginary projections of our subjective Self into everything we see there. The simplest way to gather valid factual information is by learning to observe the world mindfully, unjudgmentally, clearly, using the other-referential ventral pathways that bypass the intrusive filters of Self.

30

Value Systems for Truth, Beauty, and Reality

Humanly speaking, let us define truth, while waiting for a better definition, *as a statement of facts as they are.*

Voltaire (1694–1778)

Robert Henri's words in the epigraph for part IV are those of an artist who was sensitive to many metaphoric attributes of the temporal lobe. Its multiple networks contribute to the impression that we are seeing clearly into universal truths with a sense of profound wisdom, harmony, and unparalleled release.

How do we assign value to our systems of belief? Researchers who had once collected so-called hard data about perceptions have ventured increasingly into this soft topic area. Nowadays, they can create virtual "reality" in a laboratory setting, then test how their subjects perceive, make value judgments, and respond to this latest artificial version.

Yet, what do individual people *really* believe? Belief systems are complex because we too often vary the fixed opinions we hold about what constitutes "truth," "meaningfulness," and "reality." Biases resist inquiry, whether they are the result of one's personal experience or are cultural legacies. This makes it difficult to know what's "really" going on in someone else's brain, and especially how individuals will behave in the real world outside the laboratory (chapter 44). Poets and philosophers in the West have speculated about this fluid linguistic/experiental interface for millennia. Postmodern epistemological concepts continue to evolve, as is suggested by the following brief sampler of contributions from recent centuries.

Blaise Pascal (1623–1662) understood that "truth" had affective layers. He once said: "We know truth not only by reason, but also by the heart, and it is from this last that we know first principles." John Keats (1795–1821) reduced the issue to simpler terms. In his classic "Ode to a Grecian Urn," he said: "'Beauty is truth, truth beauty'—that is all ye know on earth, and all ye need to know."

Samuel Coleridge (1772–1834) went on to analyze the difference between what was beautiful and what was (merely) good. To Coleridge, "The Beautiful arises from the perceived harmony of an object, whether sight or sound, with the inborn and constitutive rules of the judgment and imagination: and it is always intuitive." What did he mean by intuition? He viewed it as the integrative process that had the unique capacity to create a "Unity" between the sense object, our judgment, and our imagination. Indeed, to Coleridge, this very *harmony* resulting from our intuitive functions was what distinguished the beautiful from the merely Good. He relegated "Good" to a separate category because, he said, "The Good . . . is always discursive."

Yes, one can discourse at length about what seems "good." Talk is cheap. Zen prefers silence and quiet mindful observation, not wordy discourse. In solitude, beauty strikes immediately. At deeper levels, words don't do it justice. Language falls short when we try to explain *why* we believe someone or something is beautiful. Beauty's aesthetic judgments tap universal harmonious chords, as does the essence of Zen.

William Wordsworth (1770–1850) understood the value of harmonic resonances when he observed that "we see into the life of things . . . with an eye made quiet by the power of harmony, and the deep power of joy." Yet, when the awakening of kensho taps even deeper levels, the reality it unveils is also unsentimental, cool, shorn of all prior conditioning [ZB:547–549, 570–572].

After Coleridge and Wordsworth died, England endured the Victorian era. Cultural value systems that were deemed intrinsically "good" and "true" became the ethical compass. Its needle was that formidable word "proper," the standard guide to judge the merit of each person's behavior. Accordingly, Thomas H. Huxley (1825–1895) could now state with assurance that "the whole duty of man" was to "learn what is true in order to do what is right." Shoulds and oughts prevailed.

In his early years as a mathematician, Alfred North Whitehead (1861–1947) grew up in this same culture, but went on to analyze truth differently. He came to regard all truths as "half-truths." He saw that we invented stories and applied them to the outside of things, changing them into mere "appearances." These appearances are not real, we only *think* they are real. In fact, what we humans believe is reality is only *relative*. As for the nature of *Absolute* Reality, Whitehead went on to say: "Reality is just itself, and it is nonsense to ask whether it be true or false." Real reality *is*. Just this.

Meanwhile, in the United States, Charles S. Peirce (1839–1914) was taking a liberal, pragmatic view of how truth and reality were actually being practiced. His personal perspective was relativistic, and it reflected the advent of popular opinion polls. What is truth? Writing in the *Popular Science Monthly* (1878), Pierce concluded that truth is "the opinion which is fated to be ultimately agreed to by all who investigate." What was real? To him, "the real is the object represented in this opinion."[1]

The Positive Experience Created by Fast, Efficient Processing

The flow of consciousness influences what it appears to contain. At certain times, when consciousness expands, it seems remarkably unburdened, lightweight, free-flowing. Two qualities combine to make such moments special: fluent processing and clarity of recognition (chapters 6 and 8). When cognition blends speed and clarity, their merger seems "easy on the mind." It turns out that this same combination shapes our value judgments in a positive direction. Research confirms that our aesthetic responses become more affirmative when the two ingredients join. EMG measurements show that the subjects' facial muscles now react in a *smiling* pattern overtly consistent with their shift toward positive/affective responses.[2] No longer is such a positive internal feeling concealed inside a subjective opinion.

Kensho conveys an impression of authenticity. At that moment, at the phenomenal level, the experiant comprehends it as "ultimate reality." The EMG study just cited is important for several reasons. It raises the possibility that fast, parallel processing during a state of kensho could have, *in itself*, measurable external physical manifestations. The sequences being envisioned in such an episode would unfold as follows: (1) The mental field opens up with major fresh intuitive qualities: transparent clarity, efficient processing, *and* a total release from the clutter of prior burdensome Self-centered content. (2) In combination, these additions and subtractions reinforce the entire mental experience in an affirmative direction. (3) The resulting psychophysiological attributes help transfigure the person's facial countenance in a manner that researchers can measure objectively[3] [ZB:413–418, 611–613].

Other lines of research suggest additional ways that longitudinal, well-documented EMG monitoring, performed immediately, could help identify how the state of kensho had transformed a subject's prior affective responses to a select range of stimuli used to test emotional and neutral responses [ZBR:242, 397–398].

You may be wondering, does the recent discussion of harmonic resonances have anything to do with the Path of long-range meditative training? In fact, our abstract human notions about values, truth, and reality do not condense out of thin air. They express distributed brain functions, in the course of which some temporal lobe networks play a substantial role. For example, fMRI signals from the superior portion of both temporal poles (BA 38, R > L) increase selectively when subjects insert certain kinds of richly detailed abstract conceptual knowledge into the meaning of human interpersonal behaviors.[4] When these social constructs are tested in the laboratory, they are presented as pairs of words (like *honor-brave* or *tactless-impolite*). It turns out that this superior temporal polar cortex appears to operate in the abstract without reference to an emotional valence, and that it collaborates with the allied social cognitive functions of the medial prefrontal cortex.

This general topic of harmonious interpretation continues in the next chapter.

Contemporary research into aesthetic preferences suggests that our sense of "beauty"—arising as it does from dual Self/other-referential ingredients—has multifactoral neuroimaging and cultural correlates, and these require much further study.

31

The Temporal Lobe: Harmonies of Perception and Interpretation

> After silence, that which comes nearest to expressing the inexpressible is music.
>
> Aldous Huxley (1894–1963)

> Music has charms to soothe a savage breast, to soften rocks, or bend a knotted oak.
>
> William Congreve (1670–1729)

On their own scale of values, many persons regard silence as "golden," placing it next to music (and poetry) in expressing properties of elemental beauty. Coleridge, cited earlier, viewed this beauty as an emergent property of harmonious unification. He concluded that our impression of "Beautiful" issued from a threefold intuitive act. It was a process during which we (1) integrated our perceptions of the sense object into (2) value judgments that (3) our corresponding imagination had already led us to expect.

In these three respects, our temporal lobe networks are brimful of wide-ranging patterns of expectation. Waiting templates instantly discern meaningful patterns in what we hear and see. They anticipate that these events can be pleasant or scary, harmonious or dissonant, beautiful or ugly, real or unreal.

The manifold capacities of the temporal lobe enable us to hear one single note of melody, develop its harmonic resonances, and expand them into a full-fledged organ chord. We have noted that both the temporoparietal junction (TPJ) and the superior temporal sulcus (STS) serve as an interface where visually harmonic resonances from the temporal lobe could rise to interact with the spatial savvy and symbolic resources of the parietal lobe (chapters 28 and 29).

Expert Buddhist meditators who practice a form of loving-kindness-compassion meditation show increased activation in both their right TPJ and right STS in response to sounds (chapter 9). It is not a new idea that meditation might enhance the way human beings cultivate a variety of socially adaptive intuitive processes. The ancient Taoists appreciated that their "inward training" helped to sponsor more affirmative, pleasant, and socially harmonious resonances. As a text from the fourth century B.C.E. explains:

> The true condition of the mind,
> finding calmness beneficial,
> arrives at repose.
> Neither disturb it, nor disrupt it,
> And harmony will develop naturally.[1]

Songs from Within the Musical Brain

Subtle harmonies enter into the ways we share music, language, and interpersonal relationships. In the temporal lobe, many of their resources are in overlapping regions, and their interactions extend into the frontal lobe as well. Brain imaging studies show that networks in both hemispheres engage complementary functions when we listen to music.[2]

Within the first tenth of a second after sound waves arrive, our brain begins to interpret what the waves mean musically. First it extracts the perceptual features that relate to pitch and timbre. Next it proceeds to recognize melodies and rhythms, then shifts into analyzing chord intervals. By 515 ms, we arrive at not only a sense of structure and meter but now clearly recognize the presence of harmony.[3]

Examples of the Power of Music

The Lost Chord exemplifies some intimate associations between musical harmony and temporal lobe sensibilities, as they might relate to the awesome existential resonances of kensho. Composed in 1877 at the bedside of his dying brother, this song became one of Sir Arthur Sullivan's best-known works.[4] *The Lost Chord* set to music a poem by Adelaide Porter. It spoke eloquently of one single elusive chord of organ music. When struck, it was "like the sound of a great Amen." The note's extraordinary resonances quieted all pain and sorrow, "came from the soul of the organ, and entered into mine."

An extraordinary movie documents music's primal power to soothe the savage breast. Released in 2004, the movie is entitled *The Story of the Weeping Camel.*[5] Set far off in the Gobi desert, its appeal is profound and universal. This true story centers on a young mother camel worn to a frazzle after a difficult two-day delivery. Weary and ill at ease, she refuses to recognize and nurse her new-born colt. Tragedy stalks. Finally, her shepherd sings her a plaintive song, accompanied by background music from a simple stringed instrument. The mother camel listens attentively. Tears come to her eyes—and to those of the viewers—as the strains of this music tug at her heartstrings. The melting undifferentiation releases her from her mental block, and restores her natural mothering instincts.

Camels are notoriously ill-tempered. However, Mongolian desert shepherds have known for millennia that music gentles these unruly traits. Dating from the Tang dynasty is a classic tricolor glazed statue. Despite the fact that this model camel is carrying a heavy human burden—both a plump singer and four other musicians—it still arches its head up high and is shown singing with its mouth wide open joyously joining in their music.

What Happens When We Listen to Music?

Pleasant music causes fMRI signals to increase in the ventral striatum and insula, among other positive response sites.[6] Frontal midline theta EEG power also increases. In contrast, *unpleasant* music reduces the heart rate and increases signals in the amygdala, hippocampus, parahippocampal gyrus, and both temporal poles. Patients no longer respond with negative emotions to dissonant, unpleasant music after their parahippocampal gyrus (L, R) has been surgically removed.[7] Moreover, when normal subjects respond to pleasant music, all these sites above where dissonance caused increased signals now show a strong *decrease* in such fMRI signals. This is a basic pattern. Combining both plus and minus responses, it is of fundamental importance. In this instance, it illustrates the *twofold, reciprocal* functional correlates that clarify why we "like" some music and "can't stand" other kinds. Elsewhere, it is emphasized that similar simultaneous, reciprocal increases and decreases are typical of other vital processes that shape the way our brains respond (chapters 21, 22, and 23). Discrete bilateral damage to the amygdala interferes selectively with the ability to recognize music that is emotionally sad and scary. Fortunately for the patient, happy music is spared.[8]

Music can significantly relieve the anxieties of surgical patients who require intensive care.[9] When they hear Mozart piano sonatas through earphones, their growth hormone levels increase (by 60%), their interleukin-6 levels drop (by 83%), and their serum epinephrine levels also fall (by 55%). Could similar salutary changes help to document the neuroendocrine correlates of kensho's release from anxiety? The question relates to pathways that link temporal lobe networks with the hypothalamus. For millennia, camels' responses to music have suggested that the answers merit thorough investigation [ZBR:89, 489].

Long-term musical training confers personal benefits that are increasingly well documented. Among the latest reports is the finding that musicians show more evidence of bilaterally symmetrical connectivity between their right and left visual fields than do nonmusicians.[10] Issues of nature (genes) vs. nurture (training enhances plasticity) remain to be resolved.

A fascinating fMRI study of six professional jazz pianists[11] is relevant to the kinds of intuitive free expression cultivated during long-range Zen training [ZB:638–639, 668–677]. The results illustrate the reciprocal patterns of activation and deactivation just discussed. During the pianists' spontaneous improvisations, they activated their dorsal medial frontal polar cortex (BA 10) and anterior temporal regions (BA 20–22). Simultaneously, they *deactivated* extensive regions in both their dorsolateral frontal cortex, lateral orbitofrontal cortex, and limbic system. The many limbic sites deactivated included the amygdala, entorhinal cortex, temporal pole, posterior cingulate cortex, parahippocampal gyrus, hippocampus, and hypothalamus. In a similar manner, one can envision that the Zen path could help selectively decondition the limbic system and frontal regions of their more maladaptive responses while liberating some of the most highly evolved associative functions represented farther forward in the frontal pole and temporal pole.

Commentary

Our temporal lobe offers wide-open conduits for multiple discerning interpretations. Earlier chapters emphasized that its networks engage in other-referential modes of processing, the kinds that convey visual object recognition (chapters 13, 14, and 15). Nearby are other remarkable networks that interpret many other kinds of nuanced messages [ZB:247–253, ZBR:152–157, 245–247]. Their associative functions elaborate more than rhyming coherences and musical harmonies that reach from bass through treble clefs. Their circuits also register separate wavelengths in the color spectrum and resonate with complementary colors [ZBR:410–414]. Along this ventral processing path, we render elaborate judgments automatically, without thinking, and often do so with reasonable degrees of objectivity, at least in the early milliseconds. However, we soon attach heavier emotional overtones and inhibitions during subsequent relays through our Self-centered, limbic and paralimbic networks. We can live with greater simplicity, clarity, and stability by shedding these polarizing limbic responses that infuse only rigid constraints, obsessions, and dissonances into our daily lives.[12]

The Temporal Lobe: Word Thoughts Interfere with No-Thought Processing

He who speaks doesn't know; he who knows doesn't speak.

Tao Te Ching (c. third century B.C.E.)

Better I remain silent than deceive you.

Master Yunmen Wenyan (864–949)

Zen stories often contain paradoxes and irrational statements. Trainees are slow to appreciate two simple facts: no brain overly preoccupied with Self-relational thoughts finds a comfortable home in traditional Zen, neither does an over-worked intellect full of irrelevant ideas [ZB:59–64].

What *is* valued in Zen? Skillful actions. Actions that leap spontaneously from a mindful awareness that remains clear, objective, insightful, and unselfconscious. Working with a Zen master on a koan helps Zen trainees realize the profound limitations of word language [ZBR:394–396]. Quick, fluid gestures are the body English of Zen communication, not concepts.

Silence has virtues. Schooler and colleagues observed normal subjects who were working to solve experimental tasks in the laboratory. When the subjects spoke out loud, their verbalizations distracted them, preventing them from discovering strategies that could help them find the optimal solution to the problem.[1]

How We Actively Infer Meanings while Listening to Short Stories

When someone reads aloud from a simple narrative text, we use both sides of our brain to draw subtle inferences from their description of the entire environment. In this regard, table 10 shows how the two hemispheres make different contributions when we decode meanings. Bihemispheric processing yields the requisite blended mixture of "semantic activation, integration, selection, and/or incorporation of the inferred concept."[2]

To illustrate, suppose while someone reads you a short story, you hear the particular verb that specifies the pivotal turning point of one of your inferences. At this point, fMRI signals increase in the *right* superior temporal gyrus (BA 41, 22). Perhaps later, on the other hand, you hear some other break in the coherence of the narrative, a gap that specifies a different inference. In that instance, increased signals occur first in the *left* middle and posterosuperior temporal gyrus (BA 21, 22).

Table 10
Complementary Aspects of Hemispheric Processing When Subjects Derive Influences from Simple Texts

Direction of Inference	Left Hemisphere	Right Hemisphere
Inferences predicted toward future events	Less sensitive to concepts	More sensitive to concepts
Inferences referred back toward past events	More sensitive when the prior options are simple	Less sensitive when the prior options are simple
Inferences about either future or past events	More sensitive to either option when the prior text is strongly constrained	More sensitive to either option when the prior text is weakly constrained

Adapted from S. Virtue, J. Haberman, Z. Clancy, et al. Neural activity of inferences during story comprehension. *Brain Research* 2006; 1084:104–114.

While you process this same inference, signals increase slightly later in your *left* inferior frontal gyrus and anterior insula (BA 47, 13). If your working memory is especially efficient, signals increase even more in these last two regions. In general, you will put more effort into trying to decode the inference of some subtly implied event and will generate more fMRI signals than if the event has an obvious meaning.

"No-Thought" Zen

Many habit energies and emotional pressures drive the forms of silent speech we call thoughts. In the temporal lobe, our auditory language functions are distributed chiefly in its superior portion. Our visual-object and pattern-recognition functions tend to pursue pathways in its lower portions. Bird watchers share in the all-too-human habit of attaching word labels to everything they see. This human compulsion to identify things by tagging them with word thoughts is one reason why much of the cortex in our temporal and occipital lobe cortex stays preoccupied with concepts and multitasking associations.

How can Zen training cultivate an alternative lifestyle, one that leads toward "no-thought" awareness and creative intuitions? Regular meditation helps calm those emotionally driven, highly subjective, habit energies that agitate discursive thoughts. As meditation gradually decreases the limbic pressures behind these Self-centered thoughts, it tends to "quiet the eye" and replace it with a calmer mode of evenly hovering awareness [ZBR:184–187]. This more objective awareness can serve the needs of action-oriented networks when both are deployed even-handedly. In the array of mental abilities required to be creative, being tautly integrated and staying loose are not mutually exclusive.[3]

Speculation: Perhaps flashes of insight might later be more likely to happen during quiet meditative retreats after large regions of the upper and lower temporal lobe have been relieved of their ordinary word-language chores and are less burdened by the pressures to speak. Major flashes of insight-wisdom, arriving along allocentric pathways, proceed to illuminate depths far beyond ordinary insights, and remain inexpressible in words.

Daido Loori, in his recent book, *The Zen of Creativity*, illustrates how Zen training helps to cultivate one's aesthetic sensibilities in direct ways that express the covert, ineffable dimensions of reality.[4] Long overdue is a thorough scientific study of the positive influential role that different liberal arts can have on the spiritual path by enhancing each individual's creative sensibilities.

Into the Silence; The Case of J.T.

Thirty-seven-year old Jill Taylor suddenly developed a major *left*-sided *cortical* lesion. It was a "stroke," an acute pathological process that combined the effects of hemorrhage and infarction. It compromised her *left* central areas of somatosensory function, dissolved her receptive and expressive speech functions, and damaged adjacent areas of her fronto-temporal-parietal cortex.[5] In the resulting inner silence, she then became a selfless witness to how deeply certain other people can also experience a sense of unification and inner peace. These novel episodes emerge when similar cortical deactivations on one side release functions from regions within the opposite hemisphere—now unopposed—into the field of consciousness [ZB:611; ZBR:18, 416, 467].

Our discussion in part III suggests that some (remotely) similar set of imbalances can arise transiently during kensho. However, they are being interpreted as expressing an unusual configuration of *physiological* mechanisms. These are normally more subtle. Moreover, having converged initially at the *subcortical* level, the proposal is that they first deactivate the *dorsal* thalamus, while selectively sparing its ventral tier of nuclei.

Notably, this sparing of the ventral thalamus leaves intact (a) its primary sensory contributions that are entering it directly from the internal and external landscape, and (b) its other contributions (also thought-free) that are rising from subconscious levels in the cerebellum and basal ganglia. The resulting blend could lend a variety of unusual impressions of unity to the ongoing experience [ZBR:168, 466, 357].

33

The Pregnant Meditative Pause: Introspection; Incubation

> Almost without exception, our respondents told us that the daily problem-*solving* insights come to them during this [short period of] idle time.... Most of the narratives related to problem-*finding* insight described it as occurring during an extended period of idle time, such as a vacation or sabbatical.
>
> M. Csikszentmihalyi and K. Sawyer[1]

The above point that insights arrive during idle time is accurate. It echoes the awesome moment when an organist's fingers, wandering "idly," happened to strike the great Amen of *The Lost Chord*.

One approach that social scientists use to study creativity is to interview talented subjects over 60 years old who have a long track record. Their major breakthroughs at high levels illustrate the two broad categories of our creative endeavor.[2] The first category is the kind that involves problem *solving*. The problem itself is already obvious. The seeker's task is to discover how to solve it. Usually, only a relatively short time elapses before seekers work out their solution. Clearly, most of the task-driven neuroimaging data we have discussed in these pages falls into this first short-term category: experimental subjects were given well-defined problems, and their job was to solve them.

Not so the problems in the second category. These problems are obscure, and the seekers first task *is to discover what the problems are*. A long time elapses before all the unknowns are identified, let alone solved. A personal narrative describes how such long unpredictable processes took years to evolve in the field of biomedical research.[3] Most Zen trainees also spend years of uncertainty, meandering around in a similar problem-*finding* arena, slowly discovering what Zen is, and what it is not [ZBR:7–11].

Major insightful awakenings occur unpredictably on the Path of Zen. Thus far, no formal scientific study seems to have documented the evidence often observable: *meditative practices* enhance the arrival of many smaller intuitions and insights of various sizes. The moments that illuminate the key topic of Selfhood are of two kinds. Some illustrate in an explicit manner the problems imposed by one's pejorative Self. Others illuminate ways that such personal problems can be resolved. Once you clearly realize during kensho that your Self *is* the problem, it then becomes easier to focus on ways to restructure the *I-Me-Mine*.

Introspection and Self-Analysis

As part of the ongoing process of trying to remain unattached to labels, it will be helpful briefly to return to that phrase, no-thought, in the subheading which closed the last chapter. Does a state of total "no-thought" and "no-mind" represent an accurate description of the entire objective in Zen? No. Because these phrases refer to a calm, clear analytical mind, to "an eye made quiet by the power of harmony," not to an empty-headed vacuity.

This unruffled, clear-seeing mode of mental processing sets the stage for

- an acutely focused, objective *introspection* of one's interpersonal relationships, lifestyle, and overall goals; and

- a more sustained, reflective examination of whatever minor insights might surface, enabling them to be more influential.

As the Dalai Lama says simply: "For me, analytical meditation is most helpful."[4]

Acronyms, Old and New

The mindful introspective path toward insight is ancient in origin [ZB:125–129]. One of its contemporary modifications has been called "mindfulness-based cognitive therapy" (MBCT). Back when my fellow students and I were in medical school, we were relieved to hear that the psychiatry department had just imported a "new" approach into the curriculum. It was then called "insight therapy." Thereafter, it seemed to evolve into "cognitive-behavioral therapy" (CBT), and more recently—when combined with mindfulness-based meditation—it is sometimes abbreviated MBCBT. Labels and acronyms aside, many basic principles remain the same: the little intuitions into one's interpersonal relationships, and the minor insights into larger issues, each provide important "openings." They help reformulate goals and redirect one's priorities. A stimulating teacher or therapist is a catalyst in the process of change. Still, the *major transforming factors are the internal awakenings that penetrate from within*. Introspection often discloses that various degrees of Self-dissolution occur during such insights.

On This Path of Minor Insights

The more one meditates, the more often minor insights occur. However, they do not necessarily occur *while* one is meditating. Some little intuitions smolder for hours before they ignite into lesser insights. Master Hakuin openly acknowledged how very wide-ranging insights could be.[5] Indeed, he stated that he had undergone 18 major awakenings, and had lost count of his numerous little insights.

In my experience, the regular morning meditation before breakfast is often a fertile interval when minor intuitions and lesser insights emerge. These little illuminations enter not during the immediate process of "boring into" an ordinary problem or a riddle like a koan. Instead, they arise tangentially, during open intervals of *letting go*[6] [ZBR:394–396]. This chapter's epigraph about idle time emphasizes an important point: the crucial preludes on the lengthy path toward creative insights in Zen are often the longer pauses when thoughts drop off. These are the times when one *lets go* for an extended period. Typically, these pauses occur during retreats, not while one is seated on the cushion meditating, but *later on*, unexpectedly. They tend to occur in novel settings.

Does Subconscious Incubation Enhance the Way We Generate Creative Thoughts?

How does incubating a problem enable unconscious mechanisms to sponsor creative solutions? One earlier theory was called the "fresh look" hypothesis. The phrase implied that the seeker would take off on a fresh unbiased start, simply because he or she had set the problem passively aside for a while. Dutch researchers had a different theory and devised a short-term experiment to test it.[7] Their subjects' task was to generate a long list of place names, starting with the letter *A*. The subjects performed the task, either (1) immediately after they had received this instruction; or (2) after several minutes of conscious thought; or (3) after several minutes of having been distracted in the interim. It turned out that the subjects generated the most original place names and other items after this third condition, the one which was believed to favor so-called unconscious thought. The evidence suggested that unconscious mechanisms had played an active role in developing divergent associations.

Lau and Passingham assigned their subjects tasks that were both semantic and phonological.[8] While the subjects were engaged in subliminal priming activities, fMRI signals increased in their mid-dorsolateral prefrontal cortex (BA 46). The results suggested that the frontal lobes mull over a problem, continuing to work "intelligently", without our being consciously aware of their efforts.

Incubating a Koan. Pro and Con

In Sino-Japanese Zen traditions, the koan system has served a wide variety of purposes. When Joshu Sasaki-Roshi assigns a koan to his trainees, he mentions that it is not given as an object to be understood. Left unstated are the covert ways that a koan might serve to stir the pot of subterranean brain functions, stimulating introspection in general and yielding delayed insights of various kinds and sizes.

The Zen koan has always had proponents and opponents [ZB:107–119; ZBR:61–64]. Victor Sogen-Hori's recent analysis provides one explanation for why the nature of a koan has been so difficult to understand. Historically, the koan was derived from *two* sources, not one.[9] First, and foremost was "The wordless insight of Zen." Centuries later, koans became entangled in wordy aspects of "the Chinese literary game."

- *Pro.* At the most basic level of wordless insight, the classic koan remains an unsolvable enigma. It creates a climate of unknowing, of arcane uncertainty. No literal construction of the words of a koan penetrates its layers of allusions [ZB:540–542]. These allusions resemble a kind of "insider joke."[10] They are so remote that they baffle all but the few whose mental capacities have become sufficiently open to grasp their cultural implications.

- *Con.* Many of the intellectual aspects (and associated liabilities) of the koan date from the Sung period in China (960–1126), an era that often prescribed koans in a manifestly literary context. During the so-called Literary Period, the earlier gutsy Zen poetic expressions of the Tang Dynasty gave way to vapid verses of court poetry. Moreover, many Ch'an masters began to use short "capping phrases" during what could be called a conceptual form of "koan *study*." In the course of the original Chinese capping verse game, how do the players test each other? They "apply not merely their training and poetry, but the clarity of their awakened eye."[11] In Japan, this dual approach to the koan would later become a required practice for monks in training [ZBR:458–459].

Of course, the authentic Zen masters continued to analyze their students' body English, reading between the lines of their verbal language, and often communicating with them silently by indirection and gesture. They wanted to be *shown* their trainees' whole *performance*, not simply their literary scholarship. Hori offers a concrete word example to illustrate one aspect of this dual situation.[12]

Question: What is amnesia?
  Answer: I forget.

In this instance, the trainee could respond not just with a word answer but with the shoulder shrug of an actual performance.

Prior Hints of Selflessness during Ordinary Kinds of Insight

Because this book is oriented toward selfless insight in Zen, our inquiry probes mechanisms beyond those that underlie the model of creative intuition in general. The Self/other themes developed in parts I, II, and III converged in chapters 19 and 23 on a series of working hypotheses centered on the thalamus. As the discussion evolves throughout the remainder of parts IV and V, it will point increasingly toward the meditative transformations during extraordinary states of consciousness. When Self-centeredness drops out in kensho and satori, novel insights illuminate a different dimension—*existential* wisdom. What is such unveiled wisdom? Its core is other-referential. It points to "the way all things *Really* are" when *no*-Self is intruding.

Meanwhile, the question arises: Do we also tend toward lesser degrees of selflessness? In fact, ample precedents exist. Both just before and during an ordinary insight, many persons are distantly aware that they undergo a similar, subtle inhibitory phase. Careful observation discloses that this fresh moment of insight arrives *free from their ordinary Self-attached forms of thought.*

For example, after an ordinary insight strikes, one may wonder: "Why didn't *I* think of that before?" The question is Self-explanatory. The italicized, capital *I* is the first explanation. This pejorative Self was all too often stuck in some wrong-headed approach. The second reason is embedded in the word "think." Too easily do we assume that conscious, logical thoughts are a prerequisite to solving all problems. Sight gags, déjà vu, and jazz improvisations remind us that the brain uses many quick, subconscious, automatic sources of understanding and acting.

Insight processing opens up these sources, and suspends its premature biases as it becomes less Self-encumbered. Subtle shifts occur within the right posterior parieto-occipital-temporal region and in the balances among other networks. They lead to the impression that our insight solutions seem to strike from out of the blue, and appear to arrive with no Self-referential details attached. Among these subconscious shifts are the openings through which messages from our ventral, *other*-referential pathways interact fruitfully with the inferior frontal lobe. This bottom-up consortium becomes free to explore a wide expanse of novel, abstract possibilities outside the box.

The Self-Effacing Brain

Many ambiguities and paradoxes reside along the fertile interface between Zen meditation and the brain. This writer and his readers will need both hemispheres to decode them. As our understanding of each topic evolves, so do some words and concepts used to describe this interface. Currently, the field as a whole is being referred to with the phrase contemplative neuroscience. The term "contemplative" has ecumenical connotations. The word is useful to the degree that one can begin to describe the Zen Way as involving contemplation, reflection, self-analysis, and other valuable thought-full approaches. Yet, within the core of Zen Buddhism are two noteworthy exceptions to the uniform generic applicability of "contemplative," a term that in the West might also include conventional prayer-filled thoughts and weighty spiritual ideologies.[13] The first exception occurs before kensho. The second occurs after kensho.

- Zen meditative practice emphasizes an open, clear, *bare* awareness on a Path toward selfless insight. Rinzai Zen places particular emphasis on spontaneity of action, not on discursive word thoughts and excessive verbalizations [ZB:107–109, 114–115, 122, 141]. Foyan Quingyuan (1060–1120) was one of many masters in this spare Ch'an tradition whose objections to thoughts were unmistakable.[14] "Zen practice means detaching from thoughts. This is the best way to save energy. Let go from emotional thoughts. Understand that no objective world exists. Then, you'll understand how to practice Zen."

- The two words, *selfless insight*, in the present title return us to the pivotal moment in Buddhist history. An extraordinary state of awakening occurred just before dawn beneath the Bodhi tree. The emptiness of this transforming moment lies beyond all ordinary top-down implications of what we mean when we use the verb *contemplate* [ZBR:383–386]. Yet, in no way does such an experience of insight-wisdom abandon all discerning thought processes thereafter. Instead, after this catharsis, mindful thought processes are now renewed in an exceptionally well-informed, clarified Self-effacing manner. All the old biased empathies and antipathies, the old longings and loathings, have been dissolved. In the afterglow of this brief "lightening up" the person's reflective interpretations incorporate the grace of those realizations into the reprogrammings that evolve subsequently during daily life practice. Now, a whole new series of lesser insights can develop. They are, in a sense, fresh hindsights. Their authenticity can be tested by running them through the gauntlet of the person's actual ongoing daily experiences.[15]

Having just sharpened the distinction between ordinary thoughts and insights, we turn in the next two chapters to examine what progress is being made toward understanding ordinary kinds of insight.

34

Recent, Ongoing Neuroimaging Studies of Ordinary Forms of Insight

Insights are sporadic, unpredictable, short-lived moments of exceptional thinking, during which implicit assumptions about the relevance of common knowledge to a problem must be discarded before a solution can be revealed.

Jing Luo and colleagues[1]

How does a normal brain instantly solve hard problems? This chapter and the next continue the earlier narrative [ZBR:104–105, 271–274]. Together, their pages become a progress report of the latest research on insight and creativity. In East

Asia, Niki and Luo began by using fMRI and event-related potentials to monitor subjects who were trying to solve difficult word problems and riddles. Back in 2004, their early research had suggested that the anterior cingulate gyrus could enter into some earlier sequences of breaking these linguistic impasses, leaving the right hippocampus to play a slightly later potential role.[2] It was already known that the anterior cingulate and hippocampus entered at different times into many different functions, so it became difficult to specify how and when each region might contribute during the several dynamic steps we use to solve ordinary linguistic problems [ZBR:82–85, 99–108].

In the United States, Mark Jung-Beeman, John Kounios, and colleagues were also studying insight. They began by selecting a large set of simple, three-word, association problems. Only by associating to a single (fourth) word could their subjects solve these compressed remote association tasks.[3] Had you volunteered to be one of their subjects, you would be asked to free-associate to a set of three words like these:

pine, crab, sauce.

Your task would be to think of a particular word they might (remotely) share in common. You would need to flex your imagination, and be ready to try anything, because the fourth word that solves the problem could come before any of these words, or after it.

(Answer: apple). If that sample seemed too easy, try

french, car, shoe.

(Answer: horn). Or

boot, summer, ground.

(Answer: camp).

When normal subjects see similar sets of problem words, they solve about half of them within 2 to 30 seconds. In some experiments, after the subjects vocalize their single-word answer, they must take on another responsibility. It is to specify *how* they reached the solution. Did the answer strike suddenly, as the result of insight? (they press one button, the "Aha!" button). Or did it arrive in a more deliberate manner, by incremental means? (they press the other button). Prior training ensures that they understand this crucial distinction and can press the correct "Aha!" or "non-Aha" button.

In one of the initial experiments, after the subjects failed to solve a set of problem words, they were presented visually with an extra series of cue words, and were asked to read these words aloud. Certain words were actual cues, serving as direct hints that primed the potential solution. The other words were not relevant. The researchers then added a very important technical flourish. They channeled each type of word—the real cues, or the non-cues—into the different halves of the brain. This meant that the subjects could see each type of cue in the visual hemifields of *either* their right *or* left cerebral hemisphere.

The subjects responded faster when the relevant solution cue words were directed into their *right* hemisphere. This hemisphere had a distinct processing advantage. Why was this right hemisphere advantage so intriguing? Because it was evident especially when sudden insights of the "Aha!" type had successfully solved the problem.[4]

A caveat. As chapter 7 emphasizes, many attentive functions are also represented chiefly within our right hemisphere. So then, do the faster response times on the right during these lateralized experiments mean that a special kind of insight processing is the sole reason for the solution? Not necessarily, because the responses in *all* tasks first enlist one's sharp point of facile attentive focusing. Faster, right-sided *attention* processing could also facilitate any adjacent, overlapping right-sided mechanisms of intuitive processing. That said, table 11 characterizes important (yet complementary) differences in the ways our two hemispheres function. These distinctions become apparent when subjects solve linguistic problems using ordinary kinds of insight.[5]

Monitoring Insight Processing with fMRI

This same research group then used fMRI to monitor subjects who were engaged in this task of solving similar word association problems. These were competent

Table 11
Complementary Aspects of Hemispheric Processing When Ordinary Problems Are Solved by Insight

	Left Hemisphere	Right Hemisphere
Initial processing of the problem	Ready to be more strongly activated by information that seems in context	Ready to be more weakly activated by seemingly tangential information
Vulnerability to misdirection	More	Less
Later resolution of the problem	Data less relevant initially might not be available for the final solution	Data less relevant in the initial context may prove more useful during later steps
Size of the semantic field	Smaller	Larger
Degree of semantic integration	Finer, more tightly focused	Coarser, more loosely focused
Levels of conscious participation	May be more aware of some underlying rationale	Processing occurs subconsciously, and is seemingly spontaneous

Adapted from E. Bowden, M. Jung-Beeman, M. Fleck, et al. New approaches to demystifying insight. *Trends in Cognitive Sciences* 2005; 9:322–328.

subjects who solved correctly more than half of their word problems (59%). Their button pressing also confirmed that "insight" was the basis for 56% of the correct solutions. The fMRI signals were collected during an appropriate window of time. It started 2 seconds before the button press and ended another 2 to 7 seconds after it.

In this study, the *right anterosuperior temporal gyrus* was prominent among the sites yielding increased signals (figure 4). Still, this region was even more active when the subjects *first viewed* each set of words than it became when they next proceeded to solve this word problem by insight. The researchers were already interested in this anterosuperior temporal gyrus, because prior human studies had shown it to be a polymodal association region that processed novel semantic associations [ZBR:154, 247] (table 9).

Normally, we make similar semantic associations in two situations: (1) when we comprehend language in general, and (2) when we extract meaningful themes from one sentence and apply them to another context. Notably, the increased fMRI signals arose from a large area of this right superior temporal cortex. It extended from in front of the right auditory cortex down to the midportion of the right middle temporal gyrus (BA 21, 22). Table 12 summarizes the bilateral distribution of the findings and other aspects of the fMRI study.

The Parallel EEG Study of Insight Processing

In the parallel EEG study, 128 scalp electrodes monitored the subjects' EEG responses while they were engaged in the word association task. A significant EEG finding was the burst of gamma band activity during the processing of insight solutions [ZBR:44–47]. The gamma frequencies ranged between 39 and 59 cps. This gamma burst started 0.3 second before the button press. It, too, became maximal

Table 12
Interactive Components of Semantic Processing

	Left Hemisphere	Right Hemisphere
Nature of semantic coding	A finer and more tightly focused field	A coarser and more loosely focused field
Initial semantic activations	More posteriorly in the middle and superior temporal gyrus	More posteriorly in the middle and superior temporal gyrus
Further semantic integrations	More anteriorly in the superior temporal gyrus and sulcus, and in the middle temporal gyrus	More anteriorly in the superior temporal gyrus and sulcus, and in the middle temporal gyrus
Rapid semantic selection	A more prominent role for the inferior frontal gyrus	A less prominent role for the inferior frontal gyrus

Adapted from M. Jung-Beeman. Bilateral brain processes for comprehending natural language. *Trends in Cognitive Sciences* 2005; 9:512–518.

over the same *right anterosuperior temporal region*. Was this induced gamma burst, lasting only 0.28 second, consistent with the way the solution word had abruptly emerged into some preconscious level of insight on a step up toward full conscious awareness?

An important precedent linked such induced gamma activity with the onset of meaning. In a pioneering study, Revonsuo and colleagues had used a different visual task that was *non*linguistic in nature.[6] In 1997, these Finnish researchers had shown that a major, *pre*conscious transient surge of gamma activity (40 cps) occurs in the visual association cortex over the *right* occipital and posterior parietotemporal region. This surge peaks some 400 ms *before* normal subjects go on to resolve a flat, 2-D visual scene into a meaningful 3-D coherent image. This surge also lasts for only 200 ms.

However, in the recent insight study based on word associations, a second EEG change was unexpected. It was a short burst of alpha activity (at 10 cps) that occurred even earlier and lasted only 0.75 second. It, too, was a herald, appearing only when the subsequent processing went on to solve the problem by insight. The alpha burst also anticipated, by a long interval (by some 1.4 to 0.4 seconds), the subjects' later button press, the signal chosen to report that they had just consciously reached an insight solution.

This earlier enhanced alpha activity is noteworthy for two other reasons. First, the EEGs localized it to the *right posterior parieto-occipital cortex*. Second, after this brief alpha burst, the underlying alpha activity continued on its already preexisting, slightly declining trend. Then, as this posterior alpha activity continued to fall, it dropped to its lowest level *just as the cited burst of gamma band activity rose* to reach *its* highest level in the *right superior temporal region*.

The down-up-down alpha pattern appears relevant. Also interesting is the inverse relationship between the alpha trough in the right posterior parietooccipital region and the gamma peak in the right superior temporal region. A useful rule of thumb is often applicable to such changes in alpha EEG activity: alpha is interpretable as an index. Of what? Of a physiological change in the *opposite* direction to that of the local cortical neuronal activity [ZBR:41–42, 48–50]. In short, "alpha power has come to be considered as a reverse measure of activation."[7] Accordingly, an "alpha burst" might translate into the phrase, "a brief *decrease* in local cortical functional activity." And, one might also substitute *increasing* or *higher* levels of local cortical functional activity in place of the words describing a "declining trend" or "lowest" levels of alpha. In short, the results suggest that the parieto-occipital cortex, while slowly increasing its *functional* activity, then suddenly decreased it when the gamma surge occurred.

Next to consider is what it means when an alpha burst occurs *earlier* than a gamma burst in the right hemisphere. To begin to address this question, it helps to return to table 11, and to review the columns on its right side. Here, Bowden and colleagues suggest how the *initial processing steps, the ones leading up toward an insight, diverge from insight's later steps. It is these later steps that go on to restructure the problem and resolve it.*

The general hypothesis advanced earlier by Jung-Beeman and colleagues in 2004[8] helps to articulate several psychophysiological proposals. The first two begin as follows:

- A briefly enhanced alpha EEG activity, suddenly peaking during an already downhill trend, could be consistent with *an initial weakening of some preliminary level of solution-related processing*. Why does this preliminary step remain unregistered as a conscious thought? Perhaps because a *net* decrease of local activity up in the cortex is only a surface expression of a *sub*cortical process. Perhaps it also indicates that a deeper shift has influenced the function of a corresponding region of the *right thalamus*: the right pulvinar. No electrodes are positioned down in the pulvinar to inform us how its covert thalamocortical response patterns had been changing. Nor had the later deep patterns of activity at this depth (at the moment when the alpha trough coincided with the gamma peak) yet reached a critical mass sufficient to register the bare outlines of a potential solution in any organized manner accessible to the subjects' consciousness.

- The subsequent burst of gamma activity occurs in the form of fast, synchronized neuronal oscillations. This burst could represent an increase in cortical excitation, an increase capable of integrating multiple bytes of information from over a relatively wide area. It is consistent with the solution's sudden transition toward that more integrated, conceptual form which could rise toward a more coherent level of *conscious* awareness.

In brief overview, such an alpha-gamma sequence can be viewed as one expression of the way the larger brain enters into a several-step approach to intuitive processing in general. One might envision similar elementary sequences as playing generic roles along the broad continuum of creative intuition. The first proposals to be sketched in the narrative below will be oriented toward mechanisms underlying our ordinary range of insights. They are viewed as preliminary, because they are based on pioneering experiments and on necessarily artificial conditions. Therefore, any hypotheses ventured here will need to be expanded substantially, later during part V, if we are to clarify how a *meditative* path could further enhance a person's spontaneous tendencies toward extraordinary peak experiences of insight-wisdom. Meanwhile, let the following tentative notions serve to introduce the much broader issues under discussion.

- Events that consciousness finds "meaningful" arise from patterns of brain activity that combine a mixture of inhibitory and excitatory mechanisms. Their patterns of deactivation and activation evolve at different times and at different levels:

    1. Some could express the initial faster *subcortical* arrival and processing of a mixture of impulses patterned in the pulvinar of the thalamus. As their oscillations relay through the reticular nucleus, the results may serve variously to excite/inhibit prior functions up at the cortical level. There, one *net* effect (manifested, say, as a brief alpha EEG burst) could be briefly to *interrupt* transmissions within some parts of the Self-referential dorsal path leading up through the posterior parietal cortex.

    2. Other messages gather momentum more slowly. Impulses traveling on the visual pathway through the optic radiations pursue a longer, coursing route before their messages once again enter the *temporal* cortex and stream forward along the other-referential, ventral pathway. When insightful constructs gather momentum near closure, some of their *net* excitatory functions could be surfacing as gamma peaks in the cortex of the right superior temporal region.

- Attributable to the earlier net inhibitory phase are several physiological consequences. One of the first could be to suspend some *premature* Self-centered biases within the posterior parieto-occipital networks that might have interfered with initial attempts to formulate the problem (figures 4 and 5).

- Then, with such unfruitful fixations in abeyance, fresh efforts could be made during the next excitatory phase to restructure the problem and to tap other resources that could improvise more optimal, novel solutions (chapter 31).

Recent EEG Studies of Alpha Activity during the Preparation for Linguistic Problems

Thus far, the speculations based on EEG data have combined brief, subtle local changes in the timing patterns of both alpha and gamma activities. A caveat: Can such findings, in fact, be generalized to explain some basic sequences involved in insight in general? The thesis might be more convincing if several research groups could replicate the general trend of the alpha/gamma results. How? By combining MEG and fMRI to study the sequences in detail, and by choosing different models (such as other linguistic-free versions of the "Magic Eye" task).

Meanwhile, in 2006, this same research team focused next on how alpha activity changed. This time they chose a much earlier interval. This interval spanned those 2 seconds of *preparation* just *before* their subjects viewed each word association problem.[10] Note that these subjects now took on an extra obligation.

Their additional task was to signal how *ready* they were. This signal would confirm that they now felt sufficiently attentive as well as mentally prepared to view each new set of words.

None of their word sets would be easy. Example:

bump, egg, step.

(Answer: goose)

Only 46% of these problems were solved within the standard 30-second time limit. Yet, once again, the subjects reported that a sudden "insight" was responsible for more than half of their solutions (56%).

Did a change in the subjects' earlier alpha activity during this 2-second period of preparation *predict* their capacity to solve the next word problem by insight? Yes, this early alpha activity did decrease in several regions. But which alpha frequency decreased, and where?

- The alpha activity at 9 to 10 cps was *decreased* over the midfrontal cortex.
- The alpha activity at 8 to 9 cps and 9 to 10 cps *decreased* over the left anterior temporal cortex.

In addition, alpha activity at 8 to 9 cps was substantially *decreased* over the right occipital cortex. However, this decrease occurred only before those other trials that had then resulted in *non*insight solutions. This occipital decrease raises the interesting possibility that during some of the next phases, the preliminary local increase in right occipital *neuronal* activity might actually have been *interfering* with the subjects' preparations for insight processing.

Parallel Studies of the Readiness Interval Using fMRI

EEG waves respond quickly to a task. fMRI signals take longer to respond. Given this inherent time lag, researchers need to adjust the window chosen for their fMRI measurements. Its aperture must now monitor an interval slightly later than the one corresponding to the subjects' imminent "readiness" phase during the EEG portion of the study. The researchers then made two types of fMRI comparisons:

1. In the first, they collected the fMRI signals during those preparation intervals which led to successful *(insight)* solutions. They then contrasted these data with other signals collected during a (control) interval lasting the same length of time. The control interval chosen started 15 seconds after an *un*successful attempt. In this first comparison:

- Most brain areas showed *decreased* fMRI signals during the preparation period. However,
- Readiness was associated with *increased* fMRI signals in two *posterior* temporal lobe locations: the middle temporal gyrus and the superior temporal gyrus (L > R);
- Readiness also correlated with *increased* signals in the left anterior cingulate gyrus and posterior cingulate (BA 31) region. (It is reasonable to correlate this anterior cingulate increase in fMRI signals with some of the midfrontal *decrease* in alpha activity cited with respect to the EEG data in the section above.)

The increased *posterior temporal* activity is intriguing [ZBR:154–155]. It was observed over a wide area of both the middle and the superior temporal gyrus (BA 39, 37, 22; L > R). The authors interpreted this posterior temporal activation as consistent with bilaterally enhanced preparations for semantic processing. It was speculated that the greater increase on the *left* (allowing for the issue of lateralized linguistic competence) indicated the subjects' initial readiness for stronger (prepotent) contextual associations (the kinds that might later need to be modified or abandoned.) In contrast, the *right*-sided temporal activation was viewed as in keeping with a readiness to respond by generating initially weaker and looser contextual associations. As table 11 suggests, such earlier looser processing on the right side could still remain available to "network" with other data resources, and to do so in ways that could later prove useful in helping to supply the final correct solution.

The consistent increase in anterior cingulate activities *prior* to later insight solutions was noteworthy. It suggested that some functions (among the many now attributed to the anterior cingulate) had enhanced their subjects' readiness, directly or indirectly. These cingulate functions might include its contributions to (1) suppressing extraneous thoughts, (2) selecting initially relevant (prepotent) strategies, and (3) shifting responses subsequently toward a different strategy. To the degree that this anterior cingulate gyrus served as one resource for "top-down" control, it could also participate in the ways the two brain hemispheres were better prepared—*before* the task—to express their complementary functions insightfully.

2. The authors also made a second comparison. It contrasted the fMRI data from preparatory intervals that were followed by insight solutions with equivalent data from intervals that were followed by noninsight solutions.
   - Again, the higher signal levels that would correlate with (later) insight were already more evident in the *anterior* cingulate region (BA 32, 24).

- However, fMRI signals back in those same *posterior* parts of the cingulate cortex and temporal cortex (just cited above) tended to be at lower levels during *non*insight preparations than the higher levels they had reached during insight preparations.

What is the simplest interpretation of these last two lower levels of fMRI signals in the posterior cortex? It is that the posterior cingulate gyrus and the posterior temporal cortex were substantially *less active* (and thus not as well prepared) during those earlier intervals, and that their lesser activities then contributed to the failure of the subjects' to achieve an insight solution.

A Summary of the Major Recent Experimental Findings Thus Far in This Ongoing Story

- Immediately before testing occurs, the subjects find it advantageous to be prepared [ZBR:1].

- The anterior cingulate gyrus seems to play some kind(s) of an early role in insightful responses. Note, however, that several stressful task demands are being imposed: normal subjects are anticipating that their mental prowess will soon be rigorously tested by difficult word association tests.

- Subsequently, their lateral temporal regions are activated when they successfully process these challenging linguistic tasks. This complementary insightful effort involves the posterior, middle, and superior temporal gyrus on both sides of the brain;

- During insight types of word processing, the right posterior parieto-occipital region briefly shifts toward slower wave (alpha) EEG frequencies. This occurs just *before* the right superior temporal region briefly shifts toward faster (gamma) excitatory wave activities.

With regard to these last EEG data, alpha activities have always been especially difficult to interpret [ZBR:40–53]. However, the next section reviews recent research that divides alpha and gamma waveforms into slower and faster components. The two activities have different implications. Be aware that the different reports being discussed next may describe different EEG frequencies in a nonstandard manner.

Faster and Slower Alpha Rhythms, and the Way They Change during Different Phases of Ordinary Visual Perception

Recently, alpha rhythms were monitored during the earlier and later phases of a visuospatial perceptual task.[11] The subjects' task was to indicate that they had either seen, or missed seeing, a prior visual cue. When alpha rhythms were measured during that prelude *before* the stimulus arrived, the greater alpha increase occurred in the *slower* alpha band (described here as ranging from "6–10 cps"). This increase occurred in the frontal, parietal, and occipital association areas. This preliminary increase in the slower (alpha + theta) activity predicted how successful the subjects would be in later seeing the cue.

On the other hand, *during* the later portions of these same most successful trials, alpha power then *decreased* more in the *faster* alpha band (10 to 12 cps). These alpha decreases occurred in the lateral parietal (BA 39) and occipital (BA 19) areas [ZBR:111–112].

The authors cite evidence suggesting that the preparatory *increases* in the *slower* "alpha" band (measured here between 6 and 10 cps) are associated with more efficient global attention functions as the result of "a widely activated cortical-cortical network." However, during subsequent processing, when the *faster* alpha band frequencies (10 to 12 cps) are *decreased*, they are replaced in the cortex by beta and gamma oscillations. These steps occur later as the result of cortical-*subcortical* interactions, as discussed above. These changes are correlated with the ways we process other kinds of sensorimotor, semantic, and memory-related data as their messages rise toward consciousness.

Gamma Activations and Deactivations during Visual Perception and Higher-Level Processing

Lachaux and colleagues analyzed the data from intracranial EEG electrodes recording directly from their patients' brains.[12] When their patients' task was to detect faces, gamma band activities (40 to 200 cps) responded first in the occipito-temporal electrodes (recording from the fusiform face area), and next in parietal sites. However, parts of the primary visual cortex (BA 17) also *de*activated temporarily [ZBR:112]. Once again, this total pattern suggests that normal visual processing involves a *balance* that so integrates excitation with inhibition that gamma activations are synchronized in certain regions even while gamma *de*activations in others show *de*synchronization (as discussed in chapter 37).

Similar intracerebral EEG electrodes monitored other patients who were reading words. Transient gamma band suppressions occurred in the left ventro-lateral prefrontal cortex, 500 ms after the patients had attended to each stimulus event.[13] In related studies, it was shown that only those higher gamma frequencies—between 60 and 200 cps—served to differentiate their patients' higher *psychic* functions of attention and memory from those other more *somatic* functions involved in their intention to act (motor intention).[14]

Clearly, we respond during purely visual tasks with a sequence of intricate interactions. These tasks recruit our early vanguard functions of attention into vi-

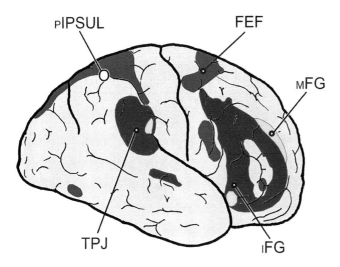

Plate 1   Lateral view of the right hemisphere
In this view, the frontal lobe is positioned on the viewer's right. The right hemisphere was chosen because the ventral ("bottom-up") subdivision of the attention system (shown in a shade of red) is distributed chiefly over the brain's right outer surface. In contrast, the dorsal ("top-down") subdivision (shown in blue) has an almost bilaterally symmetrical distribution. Both systems have only minimal medial representations (those of the ventral subdivision being represented superiorly only on the right side.) Note the two areas of overlap shown, in yellow, in the right inferior and middle frontal region. They may help coordinate the two subdivisions in ways that serve our global needs to pay attention to events on both sides of the environment.

Starting in the right frontal lobe: ɪFG, inferior frontal gyrus; ᴍFG, middle frontal gyrus; FEF, frontal eye field; ᴘIPSUL, posterior intraparietal sulcus; TPJ, temporoparietal junction (see similar distributions in figure 1). The unlabled red area in the temporal lobe is in a more anterior portion of the superior temporal sulcus (STS). The unlabled blue oval at the bottom left is in the posterior part of the middle temporal area (MTA). Its actual position is in the middle temporal gyrus, a site more superior than illustrations often suggest.

The topographical patterns represented here in schematic form are part of a larger attention network. Its fMRI signals not only increase quickly in response to conventional tasks, they also undergo slow spontaneous, coherent fluctuations of comparable amplitude. Accordingly, the figure is freely adapted both from the text and from figure 5 in M. Fox, M. Corbetta, A. Snyder, et al. Spontaneous neuronal activity distinguishes human dorsal and ventral attention systems. *Proceedings of the National Academy of Sciences U.S.A.* 2006; 103:10046–10051. See chapter 7.

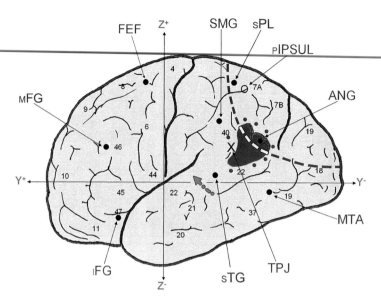

Plate 2 Directions of the two streams in a lateral view of the left hemisphere
The large red area is the *angular gyrus* (ANG) (and it includes the small circles around it). This represents the smallest of the three major cortical regions in which PET scans reveal high levels of metabolic activity even during conditions of passive rest. At right, the long, curved, red-and-white dashed line represents the general dorsal direction of the egocentric stream along the so-called *where?* pathway. The short green dashed and dotted line with a large arrowhead suggests the lateral branch of the lower allocentric stream. It rises up from below toward its representation in the *superior temporal gyrus* (sTG).

Starting at the left, in the frontal lobe: iFG, inferior frontal gyrus; MFG, middle frontal gyrus; FEF, frontal eye field; SMG, supramarginal gyrus; sPL, superior parietal lobule. pIPSUL, posterior intraparietal sulcus; MTA, middle temporal area; TPJ, temporal-parietal junction. sTG, superior temporal gyrus.

The thin, straight, crossing lines suggest the axes of the spatial coordinates. Y+ and Y− represent the opposite ends of an anteroposterior axis (from the front of the brain to the back). Z+ and Z− represent the opposite ends of a dorsal-ventral axis (top to bottom). The X and Y lines represent the kinds of standardized planes that researchers use to localize discrete brain sites in terms of their 3-D coordinates. The small numbers refer to Brodmann's areas (BA).

Plates 2 and 3 summarize schematically the nine PET scan reports condensed in the 2001 review by Gusnard and Raichle (chapter 15). These authors emphasize that the regions shown have a high active metabolism at rest that can be accurately measured with PET scans. Moreover, they are labile regions that can also become (1) *deactivated* when subjects perform overt tasks that demand outwardly oriented attention; (2) *more* activated when subjects perform Self-referential tasks under well-controlled conditions. See chapter 13.

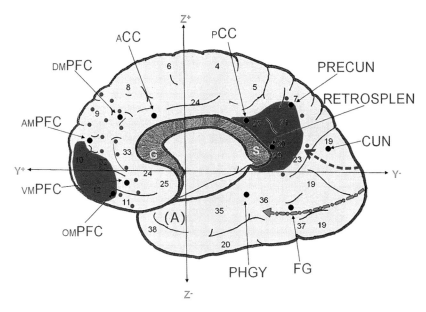

Plate 3   Directions of the two streams in a medial view of the right hemisphere
This view represents the inside surface of the *right* side of the brain. One large red area at the viewer's left (and its halo of small circles) occupies much of the medial prefrontal cortex. Here, normal subjects show high levels of metabolic activity in PET scans even under conditions of passive rest. At right, the red area represents the other major metabolic "hot spot." It lies deep in the parietal region and in front of the occipital lobe. This extensive region includes the *precuneus, retrosplenial cortex*, and the *posterior cingulate cortex*.

   The short, curved red dashed line suggests the medial course of the dorsal egocentric stream. Note, below, the longer, green arrowheaded, dashed *and* dotted line. This represents the major initial, ventral direction of the allocentric stream. It begins its medial course on the undersurface of the temporal lobe, along the lower, so-called *what?* pathway.

   Starting at the left, in the frontal lobe, are the four subdivisions of the medial prefrontal cortex, namely oMPFC, orbital medial prefrontal cortex; vMPFC, ventral medial; AMPFC, anterior medial; DMPFC, dorsal medial; ACC, anterior cingulate cortex; PCC, posterior cingulate cortex; PRECUN, precuneus; RETROSPLEN, retrosplenial cortex; CUN, cuneus; FG, fusiform gyrus; PHGY, parahippocampal gyrus. (A), the subcortical location of the amygdala.

   The gray curved area in the center is the corpus callosum. G refers to its genu; S refers to its splenium. Fibers crossing over in it enable this right hemisphere to play a predominant role in those merging functions which normally combine both to direct our attention into space and to represent individual objects out there. The lines of the vertical (Z+) and horizontal (Y−) axes are shown intersecting at their zero point, the anterior commissure. See chapter 13.

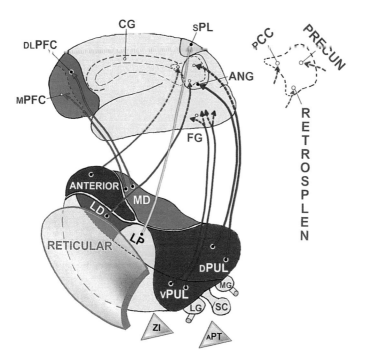

Plate 4   Thalamocortical contributions to the dorsal egocentric and ventral allocentric streams
This composite view shows the normal pathways leading from the thalamus up to the cortex. For convenience in viewing, only left-sided structures are shown. These connections rise up from the left thalamus to supply both the outside and inside of the left hemisphere. Pathways from the dorsal tier of nuclei predominate. Thus, at bottom right, one path leads from the *dorsal pulvinar* (DPUL) to the angular gyrus (ANG) on the *outer* cortical surface. A second path from this dorsal pulvinar leads up to the *precuneus* (PRECUN). Dashed lines indicate that this path projects to the *medial* parietal surface. Other projections from the *lateral posterior* (LP) nucleus supply the *superior parietal lobule* (sPL). These help to anchor each person's subliminal sensate impression of existing as a physically articulated Self-image.

In front, the *medial dorsal* (MD) thalamic nucleus projects to the prefrontal cortex, both to its outer, dorsolateral (DLPFC) and to its medial (MPFC) surfaces. The deep medial area in the back of the brain is shown enlarged at the top right. Here, two other adjacent dorsal nuclei of the limbic thalamus project to this medial surface (dashed lines). Thus, the *anterior nucleus* projects to the *posterior cingulate cortex* (PCC), and the *lateral dorsal nucleus* (LD) projects to the *retrosplenial cortex* (RETROSPLEN).

Note that relatively fewer pathways from the thalamus are shown serving the allocentric processing stream. However, messages from the *ventral pulvinar* (vPUL) are shown passing first through the region of the *fusiform gyrus* (FG) on the undersurface of the temporal lobe. These continue on their way forward through the other-referential pathways in the rest of the temporal lobe and on toward the superior temporal gyrus.

Three important inhibitory nuclei are shown, artificially detached, at the bottom. They are the *reticular nucleus*, the *zona incerta* (ZI), and the *anterior pretectal nucleus* (APT). Two relay nuclei of the thalamus are also shown at the bottom right. The *lateral geniculate nucleus* (LG) relays visual data to the occipital cortex. The *medial geniculate nucleus* (MG) relays auditory information to the auditory cortex. The *superior colliculus* (SC) in the midbrain relays its reflexive visual and related polymodal messages quickly through both the dorsal and ventral pulvinar to the cortex. Its counterpart, the inferior colliculus, plays a similar auditory role. See chapter 19.

sual information processing and advanced preparations for behavioral acts. Indeed, when MEG and fMRI monitoring are combined to study such sequential responses, their interrelationships turn out to be so complex that they resist being "grasped by naively using terms like 'activation,' or 'deactivation,' 'excitation' or 'inhibition.'"[14]

Acknowledging this caveat, suppose we would like to study the kind of everyday practical task that integrates not one, but *two* of our sensory avenues of information simultaneously. When subjects perform such dual tasks and recruit *both* visual *and* auditory modalities, it is their beta activities (at 13 to 30 cps) that correlate with faster reaction times over many regions of the cortex.[15] In these joint efforts, the frontal lobes can play an early subconscious executive role (chapter 4). Gamma responses (at 30 to 80 cps) develop early in the medial frontal regions before they become evident back in the occipital leads (at 60 to 120 cps).[16]

Commentary

Insightful problem solving is a dynamic, interactive process. Important during the immediate preparatory interval is the underlying "mental set" in the person's whole brain. Sensory association processing in the posterior regions expresses an intricate, rapidly changing sequence of thalamo ↔ cortical influences. The anterior part of the superior temporal gyrus appears to play a prominent role during the semantic processing of words. Gamma EEG activities in this large polymodal region are consistent with the way it acts to integrate meaningful higher-order semantic interpretations.

35

Alternative Ways to Study Ordinary Insight Using Neuroimaging Techniques

> Neuroimaging studies of insight should elicit restructuring, generate multiple insight events, provide accurate onset times, have the capacity for testing general and specific hypotheses, allow one to define meaningful reference states, and allow one to compare internally vs. externally triggered insights.
>
> Jing Luo and Guenther Knoblich

Insights strike suddenly. How can researchers design neuroimaging experiments to study such almost instantaneous sequences? Luo and Knoblich provide an excellent narrative review of this important topic.[1] This chapter samples some of their major points:

- When an external cue triggers an insight, the cue's arrival serves as a marker that makes it easier to follow the next sequence of events. However, when an insight is generated internally, spontaneously, it is difficult to detect time relationships.

- Each subject requires between 10 and 50 trials before sufficient data accumulate to draw conclusions from tests using event-related fMRI or event-related potentials (ERPs).

- *Restructuring* is the crucial process in insightful problem solving. Restructuring means making a big change in the deep structure of the original problem, not a superficial change.

In this regard, the authors describe some of their recent research (not yet published.) They began by presenting their subjects with *un*solvable brainteasers. (This situation is vaguely reminiscent of the plight facing Zen students who are given the unsolvable riddle of koan.) [ZBR:272–274]. Next, they provided these subjects with hints of different kinds. Only the first kind of hint provided a helpful clue, because it alone could trigger a deep structural change in the way the problem was represented. The second kind of hint might modify the way the problem was represented, but it could not yield a genuine restructuring solution. The third hint merely restated the way the problem was initially presented. fMRI monitored the subjects' response to each of the three kinds of hints.

The authors then contrast the fMRI results from the first hints with a stepwise sequence of other fMRI data. These data sets were obtained separately when their subjects were developing answers to other questions with which they were only distantly familiar. These comparisons suggested the following tentative conclusions:

- Genuine restructuring hints prompted activations in both the superior frontal gyrus (BA 8/6) and in the medial frontal gyrus (BA 8). In what way did these two lateral frontal regions appear to contribute to the solution? By helping to allocate more general kinds of top-down *executive attention toward the hints* themselves (chapter 4).

- Insightful restructuring does *not* change the way a person defines the initial spatial dimensions of the mental problem. Instead, insightful restructuring *re*-represents that problem during a later step, changing it during the final stages of problem solving.

- The anterior cingulate cortex is activated during insight problem solving. However, it is *not differentially* activated at the instant when the need arises to make a mental shift into a new response set. Incidentally, the left lateral prefrontal cortex is the region most sensitive to set shifting in the standard Wisconsin Card Sorting Task, not the anterior cingulate cortex. This lateral frontal region also becomes more activated when difficult solution cues require the person to consciously try harder.

- Brain imaging studies of insight are more difficult to conduct than are the standard behavioral studies of problem solving. Ordinary problem solving tasks, (say, of the kinds exemplified by the Wisconsin Card Sorting Task) are not appropriate as *specific* tests for insight sequences if neuroimaging techniques are being used to monitor the subjects' responses.

Results Using Ambiguous Sentences

Subsequently, the authors compared the results of fMRI monitoring during a series of different tests. In these tests, they presented their subjects visually with sentences that were either "easy" or "hard" to decode. An easy sentence was one that became meaningful as soon as it was read for the first time. An example: "The office was cool because the windows were closed." In contrast, no sentence in the hard category could be interpreted meaningfully after only one reading. (e.g.: "The haystack was important because the cloth ripped.")

A complete solution often hinged on whether an extra hint was supplied. (The authors called this a "cue.") Eight seconds later, such a cue could arrive. It could be a *confirming* cue (e.g., "air conditioned"). In this case, "air conditioned" simply confirmed the way the subjects had already interpreted the easy sentence above. Or, after an unsolved hard sentence, the next cue could be a *restructuring* cue. This restructuring cue was very different (e.g., "parachute" in the above example). The restructuring cue had the potential to remove all ambiguity from the earlier sentence, by an insightful stretch of creative imagination.

- Restructuring cues prompted unique responses. They *activated* the medial prefrontal gyrus and the left posterior middle temporal gyrus. They *deactivated* the posterior cingulate gyrus, the inferior and middle occipital gyrus on both sides, and the orbitofrontal gyrus. The authors chose to interpret the activation of the medial prefrontal gyrus as consistent with the detection of cognitive conflict. However, the activation in the left posterior temporal gyrus was viewed as consistent with a flexible interpretation of the problem.

- Unpublished data suggested that events crucially involved in restructuring could activate left-sided regions including the superior and middle prefrontal cortex and the posterior middle temporal gyrus.

- Many of the same brain regions that were activated during the major restructuring cue (e.g., "parachute") also responded to the lesser confirming type of cue (e.g., "air conditioned"). It seemed, at least in this single experiment, that "the generation of a new meaning during restructuring is achieved by a part of the brain network that is also involved in normal understanding."

- Multiple other task comparisons suggested that the anterior cingulate cortex serves as part of an early warning system. When activated, it signals that a cognitive conflict is being detected. While it notes the need for further attentional control, it does not appear to actualize the specific solution which proceeds to resolve the original problem.

- When subjects solve visual tasks involving Chinese ideograms, the lower-order functions of the visual cortex participate in an initial, tightly biased processing of the image's individual features. However, this elementary sequence is suppressed during the next regrouping. At this later time, a looser rearrangement develops, and the next higher-level functions of the visual association cortex now become more active. When these data are interpreted sequentially (along with the data showing that the occipital gyrus *deactivates* during restructuring cues), the results suggest that dynamic changes occur, *in both directions*, while visual processes continually evolve. These dynamic changes within cortical areas 17, 18, and 19 will be reflected in corresponding patterns and sequences of EEG activity during problem solving (similar interpretations were discussed in the previous chapter).

- When *external* cues are used to trigger the solution to different riddles and puzzles, the responses primarily activate the left hemisphere. Other research, based on words in the remote associates test, suggests that *internally* generated insights tend to activate networks lateralized more to the right hemisphere.

Commentary

The research on ordinary insight surveyed in these two chapters is of pioneering importance. The results are complementary. We notice that these experiments place subjects under artificial pressure to solve a particular problem within a limited time. These subjects are not idle. Harder problems prompt them to make wilder guesses, and premature biases can lead them astray. However, once the subjects are given some kind of clue, they can restructure the original problem, and proceed to realize a fresh solution.

The routine protocols followed during experimental tests of insight do not yet address the deep issues presented by so-called peak experiences. Three fundamental differences separate the current research situations from the extraordinary states of kensho-satori [ZBR:271–275].

- Kensho-satori shifts into a major alternate state of consciousness. Implicit in this dramatic "happening" is a huge physiological shift away from the conventional forms of Self-centered processing. None of the usual rules that govern conscious thought prompt a shift of such depth and scope. The shift is a sharp break with the past. No prior rational thought process had experienced, nor could imagination anticipate, such a novel reconfiguration of selfless consciousness.

- In the immediate afterglow of kensho-satori, the diminuitive *i* begins to appreciate how much experiential destructuring the *I-Me-Mine* had undergone during the previous moment [ZBR:339–341]. (see figure 7).

- Kensho-satori provides no linguistic solution comparable with the kind of conceptual literary "game" that words pose in a hard test sentence. Nor does it yield a permanent solution to the problem that it has just discovered. *Instead, it unveils the first genuine realization that the seeker is the source of his or her personal problem* (along with the realization of the way "all things really *are*"). After this brief resolution and definition of the problem of Self, the hard-slogging, day-to-day work of reconstruction can begin [ZBR:394–396]. From then on, mindful introspective attention can help to identify and resolve the residual issues that had overconditioned the emotional reactivities of the Self for so long.

36
Does Eliminating the Negative Help to Accentuate the Positive?

The art of being wise is the art of knowing what to overlook.

William James (1842–1910)

Vagal nerve stimulation can interfere with memory of negative information, an effect that may contribute to its antidepressant role.

H. Critchley and colleagues[1]

When normal people slide into a blue mood, they recall negative events more easily. During retreats, meditators commonly experience brief mood swings when negative thoughts intrude. In accord with Taoist ideas about balances inherent in Nature, it is reassuring to observe that these negative moods are normally impermanent, and one can bounce back from them into positive, upbeat moods.

Depressed patients are not so fortunate. Clinical observation suggests that their depression would lift if they could only let go of their abnormally strong tendency to recall negative thoughts. Suppose human beings could eliminate blue Mondays and banish all other dark thoughts. If our negative thoughts stopped, could that help tilt us toward a wiser, positive outlook? [ZBR:163–165, 239–247]. Maybe. If so, how?

Other things wander, not only thoughts. The term *vagus* means wandering, and it describes the meandering course pursued by the tenth cranial nerve (the vagus) on its course down each side of our neck, chest, and abdomen.

Recently, the U.S. Food and Drug Administration approved an unusual adjunct therapy: stimulation of the left vagus nerve to relieve severe, treatment-resistant depression. Most sensory fibers in this vagus nerve carry autonomic messages into the medulla that rise from our visceral organs. Even so, could such an obviously "bottom-up" mode of stimulation actually improve the rest of the brain in a severely depressed patient? The accounts that follow are cited solely as one sample of the provocative research questions now being asked. No data cited here or in chapter 51 are intended to prove that this vagal nerve approach cures all depression by exciting or inhibiting specific regions of the brain.

Critchley and colleagues report preliminary findings from one 48-year-old patient. In fact, his depression did improve during the 7 months after the vagus nerve stimulator was implanted in his neck. Still depressed (but now to a lesser degree), the patient was then monitored with fMRI while he was being stimulated intermittently. This stimulator was set to a routine cycle of 30 seconds "on," and 66 seconds "off." The *immediate* effect of this half-minute of left vagal stimulation seemed to be getting through to his frontal regions: fMRI signals increased slightly in the left dorsolateral and medial orbital frontal cortex.

Our discussion has emphasized the vital importance of inhibition, of *deactivation*, and of decreased fMRI signals. So, did stimulation also cause *decreases*? Yes. These decreases were sizable, and they occurred on *both* the right *and* left sides of the dorsal medial prefrontal cortex. Decreases also showed up in several regions elsewhere, but only on one or the other side.

Next, the patient was given the task of viewing—for 1 second—a list of random positive, negative, or neutral words. Notably, during the 66-second intervals when he received *no* stimulation, he still evidenced his usual robust undesirable tendency to encode and to remember the negative words. Moreover, during this same (unstimulated) phase while he was encoding these negative words, fMRI signals increased in his left insula, right anterior insula, right lingual gyrus, and frontal pole bilaterally.

However, it was only while the stimulator was turned "on" for 30 seconds, and while such negative words were being presented, that vagal stimulation *interfered selectively* with his initial encoding of this negatively valenced material. On these occasions, signal activity increased in his right orbital frontal cortex, right insula, left frontal pole, pons, and the ventral *medial* prefrontal cortex on both sides. Signals decreased in a portion of the left middle cingulate gyrus. Notably, vagal stimulation did not prevent the patient from remembering the other neutral and positive words that had been presented.

So what? The study points to delicate balances among multiple regions. Their patterns govern our moods, their overt expressions in our behavior, how well we remember negative events, and how efficient we are in reappraising them (chapter 23). Major interactions also govern the ways different regions of the frontal cortex influence their downstream connections in the limbic system (chapter 53). The authors' interpretations are appropriately tentative. They suggest that when left vagal stimulation enhanced the activity within *both* sides of the ventral *medial* prefrontal cortex, it was *interfering simultaneously* with the degree to which this patient was emotionally aroused by negative words. The authors postulated that this latter interference—involving the right insula and adjacent lateral regions of the orbital frontal cortex—created an offsetting influence that could have decreased the patient's abnormal tendencies to excessively encode and remember negative words. Reducing negative ruminations could tilt the net, long-term emotional balance in a more positive direction, thus lightening a patient's depression.

Nahas and colleagues monitored nine other severely depressed patients with fMRI.[2] Acute left vagal nerve stimulation generated more signals in the right insula of patients who were already more depressed. Yet, when the vagal stimulation was repeated chronically over a period of months, the patients whose depression improved were those who showed greater *de*activations in their ventral medial prefrontal cortex.

Other fMRI evidence points toward the ventral *medial* prefrontal cortex in patients who are severely depressed and unable to regulate negative moods.[3] The patients showed bilateral frontal activations when reappraising the content of negative affect, whereas their normal controls showed only increased left prefrontal signals. Moreover, the depressed patients did not normally engage their left ventro*lateral* prefrontal region when they tried to cope with their affective response by reinterpreting it. As a result, their less active ventral *medial* prefrontal cortex was unable effectively to inhibit the responses of their amygdala to negative stimuli (see chapter 53).

It is not easy to evaluate the different treatment options for severe, refractory depression. Any art in such discriminating wisdom may lie in deciding to overlook the easy option to lump all cases of depression together, and in shifting the focus instead to identifying which treatment works best for each subtype. Other recent studies have used fMRI to monitor the resting state functional connectivity of the brains in depressed patients (chapter 22). The results suggest that abnormal degrees of activity throughout a larger circuit is one guide to individualized therapy. Among its connections are links between the subgenual anterior cingulate

(BA 25), the thalamus, and the midline frontoparietal regions (the latter regions are part of the original, so-called default network)[4] (chapter 13).

Neuroimaging Correlates of Positive Psychological Well-Being

Well-being is a state involving many balanced options, not a single attribute. Drawing increasing research interest are the delicate, normal balances that regulate the interactions between different parts of our frontal lobes, anterior cingulate, and amygdala. The brain's innumerable reciprocal options often crowd very close together. For example, this area 25 just cited lies immediately below the most ventral extent of area 24 (figures 2, 5). It is in this ventral area 24 that people who report *high* levels of positive psychological well-being tend to show stronger fMRI signals when they respond to stimuli that are potentially aversive.[5] This activity translates into a positive outcome. Their buoyant personalities are less disturbed by the salient pressures of this negative information. They evaluate negative information more slowly than neutral information and respond to its valences with fewer signals in their amygdala on both sides.

The Role of the Anterior Cingulate Gyrus in Conflict Resolution

Sharp and colleagues studied 16 subjects whose ages ranged widely, from 37 to 83 years.[6] Greater anterior cingulate activity in their PET scans correlated with their greater skills in making accurate decisions during verbal tasks. Reduced anterior cingulate activities accompanied any general deficit in performance, but did not correlate with a person's calendar age.

Etkin and colleagues studied the responses of 29 healthy adults of both genders to happy or fearful facial expressions.[7] These standard faces were labeled with the words "Fear" or "Happy" in prominent red letters. Sometimes the word matched the valenced emotional expression; at other times, the faces and words were incongruent. The subjects' task was to push the correct response button that corresponded *only* with the actual emotion expressed on the face and to not be distracted by the words. Skin conductances were studied separately.

In general, during a variety of cognitive tasks, conflicting responses normally tend to activate two dorsal sites: the *dorsal* subdivision of the anterior cingulate and the *dorsal medial prefrontal* cortex that lies next to it. However, during this particular experimental paradigm for creating emotional conflict between faces and word labels:

- Increased fMRI signals in the *right amygdala* correlated with increased degrees of emotional conflict. Amygdala signals decreased when the conflict was resolved.

- Fearful and happy facial expressions activated the amygdala to the same degree.

- Greater emotional conflict increased signals in the dorsal *medial* and the dorso-*lateral* prefrontal cortex. These activations appeared consistent with the subjects making increased mental efforts to monitor the more difficult tasks.

- The *rostral anterior cingulate* was the only area in which signals increased during the *resolution* of conflicts. These activations were consistent with an *active process of conflict resolution*, not with how inherently easy the trial was. This rostral anterior cingulate activation was associated with *reduced* activities in the amygdala. Reduced skin conductance responses showed that the subjects had reduced transmissions between the amygdala and their sympathetic nervous system.

When viewed in the context of earlier studies, the data suggest that healthy subjects initially respond to threat with an unconscious activation of the amygdala. This early phase represents an adaptive, trait-related bias. However, this initial amygdala overresponsiveness can be suppressed by the rostral anterior cingulate gyrus, a suppression that is sensitive to the immediate environmental context. Notably, subjects also activate their rostral anterior cingulate gyrus when they calm their prior anxieties during the placebo response [ZBR:126–136].

Patients prone to develop severe symptoms of posttraumatic stress disorder (PTSD) tend to show less activation of their rostral anterior cingulate. This finding is interpretable as one index of their greater initial vulnerability to PTSD. In states of depression, lesser degrees of rostral anterior cingulate activity also predict the patient's poor response to subsequent antidepressant therapy. The authors draw this important conclusion: our capacity to recruit the rostral anterior cingulate helps determine how well we cope with the intrusion of negative emotional stimuli and negative emotional content.

Age and the Frontal Lobe

Grady and colleagues used fMRI to study 40 men while they performed various encoding and recognition tasks.[8] The subjects' ages ranged from the twenties to the mid-seventies. Older men displayed an interesting pattern of *decreased* fMRI signals: they showed relatively few of the expected task-induced decreases in their medial frontal and medial parietal regions. Instead, what they reduced during tasks were the fMRI signals in their *dorsolateral* prefrontal cortex. In younger age groups, this dorsolateral cortex usually shows a task-induced *increase*, interpretable then as evidence supporting a more efficient executive function in the frontal lobe. Therefore, this opposite pattern—a relative lack of *both* deactivation and activation—could help explain why irrelevant information proves more distracting to older subjects (and also why it could be to your advantage to learn to meditate when you are younger). Given how many times fMRI data have been cited in these pages, this seems an appropriate place to now sound a note of caution.

Caveat: MRI Signals in Themselves Do Not Suffice

Clinical neurology adheres to the dictum that we can interpret laboratory tests not in isolation, but only in the light of the patient's total clinical picture. The principle holds true in research. All neuroimaging data remain subject to interpretation. If structural MRI studies show a thicker cortex, this does not necessarily mean that more nerve cells reside there, and that they must all be more active. When a functional MRI scan shows a local increase in signals, one cannot necessarily conclude that only normal, healthy nerve cells are performing their normal local nerve cell functions [ZBR:188–189]. The aging brain illustrates many of these issues.

Recently, a subgroup of clinically normal adults was studied who carry the allele that places them at greater genetic risk for Alzheimer's disease. During tasks of explicit memory, many of these apparently healthy subjects already show unusually increased activations of their hippocampus and prefrontal cortex. Kircher and colleagues studied a separate group of subjects at risk, who at age 70 actually did have a mild degree of cognitive impairment.[9] At this slightly more advanced stage of dementia, their fMRI scans now showed increased activation not only in the medial temporal lobe but also in the region around the supramarginal gyrus in the inferior parietal lobule. During a longitudinal follow-up study, it was the group of subjects who earlier had shown the *most* activation of their right parahippocampal gyrus while they were encoding memories that went on during the next $2\frac{1}{2}$ years to develop substantial memory loss.

The evidence suggests that in the later decades, many normal older subjects tend to work harder to maintain seemingly normal levels of memory performance. At first, such a compensatory increase of activation is helpful. However, it may be followed later by a *decrease* in activation if structural brain degeneration supervenes and progresses, at which time a major decline in memory functions will become obvious.

The caveat when conducting longitudinal research on any subject, at any age, is that an accurate clinical history and a well-defined trajectory of functions on repeated mental status evaluations is required in order to interpret regional increases or decreases in fMRI scans and PET scans.

Implications for Kensho

The title of this chapter poses a critical question. With regard to mental balance, does eliminating the negative help accentuate the positive? Eliminating the negative does seem to help, but only after a complex sequence of interactions. During some of these steps, the rostral anterior cingulate appears to play an important role: it helps to adjust the balance among subtle emotional influences that are being mediated by the ventral medial and lateral frontal relays with the amygdala.

During a state of kensho, when all knotted legacies from the anxious past are cut off, the death of fear culminates in an impression of total deliverance [ZB:567–570, 611–613]. The studies of normal subjects by Sharp and Etkin and their colleagues are short-term experiments that underscore certain anterior cingulate functions. Because the cingulate gyrus is so complicated [ZBR:82–85], current interpretations of its roles in ordinary insights and kensho continue to be provisional.

Still, the question arises: During kensho, could impulses directed downstream from this rostral anterior cingulate gyrus suffice to extinguish—just in the amygdala—the emotional flames from the person's whole *lifetime* of primal and acquired fears? While extinction is a powerful function (chapter 53), this may be expecting too much of a cingulate → amygdala circuit per se.

Earlier, we observed that subdivisions of the anterior cingulate gyrus can be linked into networks serving attentional functions (chapter 4). Some parts of the cingulate's rostral, dorsal, ventral, and caudal regions could, therefore, be recruited to serve particular roles in attentional sequences. This category of functions could differ diametrically from those separate functional connections that the more *rostral* anterior cingulate gyrus maintains to support the Self/other role of its *medial* prefrontal and posterior cingulate neighbors (chapter 13). Our cingulate connections remain so heterogeneous[10] that no single mechanism seems likely to provide a simple explanation. In fact, some earlier studies suggested that the *dorsal* cingulate gyrus could be involved in monitoring cognitive conflict. The cited study by Etkin et al.[11] also correlated detectable degrees of emotional conflict with increased activities in the dorsal medial and dorsolateral prefrontal cortex on both right and left sides.

Therefore, it is time to update prior explanations for the impression in kensho that *all* cognitive and emotional conflict had vanished from the mental field. A plausible theory now needs to include the dissolution at several levels of the usual role that the cingulate normally plays in detecting psychic conflict in the first place. Therefore, this total dissolution of a sense of conflict could mean

- a loss of the (just cited) dorsal cingulate, medial prefrontal, and dorsolateral capacities to monitor and detect conflict;
- a reduction of the negatively biased messages from the orbitofrontal cortex. [ZB:254–255];
- a reduction in the inhibitory influence that the ventral medial prefrontal cortex has on the amygdala;

- a reduction of the resonances of fear in the amygdala and other limbic and para-limbic regions.

When we trace back these four potential mechanisms, we find that they converge on two limbic nuclei in the front part of the dorsal thalamus. Here, the anterior nucleus interacts with the cingulate gyrus, and the medial dorsal nucleus interacts with the prefrontal cortex. Both limbic nuclei can be inhibited by the GABA cap of the reticular nucleus. The resulting deactivation could contribute to the impression of an absolute death of fear during kensho (chapter 19).

37

Balancing One's Assets and Liabilities

If you think you can find one shortcut in Zen, you have already stuck your head in a bowl of glue.

Ch'an Master Ta-hui (1089–1163)[1]

In cultures constantly driven to consume, powerful limbic urges respond to the pull from attractive stimuli in the outside world. They fully engage our grasping behaviors, and take the upper hand. True, some kinds of frontal lobe function resist, and caution: "Don't get attached to alluring things out there in the environment." Yet many frontal lobe functions often don't seem to be listening. The result is a "functional imbalance," a recurrent theme in these pages.

The imbalance that causes most of our anguish is the powerful tilt toward Self-centered functions. This bias inclines us to undervalue other persons in our relationships, and it places increasingly in peril the resources in our natural environment. One optimal result of long-range meditative training is to arrive at a better balance between our Self-relational and other-relational leanings.

How does a normal brain learn to balance such habitual opposing inclinations? Looked at from the simplest physiological standpoint, its networks mesh two basic functions—excitation (+), and inhibition (−)—with a third mode of operation: *dis*inhibition. Disinhibition is the release of brain functions into an enhanced excitatory phase (+) as soon as prior inhibitory constraints (−) have been removed by inhibition (−). The term *disinhibition* can also be applied at the behavioral level. A patient who had a frontal lobe tumor provides a classic anecdote of the loss of social inhibitions. She saw the array of medical instruments in her doctor's office, could not resist the impulse to pick them up, and started using them to examine her startled neurologist.

Paradoxical Facilitation

In 1996, some neurologists might also have been surprised by its counterintuitive theme when Kapur's article first appeared. It contended that certain kinds of damage to the nervous system actually *facilitated* useful behavioral functions.[2] True, such paradoxical brain lesions are not common, and most of them restore functions barely toward normal. However, in a few instances, lesions can enhance functions to levels *above* normal.

Kapur examined some of the brain's dysfunctional imbalances between excitation and inhibition. He suggested that one remedy was to create "new sets of excitatory and inhibitory interactions." These were new pairings of *opposing* functions, new patterns that could shift the brain into a more optimal balance. Normal checks and balances are built into our hierarchy of brain functions at every level. This fact may enable lay readers to appreciate the basis for the following examples.

Artistic Talents Emerging in Adults Who Develop Frontotemporal Dementia

In 1988, Bruce Miller and colleagues graced their article with a form of documentation not seen often enough in a neurological journal. Their array of three paintings and one photograph confirmed the unusual visual skills of a few patients who were still in the *early* stages of a particular kind of dementia.[3] As chapter 28 points out, it is a disorder distinct from Alzheimer's dementia, called frontotemporal dementia (FTD), and it accounts for perhaps one quarter of the various presenile dementias.

In many FTD patients, the frontal and temporal lobe degeneration is bilateral. In one subtype, however, the atrophy shrinks the anterior temporal and basal frontal lobes, yet spares the dorsolateral frontal regions. The patients in this report were but a small sample selected from the authors' total of 69 frontotemporal dementia patients. However, these five patients' diverse visual talents were intriguing, not only because the visual abilities emerged *early* in the course of their illness but also for these other reasons:

- Their artistic impulses were expressed solely in the visual domain, never in the verbal domain.

- While they painted, the patients were recalling visual images that they reconstructed into the pictures. Word thoughts were not an intermediary step.

- Reality was the theme. Their paintings, photographs, and sculptures were *realistic* copies (lacking the kinds of abstract or symbolic content our culture associates with creativity).

- As their disease progressed, the patients became increasingly interested in the fine details of faces, objects, shapes, and sounds.

- Their visual preoccupations inclined them to be perfectionistic, and to a degree that enhanced the quality of their art.

Four of the five patients had the temporal lobe variant of frontotemporal dementia. These patients showed a "selective degeneration of the anterior temporal and orbital-frontal cortex." In contrast, two other important regions were relatively spared: first, the dorsal lateral prefrontal cortex; second, the *right* hemisphere. Note how this particular pattern enabled the innate artistic talents of the right side of the patients' brains to be preserved. The result, in the authors' words, was "an unexpected window into the artistic process."

Peering through this window at their patients' unique pattern of assets and liabilities, what did the authors see? A rare condition, one that caused a "decreased inhibition of the more posteriorly located visual systems involved with perception, thereby enhancing these patients' artistic interest and abilities." In short, the patients' condition illustrated the principle of disinhibition: The decrease of the normal inhibitory tone from their orbitofrontal and anterior temporal regions had released visual perceptive capacities farther back in their brain.

Artistic Talents in Certain Young Autistic Savants

Miller is also a coauthor in a recent paper that reviews a completely different category of disease. In this disorder of brain *development*, six young autistic savants display unusual artistic talent.[4] The unusual features of their artwork were somewhat similar to those of the FTD patients whose symptoms started much later in adult life. Among the similarities: a heightened attention to visual detail, compulsive ritualistic repetition, capacities to focus on one topic to the exclusion of other interests, and intact memory and visuospatial skills. The authors suggested that some aspects of their savants' clinical pattern might be attributable to a particular pattern of imbalance. It had caused (1) enhanced functions within the posterior neocortex, and (2) a predominance of *right* temporal lobe functions, the result of the savants having sustained a greater *loss* of left temporal lobe functions.

A recent survey reviews the general topic of why some autistic patients show enhanced perceptual functioning.[5] The article also concludes that enhanced perceptions arise in the course of an imbalance. When certain regions "overfunction" and others dysfunction, the resulting pattern includes this mixture of unusual assets and liabilities:

- Visual and auditory perception remains locally oriented.
- Low-level discriminations are enhanced.

- Complex visual tasks employ a more posterior network.

- The perception of simpler, first-order stationary stimuli is enhanced.

- The perception of complex movements is diminished.

- Information processing at a lower level remains relatively independent of higher-order operations.[6]

This pattern might begin to sound familiar. However, neither frontotemporal dementia patients nor autistic savants possess the many skills required for multiple genuinely creative insights or for episodes of insight-wisdom. Yet the reports that certain patients show distinctive artistic abilities help us to frame key questions. Further research needs to answer such questions as: Do such skills represent (1) overfunctions of certain posterior regions? (2) relative imbalances between and among the two pairs of temporal and parietal lobes? (3) certain kinds of decreased inhibition from parts of the prefrontal and anterior temporal cortex? The ultimate documentation of answers could help explain how some related functions arise in extraordinary states that transform the meditative path, and which skills enter fruitfully into creative problem solving in general.

Why Do We Get Stuck in the Matchstick Task?

Chapter 25 introduced the general topic of insight and emphasized its abrupt onset. Our first step in finding a fresh solution is to get "unstuck" from the way we had initially viewed the problem. One kind of problem-solving task uses ordinary matchsticks to construct virtual Roman numerals (e.g., I, II, IV).[7] The same task also uses matchsticks to represent two possible modes of operation $(+, -)$ as well as to represent an equals sign $(=)$. One version of the task arranges the matchsticks in combinations that represent a *false* arithmetic statement. The subject is then instructed as follows: move only *one* stick, from one position to another, so that you transform this false statement into a true statement.

Try an easy example of such a transformation. This equation is false:

$$VI = VII + I.$$

However, by moving only one match, you can convert it into a true statement: $VII = VI + I.$

Most normal subjects find the next false equation much more difficult:

$$XI = III + III.$$

Everyone gets stuck in the Roman numeral X. Why is it so hard to think outside the box and discover the answer: $VI = III + III$? Because we're conditioned to retain the original X as a tight construct. We're attached to the rigid notion that X is a whole "chunk." Once crossed in the middle, those lines seem to have a power of their own to stay crossed. It's hard to disengage from this fixation and simply shift the crossed matchstick down slightly to yield a V.

Researchers have used various matchstick tests to study patients who finally solve certain kinds of problems by insight.[8] Reverberi and colleagues began with a counterintuitive prediction. They predicted that focal damage to the lateral prefrontal cortex might actually enable some patients to perform *better* than normal controls in solving the most difficult types of matchstick tasks.[9] They allotted all subjects three minutes in which to solve each problem. Seventeen of the patients had relatively large lateral frontal lobe lesions, often bilateral. Eighteen other patients had large medial, orbital, or bilateral frontal lesions next to the midline. Cues of various types were given at various times.

The matchstick tests were rigorous. Among the 23 healthy controls, only ten (43%) managed to solve the most difficult matchstick problems. In contrast, 82% of the patients who had *lateral* frontal lobe deficits could solve the most difficult problems. Patients who had medial lesions were no more successful in solving the matchstick tests than were their controls. The conventional wisdom is that the dorsolateral frontal lobe contributes much to our intelligence. If its functions are lost, how might these strange results be explained?

The patients who had lateral frontal lobe damage showed an unusual *pattern* of potential assets and liabilities. Their wide open attitude *didn't prejudge* whether a new strategy would work. *It didn't know.* It was too simple-minded to block them from exploring a wide range of potential responses. They faced each new problem with a naive, trial-and-error approach. Knowing no answer, they were free to try anything. The authors provide the necessary cautionary note. In "real-life" situations, we direct our intelligence skillfully, reducing problems to tractable size by eliminating unlikely items. If this preliminary selection process fails, our behavior becomes highly inefficient and disorganized.[10]

The results are noteworthy for two reasons: (1) they provide intriguing parallels with the way expert jazz pianists *deactivate* the dorsolateral prefrontal cortex when they are improvising;[11] (2) they have interesting parallels with the clear non-thinking "don't know mind" that echoes down through the centuries in the teachings of Socrates, Bodhidharma, and of the later schools of Zen.[12]

Evidence That a Parietal Lobe Imbalance Contributes to Left-Sided Visual Neglect

Attentional imbalances can involve the parietal lobes. These imbalances become important to the explanation for the late epiphenomena that entered briefly during the diminuendo of kensho [ZBR:429–431, 546, chapter 96, note 13]. In 2005, Corbetta and colleagues presented preliminary fMRI data of an abnormal functional imbalance that had disabled attention.[13] Their 11 stroke patients all had *right*-sided infarctions and showed left-sided visuospatial neglect. Note that these lesions had damaged *ventral* structures: the superior temporal gyrus, frontal operculum, and insula. However, no direct damage had involved the top-down, attention-generating *dorsal* system higher up in their right or left parietal lobe, and their posterior intraparietal sulcus (pIPSUL) was spared (figures 1, 3).

The fMRI activity referable to this dorsal parietal region was the point of interest. Its signals were always stronger on the *left* side of the brain, both in relative and absolute terms, acutely and chronically. This left dorsal *hyper*activity had created an abnormal "top-down bias." How was this hyperactive imbalance manifested clinically? It directed the patients' attention off toward the *right* side of their environment. "Stuck" in the glue of events over on that right side of their external world, the patients couldn't *disengage* attention from items on this right side and redirect its focus to explore locations in their left visual fields.

The Prefrontal Cortex Helps Resolve Ambiguities

The earlier discussion in chapter 34 emphasized that our normal right hemisphere is ready to be activated by information that might first seem tangential. Goel and colleagues wondered: when patients try to make simple inferences, do right or left prefrontal lesions cause different problems?[14] Focal lesions damaged the *right* prefrontal cortex in one group of nine patients. The lesions involved the *left* prefrontal cortex in nine others. Twenty-two normal subjects, matched for age and education, served as controls. Only some of the inference tasks provided all the facts sufficient to reach a logical conclusion. Uncertainty prevailed in the others.

Damage to the *left* prefrontal cortex caused the most impairment among those patients who were provided with all the facts. In contrast, the patients who had damaged the *right* prefrontal cortex were selectively impaired when their inferences had to be based on *incomplete* information. The findings confirm that this right prefrontal cortex plays a critical role in helping us arrive at a closure when we don't yet have all the facts (tables 10 and 11). To the degree that the looser mental representations of our right hemisphere remain more flexible, they can balance the tendency of their left-sided partner to lock into tight premature conclusions.

Commentary

Yin and yang are in balance. No one is being advised to dispense with all of their frontal, temporal, or parietal lobe functions simply to enable their occipital lobes to "see more clearly" [ZB:257–259]. The intent rather is to prepare the groundwork for the next topics. In part V, the plan will be to clarify how the self-less insight-wisdom of kensho seems to draw *selectively* on patterns of exquisitely time-related sequences. These sequences involve only certain of the frontal lobes' executive and organizational capacities (table 3), only certain of the temporal lobes' allocentric capacities (table 6), and only some of the ways that other interactions of a whole brain help us process extrapersonal space (table 7) [ZBR:426–431]. In fact, the forms of excitation, inhibition, and disinhibition just discussed can be observed to reappear during successive waves of activation and deactivation as they sculpture the dynamic contours of kensho.

38

Fourth Mondo

> All is empty, clear, revealed effortlessly, naturally. Neither thinking nor imagination can ever reach this state.
>
> Master Seng-ts'an (d. 606 C.E.)

For purposes of this discussion, are you regarding intuition in the general category of cognition, and viewing insight as a form of intuition?

Yes.

What parts of the normal temporal lobe show increased fMRI signals when subjects realize that separated film clips fall into a visually coherent, meaningful sequence?

The right middle and posterior superior temporal cortex.

What parts of the normal temporal lobe show increased fMRI signals when the "mind's eye" represents visual images, and then makes meaningful associations between visual concepts?

The right fusiform gyrus on the undersurface near the temporo-occipital junction.

Why does a book about Zen Buddhism discuss patients who have visual or auditory agnosia?

Because meaning is experienced so naturally that we forget it must arise in the brain. The patients remind us that discrete damage to the temporal lobe causes visual and auditory stimuli to lose their meaning. It's useful to turn around such negative losses of meaning. It helps us consider how we might experience an enhanced version of their opposite, positive counterparts. Doing so helps envision the way some unusually *enhanced* functions within the temporal lobe could infuse the allocentric field of consciousness with extra resonances of meaning during kensho.

What do neuroimaging and EEG techniques reveal about how ordinary insight solves word association problems?

fMRI signals increase in the anterior and superior part of the right temporal region during insight solutions, in association with a localized burst of gamma EEG activity.

The more prepared the subjects were to solve problems by insight, the higher were their initial levels of fMRI signals in the posterior temporal region and in the anterior cingulate gyrus (L > R). More sophisticated MEG studies are required to interpret the complex changes in brain wave activities that unfold during the dynamic sequences of insight solutions.

What do neuroimaging and EEG techniques reveal about how ordinary insight solves difficult riddles with the aid of word hints?

Some activations of the anterior cingulate gyrus occur relatively early, signaling that cognitive difficulty is being detected. Increased responses in the superior and medial frontal gyrus are associated with the hints that go deeper, helping both to restructure a hard riddle and to sponsor its solution. Two opposite kinds of fMRI responses correlate with paying more "executive" attention to the word hints themselves. (1) activations occur in the medial prefrontal gyrus and in the posterior part of the left middle temporal gyrus, and (2) deactivations occur in the posterior cingulate gyrus, the occipital region, and in the orbitofrontal gyrus.

Does this evidence indicate that insight is a light bulb that illuminates the whole brain?

No. The data suggest that sequences of excitatory and inhibitory events unfold, sequentially, in different parts of the brain. These changes reflect the particular experimental conditions of the task system that the researchers have set up to test for insight.

Do normal precedents exist for kensho's shift into selfless insight?

Yes. Sometimes, ordinary moments of insight seem to be experienced almost anonymously.

What is the significance of the evidence that temporal lobe sites predominate during the processing of various kinds of meaningful inferences and ordinary insights?

It suggests that the brain is now placing more emphasis on other-referential attentional and processing functions, and less emphasis on pathways that are Self-referential. Moreover, comparable intrinsic shifts normally recur *slowly* in Self/other networks during passive resting conditions. In fMRI scans, these slow background cycles are manifest only several times a minute. They take the form of spontaneously fluctuating, coherent signals. Once again, when the more medial, Self-referential network is *de*activated, the lateral other-referential attentional network is simultaneously activated. These endogenous seesaw tiltings point to a slow subtle, recurrent functional antithesis. Organized normally from deeper levels, it is poised to shift these opposing networks in a reciprocal manner.

Are you again suggesting that when a major imbalance toward selflessness suddenly occurs in kensho this shift could follow a pattern similar to the kinds of normal tiltings that recur slowly and spontaneously?

Yes. Moreover, a potential fulcrum exists at the interface between the dorsal and ventral nuclei of the thalamus that can become the basis for such leveraged shifts toward selflessness and insightful processing.

Is kensho, then, "nothing special?" Or is it a "special" kind of insight?

On these pages, the answer is "yes" to both questions, depending on which perspective you prefer to use to interpret the evidence.

What does the phrase, selfless insight, mean in terms of functional anatomy?

Selfless implies that the dorsal parietofrontal pathways of the action-oriented Self are deactivated. This contributes to the dissolution of the personal sense of the *I-Me-Mine*. Insight implies that the ventral, temporofrontal, other-referential pathways are liberated into seeing all things as THEY really are. Both phenomena occur simultaneously.

Is Zen anti-intellectual?

Only to the degree that too much thinking interferes with becoming insightful.

What good is a koan?

It is an enigmatic statement, resolvable by insight. Among its multiple uses, it creates an ongoing climate of questioning and uncertainty during the long, mindful introspective quest before a novel stimulus occurs.

Part V

On the Path toward Insight-Wisdom

A perception, sudden as blinking, that subject and object are one, will lead to a deeply mysterious wordless understanding; and by this understanding will you awaken to the truth of Zen.

Zen Master Huang-po (d. 850)

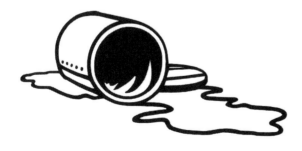

The Broken Water Bucket

Insight requires multiple analogies to illuminate its multifaceted nature.... A single metaphor may shine a spotlight, whereas many metaphors can light up the stage.

Schooler, Fallshore, and Fiore[1]

Only the person whose bucket's bottom has fallen out will be completely convinced.

Master Hongzhi Zhengjue (1091–1157)[2]

Ordinary insight is not a simple topic. Scholars invoked at least ten widely different analogies in a recent book that tried to describe what ordinary insight really is.[3] In trying to describe kensho, could one lost chord or other metaphor ever convey how much more *extra*ordinary is its flash of insight-*wisdom*?

For me, an old Japanese story about a broken water bucket can serve as an illuminating metaphor for kensho's emptiness of Self [ZB:453]. It relates the experience of a young widow, Chiyono (1223–1298).[4] In her training as a nun she was fortunate to have access to Master Wu-hsueh Tsu-yuan (1226–1286). After this Chinese master came to Japan, he later went on to found the famous Rinzai Zen temple, Engakuji, in Kamakura.

Chiyono's awakening was long-sought and elusive. At last, one moonlit night, she filled her old water bucket from a well (a well that centuries later would still bear her name). As she walked away, she saw the full moon reflected on the surface of the water. As she continued along the path, the circular bamboo strip gave way that had held together the staves of her bucket. Instantly, the bottom broke through, the moon's reflection vanished, the bucket disintegrated, and all its water drained into the soil beneath. At this moment, Chiyono experienced a sudden, penetrating flash of insight-wisdom.

She later explained it this way: "I had hoped the weak bamboo binding would hold the water bucket together. But suddenly the bottom fell out of the bucket: no more water. No more moon in the water. Emptiness in my hand!" Sometimes, in response to such an abrupt triggering sensory stimulus, the person's prior mental sets give way. All biased mental boundaries dissolve. The result of this melting undifferentiation is a total *emptiness of self*. A sudden proprioceptive surprise provides an especially effective jolt [ZB:413–414].

Chiyono then went on to complete her Buddhist training, became the first female Zen master authorized to teach in Japan, and was known thereafter as the Abbess Mugai-Nyodai. In her seventies, she was chosen to be the subject of an unusually realistic portrait statue. The carving is still venerated as an "important cultural treasure" in a Kyoto convent. Subsequently, Chiyono's episode of awakening was memorialized in a wood block print. In this, we see her portrayed beneath the full moon that still illuminates the wet earth on which rests her broken bucket. Ripe persimmons hang on nearby branches, symbolizing the long time it takes before one's practice ripens into such an awakened state. In the annals of Zen, Chiyono's story of way the moon shines on water is one of many examples that link moon metaphors and visual symbols with the emptiness of enlightenment [ZBR:432–447, 459–463].

Recently, I stumbled across an even earlier incident in which a water bucket had spilled. This happened in China, again in the context of sudden enlightenment. Tianyi Yihuai (993–1064) was a young Ch'an monk in the Yunmen school. He had fetched water from a well and was using a shoulder pole to carry the water bucket back to his temple. Suddenly, the pole broke and the water bucket crashed to the ground, triggering Tianyi's abrupt enlightenment. He too later became a Ch'an master.[5]

The two narratives suggest that the extraordinary breakthroughs into existential insight-wisdom that characterize kensho are different from our ordinary kinds of simple insight. Schooler and colleagues had posed three basic questions relating to these former *ordinary* kinds of simple insight[6]:

- What causes the early impasse, the fixation that keeps us locked inside a kind of box that resists a solution?
- What happens later, the key event that enables us to overcome this impasse?
- Having overcome the prior impasse, which specific mechanisms lead on to the sudden solution?

In this book, part IV has just considered answers to the first three questions about ordinary insight. Discussions elsewhere also addressed other aspects related to these important issues [ZB:636–677, 683–695; ZBR:394–401]. As we now turn to examine the form and content of *extraordinary* flashes of insight, we will need to pose at least two additional psychophysiological questions:

- What kinds of brief psychological changes transform the person's prior traits of character?
- What kinds of physiological changes in the brain generate the major, ongoing transformations of the person's thoughts, emotions, attitudes, and behavior?

With this preamble, the next two parts explore a series of overlapping answers at different levels to these last two questions. Part V focuses more on the kinds of attitudinal changes associated with insight-wisdom. Part VI will focus more on how the meditative path contributes to the boyancy and maturation of one's emotional life.

40

The Construction and Dissolution of Time

> Time is the number of motion . . .
>
> Aristotle (384–322 B.C.E.)

The Dissolution of Time in Kensho

All concepts of time dropped out during the taste of kensho. The mental metronome stopped ticking. The anonymous mental field experienced this total vacancy of personal "time" as an open-ended eternity. A descriptive term, *achronia*, directs attention to this gaping chasm in ongoing experience, devoid of time [ZBR:378–383]. The phrase no-self, or *anatta*, serves a similar purpose when it attempts to describe the emptiness that lacks all concepts of the *I-Me-Mine*.

Frontal Lobe Contributions to Our Normal Sense of Time

Areas at the base of the frontal lobe are among the regions that contribute to our normal autobiographical timeline.[1] Tranel and Jones compared the mental performance of seven patients who had damage in this basal forebrain region with that of 19 other patients. Eleven of these other patients had the damage in the medial temporal lobe [ZBR:412–413], and the damage in the other eight patients was elsewhere in the brain. Eighteen normals served as controls. All subjects took on the same task: lay out a year-by-year, decade-by-decade timeline of the personal events in your own life.

This task is not as artificial as it might first seem. We have each embroidered and rehearsed a fictional curriculum vitae. We polish this narrative and keep it available online to inform others. (We even bend the ear of complete strangers that we chance to meet at a party, or while traveling). We document in detail not only how many obstacles we had faced growing up but (with due modesty) how our efforts had prevailed (in spite of deep snow, et cetera, et cetera).

The patients with basal forebrain damage had the most problems with this long-term narrative task. Their timelines misplaced personal events by more than 5 years. Yes, they could remember events, but they did not know precisely *when* these events had occurred. Their most distinctive loss was in one particular aspect of *long-term* timing. It can be described as "knowing *when*, based on *years*." However, both they and the other patients whose medial temporal lobes were damaged had similar problems when they tried to retrieve other factual details about events buried in their autobiographical memories. Both groups, in short, couldn't recall other kinds of information that fell into a "knowing *what* happened" category.

Centered in this same region of the basal forebrain is its largest cholinergic nucleus: the basal nucleus of Meynert [ZB:164–169]. This major nucleus is part of the upper cluster of acetylcholine nerve cells that supplies this fast neurotransmitter to many cortical regions. Moreover, the basal forebrain carries on an extensive two-way dialogue with limbic regions. This helps to account for some of the patients' inaccuracies when they tried to reconstruct an orderly chronology of events along the timelines of their life stories.

Damage to the basal forebrain could deprive patients of the acetylcholine and related messenger systems they need to retrieve memories. Future studies could profitably examine whether some of the demented patients' timing, sequencing, and other memory deficits could respond to newer drugs that enhance cognitive functions.[2]

Many top-down contributions from the prefrontal lobes themselves contribute to the strategies we normally use to organize the timing of events that we sequence in our recent memory [ZB:557–567]. Moreover, PET scans show that we normally activate the rostral prefrontal cortex of BA 10 during tasks that require us to project timed sequences into the future (prospective memory).[3]

Right Parietal Lobe Contributions to Processing Short Intervals of Time: A "When?" Pathway

Our *acute* timing functions fall into a category different from the narrative kinds first described above. Our sense that time is ongoing right *now*—"*this* present time"—is contingent on short-term chronometer-like functions that monitor immediate cause-and-effect sequences. Such acute timing reflects a "knowing *when*, based on *seconds or less*," that serves in the background as an index of action. Indeed, it was clear to Aristotle that time was a metric of motion. We infer time sequences from the elapsed distances that things cover when they are in motion. Several recent lines of evidence suggest that such short-term timing functions enlist parts of our *right* inferior parietal lobule in their larger network.[4]

Battelli and colleagues review the functional anatomy of the same dorsal and ventral systems of attention that were first introduced in chapter 7 and summarized there in table 4. They then propose that the inferior parietal lobule on the *right side* takes on an additional role: a *specialized, bilateral metric function* [ZBR:373–374]. In particular, this *right* side appears to attend to the timing of visual relationships that arise within *both* the right and left sides of the environment.

Talented, multimodal nerve cells are disposed throughout this entire inferior parietal lobule. Their properties enable this region to co-represent environmental details in both space and time simultaneously [ZBR:374]. As one example, when we apply to language the symbolic decoding functions of this inferior lobule, they help us parse sentences effortlessly into their components, and easily discern syntactical relationships, even when their items are out of order [ZBR:149].

When transcranial magnetic stimulation (TMS) is briefly applied, it can disable a subject's right posterosuperior temporal region (figure 1). This causes a momentary block of the information that is normally relayed between the motion-and-depth-perception sensitivities down in the middle temporal area (the MTA; V5) (figure 1) and regions higher in the right inferior parietal lobule [ZBR:428–429]. The result is that the subject is briefly unable to discriminate the motions of living things. The TMS blockade has disorganized the local circuits normally used to confer both an orderly sense of structure to the timing of events and the impression that events are progressing as they unfold during the earlier milliseconds of mental processing.

Implications for Kensho

Our physical sense of Self serves as the standard axis of reference both for this normal impression that other things are moving out there, and that other things occupy a certain space at a particular distance away from us. The MTA plays a prominent role in coding for such Self-relational constructs when they arise along the dorsal egocentric pathway. Deactivation of the MTA as it joins the egocentric pathway could contribute to the reasons why kensho leaves the impression of static *non*movement.

Our usual "arrow of time" flies in one direction:

past → present → future

However, in kensho, time lacks movement. It has nowhere to "go." No arrows remain in no-time.

The inferior parietal lobule is on the lateral surface of the cortex (figure 4). Even so, its angular gyrus is one of the essential and metabolically active contributors to our normal resting Self-centered network. During kensho's major shift away from all such Self-relational processing, some metric functions of this right-sided so-called "when" pathway could share in the same deactivations that black the functions of the *medial* frontoparietal networks. The resulting short-term deficit in estimating time could contribute to the several reasons why kensho seems to drop out all arrows of time.

You might think that during such a moment of achronia, no mental capacity would remain that could still notice the fact of an arrowless interval of stasis. Yet, this curious vacancy-stasis did arise during the anonymous taste of kensho (although the vacancy was noticeable in memory only in retrospect). In the Japanese Buddhist descriptions of kensho-satori, one finds the term *fusho fumetsu*. Its sense of nonarising, nonperishing hints at the static quality within such a matrix of no-time [ZBR:360–361]. Perhaps this was one of the impressions Ch'an Master Huang-po might have been referring to obliquely when he spoke of "the Gateway of the Stillness beyond all Activity" [ZB:367].

Self-Other Discriminations in the Right Inferior Parietal Lobule

Uddin and colleagues report recent evidence confirming a greater right-sided role in Self/other judgments for a region around the right TPJ and the adjacent inferior parietal lobule.[5] Their subjects' first task was to discriminate pictures of their own faces from faces of other familiar persons. Then the investigators applied repetitive transcranial magnetic stimulation (TMS). In this experiment, they directed it to disrupt the normal functions of the right inferior parietal lobule. TMS to this right-side did disrupt the subjects' abilities to discriminate Self vs. other in this recognition task. In contrast, TMS directed to the subjects' left inferior parietal lobule did not.

To the degree that symbolic functions are deactivated more in the right angular gyrus and right medial regions during kensho and satori, then the results of their dissolution could be reflected in the greater depth of the phenomena of emptiness [ZBR:149, 204–205].

Commentary

The research cited could help account for some of the loss of both time and Self when functions are deactivated within the large right Self-referential network. Maximal degrees of deactivations in parietal and frontal regions on both sides, while still asymmetrical (R > L), might be invoked to explain the relatively greater depth of emptiness during satori.

The states of kensho and satori are brief, yet each state has the potential to transform personality traits thereafter. During the remainder of part V, before discussing how such sudden or gradual changes could transform a person's underlying attitudes, we need pause and inquire: why would anyone view such changes as manifestations consistent with "wisdom?"

Aspects of Wisdom

> Wisdom is the principal thing; therefore get wisdom: and with all thy getting get understanding.
>
> Proverbs 4:7

> Confucius barred four words from being used: No "shalls," no "musts," no "certainly's," no "I's."
>
> Analects of Confucius (551–479 B.C.E.)

Insight-Wisdom

Ancient philosophers, shrewd judges of character, knew that some positive human attributes could be carried too far. In the Buddhist context, insight-wisdom refers to the nature of insights manifest during a sudden, profound, existential "awakening." In one sense, such enlightened states of awakening might resemble the refreshing clarity that we experience normally after a good night's sleep, in that they express innate physiological capacities that everyone shares.

However, we associate the acute state of extraordinary enlightenment with its exemplar, Siddhartha Gautama (563–483 B.C.E.). Statues often show him in a sitting posture, in deep meditation. Less often recalled is another fact: Siddhartha had been on a rigorous, formative, 6-year-long spiritual quest before this sudden supremely enlightened peak experience occurred under a Bodhi tree. Only in the decades thereafter would he be known as the Buddha, meaning the "awakened one."

Such an acute state is sometimes viewed as a "spiritual illumination." It mobilizes the generic processes of intuition and ordinary insight, takes them to a novel, existential domain. Whatever descriptive words one uses, the resulting state is distinctive in form and content. One list that only partially defines its special qualities of insight-wisdom already includes 18 entries [ZB:542–544]. Further word descriptions can be added [ZBR:333–361], yet the central ingredients of this brief state remain beyond language, because they plumb the physiological coding of consciousness at the very core of the brain [ZB:627–632].

In general, the earlier Sanskrit term *prajna* refers to the sudden, flashing quality of the mental illumination that strikes during states of enlightenment. In the Zen Buddhist school that eventually flourished in Japan, *kensho* has come to refer to a substantial, but initial, state of awakening. *Satori* refers to more advanced states of transformation. The pivotal acute insights express an inherent potential to transform a person's subsequent behavior. Only when this potential is fully realized in the course of much further training does it lead to a profound emancipation from Self-centeredness and to a corresponding increase in one's innate capacities for genuine unselfconscious compassion [ZB:618 653; ZBR:396 398].

The states of kensho and satori are temporary. Similar episodes happen as happy accidents to people in all walks of life who have neither the prior benefit of meditative training nor of any spiritual inclination. Yet, when these states do arrive in the setting of decades of meditative training that includes daily life practice and frequent retreats, their sequences unfold in ways conducive to further transformations of *traits* of character. When trait changes become major in degree and endure, we associate them with rare individuals. These exemplary persons—like the historical figure of Siddhartha—seem to have evolved in a direction that represents a refined stage of ongoing human development. How do we recognize such rare persons? They show us in their behavior. They continually manifest their simplified, liberated, unselfconscious behavior. This advanced degree of "sage wisdom" exerts positive influences on others [ZB:636–677].

Compassion Tempered with Wisdom

A traditional Zen approach leads in this direction. It is often a quiet, unobtrusive, undemonstrative Path of moderation. Off the cushion, it cultivates the skillful use of simpler, down-to-earth kinds of wisdom. It replaces egocentricity with a practical, long-range, mature, ecological perspective. William James incorporated such a perspective into his definition of the term *pragmatism*. To James, pragmatism was "The attitude of looking away from first things, principles, 'categories,' supposed necessities." Instead, pragmatism meant the capacity to take a fresh long view, to look "toward last things, fruits, consequences, facts." This multidimensional perspective replaces one's adolescent Self-centered, impulsive, grasping mode. Its mature attitudes identify and defer its need for gratifications yet retain one's original childlike sense of wonder (chapters 15, 55). This perspective understands the implicit workings of the law of love; it has learned also to respect the law of unintended consequences.

Master Dogen (1200–1253) understood such everyday wisdom, and he illustrated it in his story about how another wise abbot chose to protect a wild deer. At first, the monks at this other monastery had encouraged the deer to eat grass in their garden. They were astonished when their abbot asked them to strike the deer and to drive it away. "Why would you frighten away this poor deer? Where is your compassion?" They pressed for answers. The abbot replied, "When a wild deer becomes too tame around people, it will surely be killed by the next hunter." The story illustrates the balanced objectivity that skillfully blends the warmth of compassion with true wisdom.

The Liberation Inherent in Wisdom

The wisdom we are pointing toward is the liberated form of "sage wisdom." Dropping off inappropriate shackles, it emerges spontaneously during the exceptional stage of ongoing enlightened traits [ZB:638–641]. Seneca (4 B.C.E.–65 C.E.) was a Stoic who appreciated that such wisdom could be cultivated. He once said, "Only one study really deserves the name liberal—because it makes a person free—and that is the pursuit of wisdom." Younger trainees cannot appreciate what real emancipation is until *after they have experienced* how their first kensho briefly releases them from the bondage of their overconditioning [ZB:611–613].

Immanence: Wisdom Inherent in Comprehending "The Big Picture"

During kensho, aspirants begin to comprehend the essence of an "ultimate" reality principle. Reality seems embedded entirely within and throughout their immediate experience: the whole physical universe is right *here*. *Immanence* is the descriptive term for this deep realization. The word arises from the Latin *immanere*, to remain in. A related word of Hebrew origin is Immanuel. It means God *with* us. In the Christian context, it refers to Jesus being God's manifestation within *this* world. In the Buddhist context, it means that ultimate reality is *right here, in all things*, and not elsewhere, or distant from us. Emerson once articulated how enlightened insights confer such wisdom. He said, "The invariable mark of wisdom is to see the miraculous in the common." Indeed, within such a moment, no miracle is greater than *just this*.

Should any such notion ever become too spiritually inflated and take off, Zen stands ready to throw cold water on it. As old Master Rinzai declared: "If you love the sacred and despise the ordinary, you are still bobbing in the ocean of delusion."

42

Cutting into the Layers of Self

> Behavioral psychology is the science of pulling habits out of rats.
>
> Douglas Busch

Animals show habitual behaviors. When these have close human counterparts, animal researchers can clarify how our own brain might be changing.[1] First to be studied are usually the short-term negative responses related to fear. However, positive affective responses also can be correlated with a sequence of neurochemical changes in the brain. For example, when animals eagerly anticipate being fed their next meal, the dopamine system is activated in their ventral striatum. Then, while they are eating pleasurable substances, they activate the receptors for opioids and GABA in their ventral striatum, amygdala, and orbitofrontal cortex.

Becoming Released from the Burdensome Layers of the Self

What psychological role does our *Me* serve in the human triad of Self? We are sentient creatures easily threatened. Things harm *Me*. Events bruise and batter *Me*. The Me is our *fearful* Self. Me is the pronoun cast in this vulnerable role. Research in rats and lower primates suggests how humans might minimize some elementary limbic contributions that create this fearful Self [ZBR:116–123]. Animal research provides other hints: how to diminish my Self's strong instincts to hold on like a pit bull, tightly attached to any material possession and opinion I believe is *Mine*; how to become less angry when my turf is threatened.

But what about positive experiences? Can someone who has been shorn of Self experience an affirmative impression at that same moment? Yes, for several reasons. Because a profound *release* arrives during the very act of cutting off the pejorative layers of the *I-Me-Mine*, and it contributes to the net positive sense of experiencing a great Amen. A release from what? From the vast mental superstructure that had not only overconditioned our past, multitasked our present, but mortgaged us to an anxiety-ridden future.

True, other primate societies create complex psychological problems. Yet, few societal burdens match the layers of psychic complexities that "civilized" human societies impose daily on each Self. This helps explain why kensho's sudden release from the weight of all prior overconditioning enters experience as a profound "lightening up." No burden of thoughts that you could create willfully, when lifted from the *top* of your psyche, would lead to such release. Instead, when kensho liberates the unconscious, it is the convictions at deep psychological layers that drop out of the bottom of the bucket (chapter 19).

Whittling off Limbic Drives Incrementally

Zen has already been shaving off the layers of the psyche. Incremental deconditioning was taking place during the early years of meditative training. Mindful introspection identified one's simpler Self-centered impulses and counterproductive attachments. Found wanting, they were whittled off, and tended gradually to disappear [ZBR:260–265]. Long-term meditative practice also shaves off the unfruitful impulses that drive the psyche from below, helping to conserve and reprogram their misdirected habit energies. Gradually, the axis of one's ethical value system begins to tilt. In which direction? Outward, centrifugally, toward *other persons' needs*.

How vigorously did old hidden cravings drive our earlier behavior? We can observe the raw power concealed in our own roots of desire nakedly displayed in the cravings of drug addicts [ZBR:251–260]. Addicted cravings persist despite the negative personal and social consequences of taking habit-forming drugs. Recently, *former* drug users were studied in the effort to clarify which underlying mechanisms caused their earlier substance abuse.[2] Did their social behavior seem to have recovered? Yes, they had all stayed "clean." Did their brain recover? No. Long after their drug use ceased, the subtlest drug cues still activated their amygdala and ventral putamen.

Unstated in Zen is a major premise of long-range meditative training: diminishing the unfruitful influences that the amygdala has on other regions, higher and lower (part VII). Yet, these personal liberations usually evolve at a glacial pace, much too subtly to seem practical, recognized more in hindsight than at the time. On the background of such incremental change, could a deep crevasse open up suddenly, an event that cuts through every knotted problem in the psyche, from top to bottom?

The Ancient Sword Cut

Antiquity witnessed the swift efficiency of a sword slash. The theme reappeared in a legend about Alexander the Great (356–323 B.C.E.). In this legend, he was confronted by a thick rope that had been tied into an intricate knot by Gordius, a minor king in ancient Phrygia. Why would any Gordian knot—real or mythological—pose a challenge for Alexander? Because an oracle had foreseen events and passed along the word: only that person destined to become the future ruler of Asia could untie this knot.

At first, would Alexander try to solve his visuospatial task at a purely cognitive level? Maybe. Zen meditators also get stuck in a headful of logical thoughts, wrestling with their unsolvable koan. Alexander solved this knotty problem with one swift sword slash. It was a creative solution, yet one not without parallel in antiquity. In certain respects, it was comparable with an eventful moment two centuries earlier. As that day dawned, supreme enlightenment struck another man beneath a Bodhi tree, and Asia would open up to his teachings thereafter [ZB:668–677].

In the mythology of ancient Mahayana Buddhism, Manjusuri would be the Bodhisattva designated to wield that sword cut of existential insight-wisdom. It is a clean cut, severing all tangled layers of the *I-Me-Mine*, from top to bottom. The cut serves as the incisive agent for prajna's extraordinary state of flashing mental illumination. The way it deeply deconditions the Self is accomplished neither by pious religious thoughts alone nor by little insights that scratch only the surface during ordinary kinds of cognitive-behavioral therapy.

Later, during the sixth century C.E., when the legendary Buddhist monk Bodhidharma traveled north from India, he brought to China the austere ingredients of a dedicated approach to meditation. The Chinese had already appreciated that meditation was a useful Way—a Path, a Tao—that could help cultivate enlightened wisdom. Four striking statements summarize the teachings of the young Ch'an Buddhist sect during its early development. The quatrain illustrates how this direct flash of insight-wisdom differs from ordinary factual knowledge [ZB:8].

- This wisdom is transmitted independently of any prior knowledge the person might have obtained from the old scriptures.
- It does not depend on words and letters.
- It impacts the human psyche directly.
- Its deep insight illuminates one's essential nature, inspiring the person to be further transformed, as was the Buddha.

This school later spread from the Chinese mainland, and became the school we know as Zen by the way the Japanese pronounced the word, Ch'an. When Kobori-Roshi demonstrated the nature of Rinzai Zen to me, his gesture showed that a cut (J: *kire*) was implicit in the process of kensho. It was a cut intended to sever the pejorative Self of all maladaptive attachments [ZB:109].

43

Striking at the Roots of Overconditioned Attitudes

> There are a thousand hacking at the branches of evil to one who is striking at the root.
> Henry Thoreau (1817–1862)

For most of us, having grudgingly acknowledged a few imperfections, it would suffice to trim only a few branches of each dysfunctional *I*, *Me*, and *Mine*. A snip here, a little more there. It's hard to strike off the deep roots of Selfhood.

Zen probes deeper. It will have a major lasting personal influence on the relatively few who, like Thoreau, devote solitary hours to expose and to strike off the deep roots that cause their suffering. We resist. Root pruning hurts. It requires courage and fortitude to stay this long course of Self-sacrifice. For those who persist, and then happen to "let go" during a moment of idle time, an unusual flash of mental illumination can transform consciousness.

In the immediate afterglow, one of kensho's several realizations might then arrive transparently clear: *if a person could maintain this same selfless state, such a perspective could serve as a basis for all ethical behavior.*

An Ethical Basis for Zen Buddhist Training?

A Utopian message. It seemed new to me [ZB:645–648]. However, the belief that Zen Buddhism had a deeply ethical core was an age-old realization. The sixth Zen patriarch, Hui-Neng (638–713), characterized this original self-nature as "without error, disturbance, and ignorance." Ch'an Master Baizang (720–814) described the person who had "truly cut off the passions" as "One who lets the world be as it is, always acting in countless situations with clear rectitude."[1] In Japan, Master Eisai (1141–1215) appreciated the ethical nature of this same basic principle. He said that enlightenment could set disciplined rules for the person's conduct, and establish precepts that left no room for confusing good with evil. Still later, the Rinzai master Bunan Shido (1602–1676) phrased this realization in the following way:

> Die while alive.
> Thoroughly die.
> Then just do as you will,
> And all is right.[2]

Is this just an example of overbeliefs and misplaced idealism? How could any brief cutting off of Self on a Path of Self-negation inspire such lofty notions of universal truths and ethical behavior?

The roots of Ch'an Buddhism grew in a cultural soil already richly tilled. In China, qualities of personal character had been emphasized since the era of Confucius (c. 551–479 B.C.E.). Permeating the social compact was a universal sense of obligation among individuals at all levels. At the historical core of authentic Zen training is a mindful, introspective path of character development. Its approach is founded on the ancient Indian Buddhist values of restraint and renunciation (Skt: *shila*). Zen Buddhism is not a quick fix. "Dharma-bum," substance abuse, varieties of sociopathic behavior do not enter into the Zen under discussion [ZBR:291–302].

Inherent in this Buddhist Path is the artful cultivation of ordinary common sense, morality, and ethical behavior during one's daily life. Living Zen practices are designed to cultivate personal qualities of clarity, wisdom, compassion, rectitude, and courage. The serious aspirant voluntarily renounces situations that could invite unfruitful behaviors, including forms of self-indulgence, spiritual materialism, and the use of intoxicants.

After a long preamble of meditative training within such an enriched cultural setting, what happens when kensho happens to strike off the roots of the Self? The impression of errorless rectitude unfolds automatically. It is the brief realization that no evil conduct could possibly arise in a world so ideal, a domain so shorn of pejorative subjectivities.

This might seem to be a startling claim of Pollyannaish dimensions. Yet every year such a curious realization is introduced to a few awakened trainees who represent a wide range of religious disciplines. What operational principle could give rise to such preposterous notions of omniscience and infallibility? In the clarity of the immediate afterglow, the rationale seems straightforward: on so calm a horizon that continually expresses our intrinsic self-nature, no potential seems to exist for high waves and "wrong" actions to arise. *Continually?* There's the rub.

Doubts gather momentum. And on the printed page, the words invite a reader's instant disbelief, because the obvious problem is that kensho and related peak experiences are *transient* states. Their affirmative residues dwindle. Fallible human beings in every century succumb to impulsive behaviors after having emerged from a transiently enlightened state. As Emerson once observed, "our faith comes in moments; our vice is habitual." Doubts may lead others toward a secondhand misunderstanding of the matter-of-fact, empirical nature, and particular timing of this brief realization if its word description is viewed out of its momentary context.[3]

Redefining the Root of Freedom

The layers of meaning in words continue to cause misunderstandings. Consider the statement by Ajahn Amaro, a monk in the Theravada Buddhist tradition. Recently, he described how he responds when people ask him: "How do enlightened people act?" He replies, "They act like perfect anarchists."[4]

Fortunately, the interview allows him to clarify this interpretation. He goes on to point to the Greek root of *archist*, a word meaning "rule." Following this interpretation, what he's actually saying is that enlightened individuals are no longer held in the rigid grip of any fixed rule or law. Instead, "now totally freed and unfettered, completely unbound," they *are* "an inclination guided by infinite wisdom and infinite kindness." This means that "their actions in the world are immensely powerful, but not guided by ego's concerns." To *be* an inclination is a useful concept, because such a leaning has neurophysiological origins. It expresses the enlightened person's gentle tilt toward unselfconscious behavior. In short, while enlightened individuals might first appear to be iconoclastic, their inclinations manifest degrees of deep selfless wisdom and compassion that predispose them to act toward others in beneficial ways [ZB:638–645; ZB:668–677].

Adopting Flexible Rules

The Soto Zen master Shunryu Suzuki had a favorite phrase: "not always so." Indeed, he said, "'I don't know' is the first principle."[5] He was not saying that Zen encourages a not-knowing ignorance. By "I don't know," he meant that it is a basic Zen practice *not* to be trapped into certainty by rules or by the apparent truthiness of words. Similarly, to Daisetz Suzuki, living Zen meant "not to be bound by rules, but to be creating one's own rules." Our own story of visual illumination in the West would have been delayed had not Thomas Edison shown a similar readiness to break with convention. Indeed, one of the inventor's favorite expressions was: "There ain't no rules around here! We're trying to accomplish something!" The Zen koan is another reminder that one's logical, conventional thoughts do not solve all problems.

Zen paradoxes are unsettling. Gradually, its students learn to reconcile Zen's curious mixture of tradition and iconoclasm [ZB:678]. In fact, similar paradoxical qualities are inherent among persons who practice biomedical research. Thomas Kuhn pointed to this reconciliation when he described a successful research scientist as someone who "must simultaneously display the characteristics *both* of the traditionalist and of the iconoclast."[6] Clearly, if you're conducting creative laboratory research, it helps to balance your maverick inclinations with the skillful means and ethical restraints inherent in simple horse sense. The same flexible approach holds true of the earthy, practical empiricism that resides in everyday living Zen.

Redefining Inclinations in the Nucleus Accumbens

The nucleus accumbens is a part of the basal ganglia. It occupies a region called the ventral striatum, lying close to the midline around the front of the third ventricle. The term *accumbens* (Latin, "to recline at table") comes from the way this small mass of gray matter might seem to "lean" toward the midline of the septum [ZBR:79–82]. Energized by its rich dopamine supply from the ventral midbrain, the nucleus accumbens occupies a key motivational interface. It is poised to infuse affective messages from the limbic system into motor systems that express our behavior.

If you were a Roman, reclining at a banquet that offered the accumbens strong appetitive stimuli, your greedier "inclinations" could encourage you to lean forward, approach things, reach out, and grab them. But, suppose your accumbens were to receive an aversive message. Now it could contribute to very different avoidance behaviors, enabling you to recoil. Individuals who experience more negative, fearful emotional responses release more dopamine into their nucleus accumbens and ventral caudate nucleus.[7] In adolescents, the accumbens is activated more during reward-seeking behaviors than is its counterbalancing neighbor, the orbitofrontal cortex.[8] This imbalance between the two regions could further incline impulsive adolescents to satisfy their immediate, risky needs rather than adopt the distant long-term goals that evolve as they become more mature. In adult rats, the core of the accumbens helps the animal shift into and maintain novel behavioral strategies. The outer shell contributes to the way the rat learns which incoming stimuli are irrelevant.[9]

Many studies show that the ventral striatum plays an important role in drug addiction [ZBR:251–255]. How? Recent fMRI studies suggest that the accumbens helps maintain an intimate sense of what we *expect might happen next*.[10] Indeed, let this next stimulus fall only slightly short of our expectations and the accumbens becomes activated. When the accumbens is tested in a classical Pavlovian conditioning system, it responds sensitively to both an appetitive (+) stimulus (a $5 reward) and to an aversive (−) stimulus (an electrical shock to the left index finger). The accumbens has this flexibility to tilt in either direction. Research needs to clarify precisely how meditation influences this tilt.

How do we attach such a plus or minus, "good-or-bad" affective value to stimuli of either kind? We seem to refer to a value scale of personal beliefs. Each scale extends from dollars-pleasant-desirable (+) at one end, to shock-unpleasant-undesirable (−) at the other. Many plus/minus messages about valence relay from the amygdala and orbitofrontal cortex over to our ventral striatum. This interactive circuit suggests at least two basic mechanisms that can enable meditative training to strike off the roots of our overconditionings and begin to "gentle" our responses. It can (1) reduce the positive and negative coding biases that are implicit in this scale of valences, and (2) reduce the overall strength of our nucleus accumbens–dopamine pathways [ZBR:116–120]. Emotional zero lies between the two extremes of + and −.

Several other circuits can nourish the roots of our excessive longings for positive rewards. These potential sources of attachments become evident when fMRI is used to monitor subjects who are performing a simple task. They extract information from their anterior cingulate and medial prefrontal cortex that predicts what their next actions will be[11] (chapter 53).

Qualifications on How Feasible It Is to Test Inclinations during the Immediate Post-Kensho Period

Our inclinations have widespread origins in the brain's systems of checks and balances. It will be emphasized here that valenced messages from the right amygdala contribute to our implicit moral attitudes, inclining us to act unconsciously in biased ways. The amygdala relays its stimulus-reinforcement associations up to the ventral medial orbitofrontal cortex, where they will then be processed during higher-levels of decision-making and response-selection.[12]

No similar study of fMRI sequential activations will be easy to design, conduct, and interpret in the immediate, post-kensho period. Lifelong layers of personal conditioning complicate the interpretation of each individual meditator's fMRI signals. For example, normal subjects are already inclined to be apprehensive witnesses *before* they see test pictures. Why? Because they anticipate that they will soon encounter some images that are strongly negatively valenced. This expectation shifts them into a guarded, "better-safe-than-sorry" mode. Their negative bias generates unnatural *baseline* signals that resemble the patterns seen when they are certain the next picture will be unpleasant.[13]

Other normal subjects begin with an innate psychophysiological bias. They are temperamentally inclined to be pessimists. This trait is associated not only with more fMRI signals in their insula on both sides but also with more signals in the right inferior frontal gyrus, medial thalamus, and the red nucleus down in their midbrain. Will kensho's immediate residues of *fearlessness* dissolve all such signals that represent *this* particular person's pessimistic trait? Without ample longitudinal baseline data, researchers won't know how each individual meditator's preexisting personality trait has been influenced and reshaped by the psychophysiological changes that had just occurred during kensho. So, how testable are hypotheses about kensho? Whatever the answer will be, one qualification is clear: Granting agencies must provide full support for longitudinal studies of meditative training, enabling researchers to measure sequential trait changes in *individual meditators* over a minimum of 5 years, not 5 months (see chapter 55).

Meanwhile, we continue to rely on the frontal cortex to manage networks intelligently, to fine tune our civilized needs for rules in a flexible balanced manner with those creative freedoms that sense when convention needs to be overruled. How do our prefrontal regions (medial, orbital, polar, and dorsolateral) know when to excite or inhibit the valenced responses that arise from the limbic system and other parts of our brains? These pressing questions address issues now drawing intense scientific, social, religious, ethical, medical-legal, philosophical, and political interest. The next chapter considers new brain imaging approaches. They reveal how our brain tilts its psyche/soma balances to enable mere shoulds to become shalls, oughts to become musts, and inclinations to translate into overt acts.

44

Neuroimaging Our Representations of Shoulds and Oughts

> A moral being is one who is capable of reflecting on his past actions and their motives—of approving of some and disapproving of others.
> Charles Darwin (1809–1882)

Darwin's Victorian era had ample reason to examine its moral standards. In our era, whose actions and motives remain pure and beyond reproach? Recently, a field called "moral cognition" has gained momentum. Reminding us that "shoulds" *ought* to govern our social behaviors, its findings suggest that we make value judgments about "good" and "bad" in widely distributed systems at multiple levels in the brain [ZBR:398–399]. Every day, headlines confirm that emotions drive peoples' actions beyond their full conscious control. Is brain imaging now so sensitive that it can detect automatic moral beliefs and attitudes, find hidden biases that shape how we *really* think and usually behave?

Testing for Covert Emotional Associations

One way to answer this question is to measure how we respond to an Implicit Association Test (IAT). Fast reaction times on the IAT reflect how we feel, deeply, that certain actions are moral or immoral. In contrast, slow reaction times suggest that our responses are ambivalent and/or deliberately thought out. Consider the big differences between the ways we respond to flowers vs. bugs. Since childhood, we've been conditioned to associate flowers with good attributes, insects with bad. Tests now show that we react faster when flower is paired with "good" than when some researcher presents us with a test that pairs flower with "bad."

Similar implicit association responses formed the basis for the fMRI study by Luo and colleagues.[1] The results are summarized in table 13. Their subjects viewed a color photograph for 2 seconds. Some IAT pictures illustrated a legal behavior; others showed an illegal behavior. The photographs showing legal acts were presented at two levels of intensity. Half of the legal actions were highly arousing (e.g., skydiving). The other half were less so (e.g., playing the guitar). Among the illegal behaviors, half were also highly arousing in nature (e.g., the

Table 13
Some Neural Correlates of Subconscious Moral Inclinations

	Congruent Decision	*Incongruent Decision*
Examples of paired concepts based on Implicit Association Test photographs	Bad animal paired with moral transgression	Good animal paired with moral transgression
Degree of cognitive-moral conflict	0	+
Reaction times (ms)	Shorter ($\pm$700)	Longer ($\pm$760)
Increased signal activity in precuneus, insula, anterior cingulate (BA 25), ventrolateral frontal gyrus (BA 47, premotor cortex (BA 6), and caudate nucleus	Less marked	More marked
Role of the right amygdala	Contributes to the formations of more intensely valenced stimulus-reinforcement associations	
Role of the left ventromedial orbitofrontal cortex (BA 10)	Contributes to higher-level decision-making and response selection at higher levels of salience	

After Q. Luo, M. Nakic, T. Wheatly, et al. The neural basis of implicit moral attitude—an IAT study using event-related fMRI. *Neuroimage* 2006; 30:1449–1457.

scenes included guns and knives in acts of interpersonal violence). The other half were less arousing, but still illegal, because the acts of vandalism shown were causing property damage. The control pictures were relatively tame (e.g., showing a snake or a puppy.)

During one phase of the study, the subjects' task was to respond to *congruent* pairs of two types. When legal behaviors were paired with "good" animals, the subjects confirmed that the two topics matched by pressing on a button with the left hand. And when illegal behaviors were paired with "bad" animals, they responded to this congruent match with a right-hand button press.

However, in a separate phase, the subjects were presented with *incongruent* pairs. In such a mismatch, illegal behaviors were paired with "good" animals; legal behaviors were paired with "bad" animals. Incongruent tasks confront a subject with conflicting perceptions, attitudes, and actions. Yet, even though the experimental design was complex, these normal subjects made few errors (1.62%).

The results illustrate that normal healthy adults are biased to respond with automatic negative associations to any behavior they believe is illegal and immoral. Illegal stimuli drew faster responses than did legal stimuli. Congruent trials, having shared the same underlying conceptual theme (e.g., moral transgressions paired with bad animals), were also responded to more quickly than were the mismatched, incongruent sets.

fMRI Correlates of IAT Responses

Incongruent tasks require subjects to overrule their basic inclinations to make a particular motor response. During such incongruent situations, fMRI signals increased both in the left anterior cingulate gyrus (BA 24), and in the region where this gyrus extends under the bend of the corpus callosum (BA 25) (figures 2, 5). Signals also increased in the right ventrolateral frontal gyrus (BA 47), in the premotor cortex on both sides (BA 6), and in the left caudate nucleus (a part of the basal ganglia also known as the dorsal striatum) [ZBR:248, 280].

What role(s) did the anterior cingulate gyrus play in this whole response? It was believed to participate at the level of monitoring goal-directed behavior, especially when conflicts arose between a cognitive option and an emotional option. Subsequent interactions between the anterior cingulate and the ventrolateral frontal cortex were viewed as a resource that provided higher executive control over the motor responses that were being mediated by the caudate nucleus.

fMRI signals also increased within the right amygdala. This finding suggested that the amygdala contributes emotionally valenced information (the "automatic" moral attitude) that helps responses tilt in alternative directions (+/−) during the IAT task. Signals increased in the left *medial* orbitofrontal cortex when scenes showed extreme degrees of interpersonal violence. The evidence suggested that this left medial orbital region could be helping to select the most appropriate responses to whatever kinds and degrees of reinforcement might be needed. Both the right amygdala and this left medial orbitofrontal region appeared to contribute to the "emotive strength" (the reward/punishment value) that the subject developed—automatically—to each picture that was being seen.

The responses to illegal stimuli generated increased fMRI signals in the motor and premotor cortex, in the superior temporal regions (BA 41, 22, L > R), and in the right amygdala. Once again, the data were consistent with a meaningful interpretive role for the superior temporal region. This helped the witnessing subject interpret what was being intended by a given act, a decision that could then be used to shape his or her moral reasoning.

The Origins of an Implicit Moral Attitude

How do our experiences gradually condition us to develop such an implicit moral attitude? The authors suggest three factors that enter in. Let's begin with simple words, followed by the complicated terms used in standard psychology.

- We're tempted—a stimulus/reinforcement association is activated.
- We're informed that to act would be immoral—a moral transgression/negative valence association is represented.
- We're informed about the potential consequences—a negative valence expectancy is more strongly represented than is a positive one.

Research tends first to study the negative aspects of "moral cognition" and "social cognition." It's easier to document the hard-edged, negative valences of a rigid Calvinistic attitude than the softer affirmative responses of altruism, kindness, good will, and forgiveness. Ideally, long-term meditators will be tested for the kinds of softer IAT qualities that nourish the social compact during equally rigorous fMRI studies in the future.

Testing for Other Biased Attitudes

Meanwhile, a separate fMRI study from the National Institutes of Health also made use of the Implicit Association Test.[2] Knutson and colleagues detected the racial and gender attitudinal biases in 20 normal subjects. When these subjects viewed pictures that were congruent with (and therefore confirmed) their own covert biased associations, fMRI signals increased in their anterior medial prefrontal cortex and in their rostral anterior cingulate cortex. In contrast, signals increased in the dorsolateral prefrontal cortex when their visual associations were incongruent with (and did not match) their preexisting stereotypes. Implicit, stereotyped, gender biases also activated the amygdala.

In brief, this study suggests that our anterior medial prefrontal cortex participates in the ways we represent stereotyped (politically incorrect) attitudes, whereas our dorsolateral prefrontal cortex functions to counter and overcome such stereotypes. This dorsolateral convexity helps supply executive contributions (of political correctness) essential to the governing of our moral behavior. Its countless associations can provide more *objective* evaluations that have access to high levels of native, empirical intelligence. Acting in concert with the frontal polar and orbital cortex, all four frontal association regions help us balance unfruitful instincts and restrain impulsive emotional drives.

Buddhism uses a specific technical term, *moksha*, to refer to the abrupt release from such worldly bonds during kensho-satori. This transient release refers to the unconditioning of those weighty layers of Self-consciousness that were entangled in our elaborate web of overconditioned, maladaptive dos and don'ts. As the last chapter notes, this deprogramming is remarkably selective. One's native virtues and authentic ethical sensibilities persist. The liberated, selfless, intuitive human compass still comprehends in which direction lies true North. Future research needs to specify which objective capacities enable this affirmative moral compass to continually express its rectitude in ongoing thought and deed, even though many rootlets of its emotional subjectivities had been severed, dissolved, or bypassed.

45

Distinctions between Intuitive Mind Reading, Simple Empathy, and Compassion

> The capacity to understand other people's emotions by sharing their affective states is fundamentally different in nature from the capacity to mentalize.
>
> Tania Singer[1]

Babies have an innate, *reflexive* capacity to share other persons' simple emotions and sensations. However, our more cognitive, intuitive mind-reading skills do not begin to develop until around the age of 4 years. These skills enable us to understand others' intentions, attitudes and beliefs. Table 14 summarizes some elementary contrasts between the earlier forms of simple empathy and the later capacities for intuitive mind reading. A wide variety of executive functions enables the regions cited on both sides of the table to blend the two kinds of functions in a practical manner.

Table 14
Distinctions between Intuitive Mind Reading and Empathy

	Intuitive Mind Reading (Includes "Theory of Mind" and "Mentalizing")	Simple Empathy
Descriptors	Capacity to understand others' desires, intentions, attitudes, and beliefs	Capacity to share others' simpler feelings (emotions and sensations)
Major regions of origin	Lateral temporal lobe and prefrontal cortex	Sensorimotor cortex, limbic and paralimbic systems
Subdivisions	Temporal poles; posterior superior temporal sulcus (STS); medial prefrontal cortex (MPFC)	Anterior insula, rostral anterior cingulate cortex, secondary somatosensory cortex, amygdala (are activated when others are perceived to be in pain or are fearful)
Developmental trajectory	Mentalizing develops at around age 4 years; intuitive functions tend to mature later and to decline earlier	Newborns already engage, reflexly, in "contagious crying"; empathic functions tend to mature earlier and decline later
Commentary	Observation of others' actions also stimulates representations in the so-called mirror neuron system	More complex levels of empathy also go on to develop a perspective on the psychic origins of others' distress
Deficits that might have potential clinical correlations	Autism	Criminal psychopathology

Adapted from T. Singer. The neuronal basis and ontogeny of empathy and mind reading: Review of literature and implications for future research. *Neuroscience and Biobehavioral Reviews* 2006; 30:855–863.

However, no simple formula specifies how the *gross* structure and gross function of the normal brain enables healthy children and adolescents to develop into mature adults (chapters 15, 55). Some evidence even suggests that during two crucial decades, from age 10 to age 30, gray matter volumes decline in the frontoparietal cortex, as does the power of the theta (3.5 to 7 cps) and delta (0.5 to 3 cps) bands in the EEG.[2]

On the other hand, fMRI studies have contrasted the different ways normal adolescents and adults think, both about another person's mental intentions and about simple cause-and-effect physical events.[3] The *medial* prefrontal cortex of the 19 adolescents (ages 12 to 18 years) was activated more when they interpreted intentions. In contrast, 10 adults (ages 22 to 38) used a different interpretive strategy. It depended more on activating lateral cortex farther back in their *right* superior temporal sulcus (STS). This STS becomes of interest to meditators in regard both to its associations with empathy (chapter 9) and insight (chapter 34).

Our simpler forms of normal adult empathy have other fMRI correlates, as the next chapter will illustrate. Yet these elementary degrees of empathy must become much more highly refined before they approach the advanced levels of skill expressed during authentic compassion. Buddhism reserves the technical term *karuna* for such extraordinary levels of compassion. In these most highly refined manifestations, karuna enables us to correctly perceive a situation, sense deeply how it would affect us, project our interior feelings sympathetically toward others, and then reach out *selflessly* to improve the situation in the most appropriate way. Note: Compassion at this highest level, while remaining *unself*conscious, operates dispassionately with consummate wisdom and skill.

46

Empathy, Forgivability, and the Responses of the Medial Prefrontal Cortex

What wisdom can you find that is greater than kindness?
                                   Jean Jacques Rousseau (1712–1778)

When the Dalai Lama says my religion is "kindness," he is expressing an unusual capacity to respond with empathy and to forgive others that appears to manifest a rare level of wisdom. Lee and colleagues in Sheffield, England conducted an experiment of interest in this regard, although it was designed with a very different purpose in mind. Their original goal was to show how the normal brain responds differently to social situations than does the schizophrenic brain.[1]

They compared 14 normal controls with an equal number of acute schizophrenic patients who went on subsequently to improve. All subjects first read an interpersonal social scenario for 16 seconds, then responded by finger presses to each of its several potential options. The scenarios illustrated three general themes. The first involved the simplest kind of social reasoning, and evoked the subjects' fastest responses. During the two other scenarios, the subjects had either to make empathic judgments, or to choose which of two crimes was the "more forgivable." These other responses were slower.

Normally, we recruit multiple regions when we respond with empathy [ZBR:267–269, 535]. In this study, the normal subjects also increased their fMRI signals during empathic judgments in many sites: in the medial prefrontal cortex (BA 10) and inferior frontal gyrus (BA 45) on both sides; in both their middle temporal gyrus (BA 21), left angular gyrus (BA 39), and right posterior fusiform gyrus (BA 19), as well as in the thalamus, precuneus, and cuneus.

Initially, when the schizophrenic patients' symptoms were more acute, their judgments showed less empathy, and they showed *less* activity in all the above regions than did their controls. Moreover, they also failed to activate the thalamus.

When the normal control subjects made forgivability judgments, signals increased both in their medial prefrontal cortex (BA 10) and superior frontal gyrus (BA 8, 9) on both sides, as well as in the right middle frontal gyrus (BA 8). Signals also increased in their posterior cingulate (BA 23), cuneus (BA 19), thalamus, and over a wide inferior temporal region. This included the lingual and posterior fusiform gyrus.

The Follow-up Study

Several points of interest serve as a preamble in order to interpret the second set of data on the recovering schizophrenic patients. Not only had their acute symptoms and behavior improved, but documented improvements also occurred in their psychological test scores, social functioning scores, and in the depth of their insight into the nature of their illness. In this clinical context, how is "insight" defined? Insight means how well these patients complied with treatment, recognized that they were ill, and could label their own individual psychotic phenomena as symptoms caused by their illness. (How healthy are many contemporary societies, when judged by such standards of mental hygiene?)

After the patients had partially recovered from their acute psychotic episode, their fMRI data during empathic judgments now showed greater increases in activation in the left medial prefrontal cortex (BA 10/9), the right fusiform gyrus (BA 19), the posterior medial temporal area (BA 37), the lingual gyri (BA 18), and the left supramarginal gyrus (BA 40). Moreover, during the second set of improved forgivability judgments, the patients showed increased left-sided signals in the medial prefrontal cortex (BA 10/9), as well as in the cuneus and precuneus (BA 18/7), the posterior middle temporal area (BA 37), and the paracentral lobule (BA 31).

Which region showed the most obvious increase in signals that correlated consistently with the patients' clinical recovery? It was the *left medial* prefrontal cortex. The right lingual gyrus and the cuneus were two other regions that, with recovery, showed substantial increases in signals during both empathic and forgivability judgments.

This interesting, two-phase study combines clinical, psychological, and neuroimaging documentation with fMRI signals measured during responses to a simplified, three-scenario structured task. Prominent among the findings are the association between empathy, forgivability, and the medial prefrontal cortex.

Suitably modified, similar experimental designs could be used in longitudinal studies to test whether individual long-term meditators do become kinder and more humane persons who manifest empathy, compassion, and forgive gross social errors in other persons.

47

Rigorous Retreats, and the Supporting Influence of a Friendly Hand

> Young monk: I don't see the gift in my suffering!
> Old monk: That gift wrapping. Remove it ...![1]

> Tell me and I forget. Teach me and I remember.
> Involve me and I learn.
>
> Benjamin Franklin (1706–1790)

Thus far, trying to describe Zen, we have used words on a printed page that portray it as a mindful, introspective meditative Path of deconditioning your own Self and reprogramming it. Much more is involved. Most formal talks in the zendo after sitting will be forgotten, as will most of the words you have read. Certain private interviews with your teacher remain memorable. Yet, when do you start learning what Zen is, and who *you* really are? Only when you wholeheartedly involve yourSelf in a Zen retreat.

Retreats are rigorous. You are losing sleep, your body aches, you become frustrated, bored [ZB:235–240]. Meanwhile, your brain is undergoing subterranean stress responses. The ways these responses surface in the form of little "quickenings" provide us with clues to the mechanisms causing the later states. These major states are transformations of consciousness. Will you decide to join the cadre of a motivated support group, voluntarily exposing your vulnerable psyche and soma to such stresses, *if* the cost-benefit ratio seems worthwhile? You should. You ought to. *Will* you?

The Stick-Carrot Ratio

For many centuries, Zen teachers have acquired a justified reputation for afflicting the overly comfortable with varieties of tough love. Learning proceeds not through positive rewards alone. Some cultural norms do tilt the cost-benefit ratio in a more rigorous direction, one that makes allowances for techniques now called "altruistic punishment."[2] Seymour and colleagues explore the general topic of such tough, altruistic behavior. They define it in formal terms as an action that involves some degree of personal cost to the one who does the punishing. At least when assessed by PET scans, such behaviors do increase the energy cost in the basal ganglia because they increase the activity of the punisher's caudate and putamen.

Looking back from the vantage point of our twenty-first century, Master Lin-Chi I-shuan's conduct in ninth-century China often seems to have been intended to rattle the cages and shake everyone's comfort level. That especially rigorous Ch'an school (it would later evolve into Rinzai Zen) reflected both his own hard-nosed personality, that of his teacher, and the cultural vigor of the Tang dynasty. Today, knowing more about the biology of stress and strain, we appreciate how some stress responses have beneficial results, especially when they are individualized, timed, and calibrated with care [ZB:235–240; ZBR:113–116]. More advantageous in the West today is often a blending of retreat styles, one that softens an ancient oriental boot camp approach with some gentler methods imported from the Soto Zen and the Theravada schools of Buddhism.

Comforting the Afflicted

Whichever styles one volunteers to endure during formal retreats, it still proves difficult to stick to one's own daily routine of sitting meditation at home. Fortunate are the meditators who are sustained on this Path by the genuine close support both from within their own family, from like-minded members of their sangha, and from an authentic teacher [ZB:119–125; ZBR:64–69]. Does the support from a significant other person reduce one's stress responses during difficult situations?

Coan and colleagues used fMRI to monitor how married women responded under the threat of an impending electric shock.[3] When each wife held her own husband's hand, her emotional and behavioral responses to threat were less pervasive than when she held no hand at all, or merely held the hand of some anonymous male researcher. The quality of the relationship between each husband and wife was very important. The higher it was, once the wife held her own husband's hand, the more she reduced the threat-related neural activation in her right anterior insula, superior frontal gyrus, and hypothalamus.

48

Show Me

> I come from a state that raises corn, and cotton, and cockleburs, and Democrats, and frothy eloquence neither convinces nor satisfies me.
> I am from Missouri. You have got to show me.
> Willard D. Vandiver (1854–1932)[1]

Willard Vandiver, U.S. representative from Missouri, made these remarks over a century ago. Little could he guess at the time that his phrase," Show me" would later become his state motto, and be enshrined on its license plates (let alone wind up on this page as an example of an important principle in Zen).

How does a Zen master test the depth of his students' brief awakenings, and of their ongoing maturity on the Path? He challenges them to *act*. He tests the way they react to arcane, *show*-me situations. "*Show me* how you look at this flower!" "*Show me* your original face!" "*Where* is one?"

A Zen master wants no frothy eloquence. He's all too familiar with your old biased words, has seen your other, stereotyped behaviors. He's not interested in these. He's looking for something new. He's watching for your instant motor response. He's paying attention during those first 500 event-related milliseconds of your body English. He wants to be shown hard evidence that you have been deconditioning your rigid ways of thinking and acting. If so, your movements will arise instantly, flow freely. Long years of authentic Zen training cultivate brisk, fluid actions arising from liberated sensorimotor pathways, not navel-gazing apathy or metaphysical speculation [ZB:668–677].

Your Zen master wants to see you *manifest* enlightened Zen behavior. To you, he's saying "*Show me*" responses that are

- expressed from a foundation of poise;

- spontaneous, with no initial hesitation;

- quickly executed;

- simple but efficient;

- highly creative;

- improvisational, yet sufficient to resolve the immediate situation;

- so selflessly motivated that they also resolve the big picture as well;

- liberated from discursive thoughts and emotional preoccupations.

Actions speak louder than words. Emotions and motivations are two terms both sharing the fruitful concept of *motion*. Can skillful movements show that we had let go of discursive thoughts, rechanneled their restless energies, entered a "no-thought" awareness, yet spared all the practical attributes of useful cognition?

Instinctual, Emotional, and Cognitive Aspects of Our Motivational Drives

A training program must be well-balanced to sponsor such liberated behavior. A practical program of meditation needs to do more than harness one's unfruitful motivational drives and emotions. It needs to *redirect* the vital energies that had sponsored one's previously overactive approach and withdrawal behaviors [ZBR:244–245]. True, the word "motive" does include a cognitive connotation, a shade of meaning that might mislead someone into thinking that only conscious thoughts drive all motivations. However, motivational drives have covert subcortical origins that are deeply instinctual and emotional.

Neurological damage in patients usually produces negative signs of deficit. At the conceptual level, these negative signs can be "turned around" to illustrate useful principles. For example, patients show *decreased* spontaneous movements in several abnormal neurological conditions. Textbooks use the term *abulia* to describe one such clinical state.[2] Typically, abulic patients show a severe slowing that affects *both* their psyche and soma. Not only are their spontaneous movements and speech "de-energized" in a sense but they also show a marked poverty of ideation and emotional reactivity. The disorder, called *akinetic mutism*, manifests extreme degrees of such mental and physical inertia.

Habib has surveyed the several different neurological disorders that seem to dissolve patients' "motivational energies."[3] The case reports suggest that the lesions in such patients have interrupted various sites from the brainstem up through the cerebrum. Linked by a series of looping circuits, the several regions in the cerebrum include the anterior cingulate gyrus, nucleus accumbens, medial caudate nucleus, the ventral part of the globus pallidus, and the frontal cortex together with its connections with the medial dorsal nucleus of the thalamus. Many of the same levels receive their supply of dopamine from the nerve cells of the substantia nigra and ventral tegmental area in the midbrain [ZB:197–201, 674–676].

One heroic challenge in the future will be to discover how an appropriate array of selectively balanced changes among diverse receptors within such large networks can reinforce our natural trends toward emotional maturity, reprogramming meditators' behaviors toward spontaneous simplicity, stability, and compassion [ZB:691–695]. The meditative transformations of consciousness seem capable of rechanneling energies toward these worthwhile human qualities.

49

Fifth Mondo

Let go of all your previous imaginings, opinions, interpretations, worldly knowledge, intellectualism, Self-centeredness, and competitiveness; become like a dead tree, like cold ashes. At the point when your feelings and views are all gone, and your mind is left clean and naked, then you open up into Zen realization.

Master Yuan-wu (1063–1135)[1]

What is special about the insight-wisdom of kensho?

It strikes selflessly, in the absence of time and fear, during an alternate state that transforms consciousness and liberates the *I-Me-Mine* of its prior over-conditionings.

What is so special about a Zen master?

The Zen master is an exemplar who inspires you to endure the long meditative path toward such states, who supports you during its rigors, and confirms that while you may arrive at some milestones along the way, you are still on an endless journey, in good company. As for progress, he wants to be *shown*.

How does the brain change during natural development in ways that enable teenagers to mature into adults?

We seem to be using some Self-referential action-oriented, frontoparietal networks less and some other-referential, frontotemporal networks more.

How does this gradual developmental trajectory relate to the thesis that insight matures substantially during an allocentric mode of processing at the same instant that Self-centeredness drops off?

Words imperfectly describe the events that enter experience during this state. No-I corresponds with its personal selflessness (*anatta*). When insight-wisdom arises in this context, its realizations include emptiness (*shunyata*) [ZBR:383–386], and the comprehension of immanent Reality. This moment of Oneness confers the impression that all things are interrelated perfectly and eternally (*suchness*) [ZBR:361–371].

Part VI

Toward Emotional Maturity

Don't be afraid to abandon your faults.

Confucius (551–479 B.C.E.)

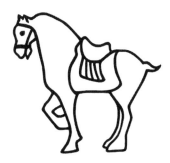

On Learning about the Emotions

> Our intelligence can function reliably only when it is removed from the influences of strong emotional impulses.
>
> Sigmund Freud (1856–1939)

Emotions prevent us from seeing the world clearly. When someone gets angry, we used to say they were "flying off the handle," or "getting all riled up." More recently, we say they are "losing it."

I'm partial to the phrase, "getting all riled up." To me, riled conveys both that excessively fast turbulent flow and the turbid sediment it stirs up from the bottom. Our vision gets blurred when these fast-moving events carry us away.

Myokyo-ni emphasized that Zen training involves becoming familiar with our own emotions. Mindful introspection soon identifies the two main fires that inflame our emotions as greed and hatred. These emotions move us. Their longings lead to approach behaviors, and their loathings to avoidance behaviors [ZB:347–352]. In the next chapters, we survey recent research that clarifies how emotions arise, and consider the advantages of examining emotions in a matter-of-fact manner while patiently enduring them.

Modulating the Emotions

> It is commendable to get angry at the right things and with the right people and in the right way and at the right time and for the right length of time.
>
> Aristotle (384–322 B.C.E.)

Anger is okay, so long as it follows Aristotle's logic. So are our other emotions, after we learn to modulate them. *Modulation* is another word that has musical connotations. Its Latin roots refer to the ways we convey shades of meaning when we sing or play an instrument. We do so by adjusting our pitch, key, or volume. Musicians are said to be "in the groove" when they modulate intuitively and unselfconsciously, skillfully blending sensibilities that are instinctual, emotional, and cognitive. In the Orient, it was appreciated that mental functions were not purely cognitive, but were rather infused with affective sensibilities, one reason given for the way that the old Sino-Japanese word *shin* translates as both heart and mind.

A Zen Commentary on the Emotions

Rarely surpassed is the spirited form of the horses created by Chinese artists during the golden age of Zen in the Tang Dynasty (618–907). Myokyo-ni used to say that Zen training resembles the optimal way you approach the training of a spirited horse. The objective is not to break its spirit, but to *gentle* the wild quality of its energies, enabling their innate powers to be rechanneled more fruitfully. Emotional events come and go in daily life, serving the meditator as a focus for practical introspections on impermanence. When Myokyo-ni continued to be upset emotionally by someone or something, her teacher reminded her to question herself: If I had but five more minutes left to live, would this still be worth getting mad over?

Fear

Fear is our most potent emotion [ZBR:243–247]. The amygdala is the gateway through which fear relays its negative valence to be processed up and down the neuraxis into aversive conditioning responses. Subjects who are chronically and severely afraid of spiders have volunteered to watch film clips of spiders. Instantly they respond with increased fMRI signals both in their dorsolateral frontal cortex (regarded as a secondary coping strategy) and in their parahippocampal gyrus (viewed as a reactivation of memory sites) [ZBR:93]. On the other hand, an *anticipatory* anxiety develops in other spider-phobic subjects while they are waiting, apprehensively, knowing that they will soon see a spider.[1] This expectant fear coincides with increased fMRI signals in their dorsal anterior cingulate cortex, insula, thalamus, and visual association regions.

Sadness

Sadness is different. Sadness is categorized among the higher sentiments. Its burden falls especially heavily on patients who suffer from depression (chapter 36). After damage to the amygdala on both sides, patients cannot accurately recognize sad expressions in pictures of other persons' faces [ZBR:92]. Furthermore, among normal observers, the more empathetic are sensitive to certain slight changes in pupil size that can appear when facial photographs express different emotions.[2] To sensitive subjects, smaller pupils are equivalent subconsciously to enhanced expressions of sadness (but not to different expressions conveying fear, surprise, or disgust.)

When normal subjects recall sad episodes, they increase fMRI signals in the lateral orbitofrontal and adjacent ventrolateral regions of their frontal cortex [ZBR:165]. On the other hand, recent studies of young monozygote twins could not consistently correlate episodes of recalled sadness with sources in particular frontal regions,[3] despite evidence that twins' frontal lobe volumes are highly (90% to 95%) inheritable.[4]

The question arises: What can be learned from subjects who choose, voluntarily, to recall a given emotion?

Recalling Anger and Other Emotions

When emotional responses strike spontaneously, they "feel" stronger and different from those we recall voluntarily, chiefly because spontaneous events first unfold naturally in distinctive, primary physiological patterns inside the brain. Corresponding physiological changes out in the body feed back their secondary contributions into the brain. Accordingly, when we get angry and then feel "hot under the collar," it is because the earlier central nervous system events that first influence the hypothalamus prompt the secondary sympathetic nervous system discharges that cause an obvious flushing of the skin.

Anger has a distinctive physiological profile. Forty-three subjects closed their eyes, then rated how intense their emotions became when they chose to relive the experience of a specific emotional episode that was characterized either by fear, anger, sadness, or happiness.[5] The anger pattern was consistent with sympathetic nervous system activation. It increased the heart rate but caused relatively few changes in the variability of the heart rate. The increased heart rates during the three other emotions were associated with actual decreases in the variability of the heart rate.

An extensive literature in recent decades correlates heart rate variabilities with multiple psychological and physiological parameters.[6] For our present purposes, it is sufficient to note why this is a tricky area to evaluate: (1) One's breathing rate influences one's heart rate through complex neural and vascular mechanisms that chiefly converge on the vagus nerve. (2) The vagal *motor* fibers that slow the heart rate during inspiration are well-insulated with myelin and conduct impulses quickly. They arise in the medulla at a site appropriately named the *nucleus ambiguus*. (3) In contrast, the other vagal motor fibers that mediate the heart response during classical conditioning are poorly insulated. They originate in the dorsal motor nucleus of the medulla. (4) Most fibers in the vagus return *sensory* messages from the viscera to the nucleus of the solitary tract in the medulla [ZB:165, 229].

A Commentary on the Psychophysiological Changes Associated with Slow Breathing Rates

Slow, regular breathing has long been useful in decreasing the anxiety and pain associated with childbirth. Slow-paced breathing also decreases the response to experimental threat and increases the amplitude of those normal heartbeat irregularities that are linked to one's breathing cycle (respiratory sinus arrhythmia).[7] Paced breathing at slow rates around four to six times a minute results in the highest amplitudes of this heart rate variability. Experienced Zen meditators breathe at such slow rates [ZB:94–95]. At these slow rates, both parasympathetic and sympathetic mechanisms overlap in complex ways (e.g., in support of the reflexes that regulate both blood volume and blood pressure. The term *positive resonance* is used when different mechanisms overlap and reinforce each other.)

Each person has a particular low breathing rate (around six breaths per minute) at which paced biofeedback has the greatest effect on heart rate variability.[8] It is speculated that biofeedback-assisted breathing at this optimum resonant frequency "stimulates and exercises autonomic reflexes," renders them "more efficient," and helps restore an appropriate balance between the sympathetic and parasympathetic systems. Preliminary clinical trials suggest that biofeedback procedures can improve both the pulmonary gas exchange and the psychological profile of depressed patients.[9] On the other hand, a skeptic might suggest the need to rigorously control for the positive placebo effects inherent in such biofeedback procedures. Moreover, supervised programs of vigorous exercise also have salutary physiological effects on one's psyche, autonomic nervous system, and cardiovascular-pulmonary functions. Finally, but not incidentally, concentrative meditation has recently been proposed as a way that might help meditators arrive at their optimum "resonant peak."[10]

A Commercial Device for Relieving Emotional Stress

When Freud spoke about the adverse influence of "strong emotional impulses," no handheld electronic device was on the commercial horizon that promised to relieve such stressful influences.[11] Now, simply by spending $299 and placing a finger in the infrared pulse sensor of a "StressEraser," the changes in one's pulse rate can be subjected to an algorithm that transforms them into peaks and valleys on an accompanying screen. This visual "feedback on each individual wave in real time" anticipates the degree of one's respiratory-induced sinus arrhythmia. These words imply that the peak of each wave is now calculated to predict the moment just before the heart rate begins to fall secondary to a fresh burst of vagal nerve discharges. Large, tall respiratory sinus arrhythmia waves indicate greater degrees of heart rate variability and suggest the presence of greater degrees of (pacifying) parasympathetic/vagal tone. When large, high, smooth waves of respiratory sinus arrhythmia appear, they are said to indicate an advanced stage when that user's changing heart rate and respiration are covarying "in a synchronous phase relationship."

In theory, having this immediate feedback—"a window into vagus nerve activity"—enables one to visualize how properly to modulate one's own breathing. Theoretically, with the aid of this biofeedback "BreathWave" approach, one becomes able to so synchronize outbreaths that they enhance vagal nerve discharges, activate the relaxation response, calm the mind, and relax the body. At least, this is the claim of the company that markets the device. Their brochure cautions that both a calm mind *and* a particular breathing pattern (usually between 4.5 and 7.0 breaths per minute) are prerequisites for engaging one's own relaxation response. For novice meditators, having a visual wave peak could enable them to time their inhalations and exhalations in greater synchrony with their individual vagal tone, and to align their accompanying thoughts, breath countings, or mantra accordingly.

Commercial aspects and temporary usefulness aside, the relationships among slower breathing rates, slowing pulse rates, and vagal tone are well-known.[12] For example, the heart rate variabilities of parasympathetic origin correlate in a different context with fMRI signals arising in the ventral part of the left anterior cingulate gyrus [ZBR:84]. Tendencies to enhance sinus arrhythmia are also reported in association with increased vagal tone during "transcending" episodes in transcendental meditation (TM) practice [ZBR:50–51]. During Zen meditation, changes in heart rate variability correlate with greater degrees of frontal midline theta activities and with suggestions of lesser degrees of engagement of the sympathetic nervous system [ZBR:51–53]. That said, unless stringent placebo controls are used, it could take years to sort out the validity of the recent claims and counterclaims relating to the use of biofeedback to monitor heart rate variability.

The Wandering Tenth Nerve (Continued): Its Origin in the Medulla

In the interim, a provocative study of long-term meditators focuses interest on the plasticity of vagal nerve cells around their site of origin in the upper medulla. Peter Vestergaard-Poulson and his Danish colleagues at Aarhus University used structural MRI to study ten experienced meditators.[13] These subjects had each practiced Buddhist styles of meditation with the same teacher for a total of 8000 to 35,000 hours over a period of 15 to 31 years.

The meditators' upper medulla showed a significant increase in density. The area involved was larger on the left side, and it extended upward along the dorsal aspect of the medulla. This general location happens to correspond with several groups of vagal nerve cell bodies: those of the nucleus of the solitary tract, the dorsal motor nucleus, and the nucleus ambiguus [ZB:165]. The mechanisms responsible for this intriguing finding remain to be clarified as do their functional correlates.

Our frontal eye fields (FEFs) can hold attention either on pleasant scenes or unpleasant scenes. On which topic shall we choose to fix our attention? The choice determines how much and what kinds of fMRI activation our brain develops in response to emotional images.[14]

Meditation has offered for millennia a low-tech way to reduce the emotional overload. Thich Nhat Hanh reminds us that we can always choose which image to view on our own internal TV screen. Do we want a peaceful channel? We can turn to a peaceful channel. Do we wish to reinforce our longings for news? We can stay tuned to the litany of woe on channel TV. We make up our own minds.

In the next chapter, we consider additional ways that meditative training helps to dissolve fearful responses at various stages along the Path of Zen.

52

How Could the Long-Term Meditative Path Modulate the Emotions?

To conquer fear is the beginning of wisdom.

Bertrand Russell (1872 1970)

Anger is never without a Reason, but seldom with a good one.

Benjamin Franklin (1706–1780)

Tracing the Normal Pathways of Fear and Anger

Emotions shape our earliest perceptions. Luo and colleagues at the National Institute of Mental Health conducted a classic study of how first we respond to an emotion seen expressed on another person's face.[1] They monitored normal subjects using a new technique. It combined magnetoencephalography (MEG) and synthetic aperture magnetometry with a "sliding window analysis." Its sensitivities helped them detect (1) where in the brain the gamma frequency response arose, (2) when this gamma response began, (3) when it reached its peak, and (4) how long it lasted.

Their fifteen subjects, both male and female, viewed pictures of faces for a mere 0.3 second (300 ms). The faces expressed fear or anger or were emotionally neutral. The neutral faces evoked the expected MEG visual response in both sides of the occipital/temporal cortex [ZBR:45, 182, 189, 246]. This neutral response be-

Table 15
Gamma Synchronization Responses in Emotional Processing Pathways

	Fear Pathway (ms)				Anger Pathway (ms)			
	Onset	Peak	Duration	Side	Onset	Peak	Duration	Side
Amygdala	25	235	280	R	155	215	110	L
Occipitotemporal cortex (BA 17–19, 37)	45	145	260	Both	25	145	270	Both
Inferior frontal gyrus (BA 47)	205	245	110	R	—	—	—	—
Anterior cingulate gyrus (BA 32)	—	—	—	—	165	225	110	R
Orbitofrontal cortex (BA 10)	—	—	—	—	175	205	60	L

Adapted from table 1 of Q. Luo, T. Holroyd, M. Jones, et al. Neural dynamics for facial threat processing as revealed by gamma band synchronization using MEG. *NeuroImage* 2007; 34:839–847.
The numbers show how quickly normal subjects respond with event-related gamma wave synchronizations to pictures of faces during MEG monitoring.

gan some 30 to 40 ms after the onset of the facial picture stimulus, and it lasted some 270 to 280 ms.

Ancient texts can be interpreted to suggest that the Pali term *manasikara* could correspond with the first critical milliseconds when preattention's sharp point impales an object and selects it for further cognitive scrutiny.[2] Table 15 suggests that this reflexive act involves much more than our usual knee-jerk responses to the tap of a reflex hammer. Indeed, the subcortical gamma response arises not from our emotionally neutral circuits, but from a discriminating pathway. Its hard-wiring has already been shaped by evolution and confirmed during overconditioning. It *recognizes* that a fearful face poses a threat more serious than an angry face. Table 15 summarizes significant steps in the way we process the separate emotions of anger and fear.

Fear

At the top left of table 15, notice how quickly our subcortical pathway responds to fear. Gamma responses appear in the amygdala as early as 25 ms, especially on the right side. In this report, gamma synchrony was not detected as reaching the inferior frontal gyrus until later, at 205 ms, also on the right side.

Relatively coarse visual information could be transmitted during the upslope of the first wave of subcortical messages as they pass from the colliculus through the pulvinar to the amygdala. However, the peak of this amygdala response does not occur until 235 ms. By then, the amygdala could also have been receiving fresh, recurrent waves of finer-grained information from the occipito-temporal cortex, because this region's earlier peak had already been reached at 145 ms, during which time it could have supplied such cortically refined input (chapter 4).

Anger

In contrast, the right-side columns of table 15 show that an angry face does not prompt the observer's amygdala to respond until much later, at about 155 ms. Anger responses then relay forward to involve both the anterior cingulate gyrus (165 ms) and the orbitofrontal cortex (175 ms). In these subjects, anger responses arose predominantly on the left side. In the amygdala, anger responses did not persist as long as did the responses to fear.

Intricate circuits lead into the amygdala and relay messages back and forth between the amygdala and the cortex. We are still learning how these pathways function to moderate human behavior [ZBR:88–94]. (See the updated section on the amygdala in part VII.)

The Prevalence of Attacks of Panic and Anger

Tragic events on land and sea triggered waves of anxiety around the world as the new millennium began. Fear and anger remain pervasive. People have anxiety attacks, and get riled up more often than we realize. Recently, some 9282 subjects were surveyed face-to-face with the aid of a WHO-structured interview.[3] At least one person in five (22.7%) had experienced isolated panic attacks during their lifetime, most of which attacks were moderate or severe in degree.

In the same survey, the lifetime prevalence of intermittent episodes of explosive anger was 7.3%.[4] Anger attacks began in adolescence at the average age of 14 years. Only 28.8% of the subjects had received treatment for their anger outbursts. However, the episodes of explosive anger had significant consequences. In the course of their average of 43 such lifetime attacks, the average property damage reached a total of $1359, and some person had been injured 77% of the time.

Implications of the Dissolution of Fear during Kensho

Investigators interested in human emotions have yet to take full advantage of how thoroughly fear drops out during kensho. Many ancient statues of Buddha show a particular *mudra*, or position of the hand. In the *abhayamudra*, the Buddha's right hand is extended, facing away from his torso at waist height, and the fingers are held close together. This gesture can be translated as total fearlessness [ZB:567–570]. Fearlessness is not to be confused with any egocentric notion of invincibility. Rather, it signifies the complete absence of fear per se. When Self-centeredness vanishes in kensho, fear drops out along with every trace of the defense behavior associated with it.

Our normal sense of fear arises within networks into the amygdala that soon link it with the frontal cortex, the hypothalamus, and the central gray region of the midbrain. How do fear (and other emotions) gradually become less overwhelming on the long meditative path, then briefly dissolve during kensho? The sensitive new MEG techniques just discussed make it theoretically possible to test several working hypotheses. However: such data need to be collected individually, longitudinally, and multidimensionally, with special reference to where each meditator is on his or her *long ongoing path* of meditative practice. Clearly, in such a project, investigators must remain on call during retreats. Time is of the essence. Researchers must be poised to react quickly (to respond like emergency room personnel). They must also be certain how many seconds, minutes, or hours have elapsed between the flash of kensho and the time that their first MEG, fMRI, and other multidisciplinary measurements are being performed.

Tests of Working Hypotheses for Kensho

By way of concrete illustrations, let us begin with an advanced, mature, adult meditator who is enrolled in such a longitudinal, well-controlled study. Suppose that during a retreat, this meditator happens to awaken suddenly into an authentic state of kensho. One testable hypothesis could be that transmissions were interrupted through *both* the fast and the slower fear pathways *during* this state. One further possibility might be that the person's earlier *sub*cortical pathways (assumed here to be relatively more hard-wired) were the more resistant to such interruptions. If so, then the peak amplitude and duration of the gamma response to fear at the *cortical* level (say in the inferior or medial frontal gyrus on the right side) could show the relatively greater reduction when compared with this same meditator's *prior* series of MEG observations and related measurements.

Suppose next that a different meditator was farther along on the Path, in the direction of the ongoing *stage* of enlightened traits [ZB:637–641; ZBR:394–396]. Perhaps in this case, the person had been in regular practice for several decades, and had already experienced one or more authentic awakenings into kensho-satori. Note that in this more advanced situation, *prior to this latest retreat*, some of that person's *baseline* responses already could have shown reduced MEG fear responses in the gamma band, perhaps both in the (fast) subcortical pathways *and* in the (slower) cortical pathways. Therefore, whatever *new* changes might be superimposed during this advanced meditator's latest developing state of kensho or satori would need to be interpreted *with reference to* those earlier, well-documented *trait* changes that had already reduced his or her baseline responses. Repeated baseline testings before each major retreat are essential (chapter 15).

Recent behavioral studies monitored the emotional responses of a patient who had sustained a major thalamic lesion centered on his left pulvinar.[5] This patient recognized no fearful facial expressions when pictures of faces appeared in his opposite (right) visual field. Collateral evidence suggested that his damaged left *medial* pulvinar had disrupted the fear recognition messages along two pathways: (1) the slower, more conscious, occipital-temporal-amygdala route, and (2) the faster, subconscious, colliculo-pulvinar-amygdala route.

Improved techniques can now monitor not just our fear and anger pathways, but also the disgust pathway to the insula, (and such other higher sentiments as contempt and sadness). These techniques will become important tools in the future for those research groups, meditators, and granting agencies who remain committed to this worthwhile project of defining how and where the long-term meditative Path influences the emotions. These techniques now appear to be sufficiently sensitive to document three kinds of distinctive changes on the meditative Path.

- They can detect the residues of the overt short-term dissolution of emotions that had occurred during an episode of kensho only minutes before.
- They can detect residues of the subtle ways that meditative practices incrementally transform and modulate our previous overconditioned behaviors and attitudes [ZBR:240–247]. These changes set the stage for the gradual arrival of random insights of various kinds and sizes.
- fMRI monitoring can detect a crucial two-phase executive sequence.[6] During these two steps, normal subjects first use their frontal-polar regions (BA 10) to briefly suppress and defuse their disturbing emotional memories (chapter 4).

1. One of these cognitive control pathways acts through the right inferior frontal gyrus (iFG). How does this pathway reduce the emotional burden of the incoming sensory messages that disturb our working memory functions? By deactivating their sequences as they ascend through the fusiform gyrus and the pulvinar.

2. The second pathway for cognitive control proceeds through the right *medial* frontal gyrus (DMPFC in figure 2). It reduces the activity of the limbic components that represent and retrieve memories at the level of the hippocampus and amygdala.

The next chapter considers ways that meditative training can help us use such pathways to whittle away at our overconditioned responses.

Newer Views of Extinction

How much there is in the world I do not want.

Socrates (469–399 B.C.E.)

The extinction of fear and extinction in general is considered to be inhibitory learning.

Barad, Gean, and Lutz[1]

Trainees on the meditative path begin to shed their previous "wants" [ZBR:260–265]. In psychology, extinction means that you unlearn prior behaviors that had been conditioned.[2] Everyone has been conditioned, both for better and for worse. Therefore, if extinction is to simplify our lives, it must be *selective*. Will marriages, families, friendships, jobs succeed or fail? Too often, the outcome is uncertain. It hinges on whether we had exchanged old unskillful habits for social skills that were more adaptive, learned to say what needed to be said, and behaved more skillfully [ZB:327–334]. Yet, hard as we tried to shed counterproductive behavior patterns, they still tended to return.

How can we finally quench the smoldering fires of those old conditioned responses? There's no simple answer. Established behaviors are hard to get rid of. Their barbed hooks are embedded too deeply and have too many sensory and motor points of attachment. Moreover, multiple mechanisms are included within the process of extinction itself. Among them are selective inattention, inhibition of response, the block of nonreward, and secondary reinforcement. Given all these variables, it is no wonder that the ingredients of extinction prove notoriously difficult to untangle.[3]

Evolving Views of Nirvana

The notion of "nirvana" has confused people for millennia [ZB:579–584]. *Nirvana* is an old Sanskrit term. The early Indian Buddhists used it as a metaphor to refer to the major, permanent extinction of the egocentric Self. In this usage, extinction implied that the fires of their deluded yearnings and aversions were finally extinguished. The white-hot flames of emotion were blown out that had consumed them with longings and loathings.

Centuries later, Ivan Pavlov (1849–1936) conducted a series of classic studies of such opposing behavioral phenomena. Phrases such as "appetitive conditioning" or "fear conditioning" have since been used to describe his experimental techniques. Pavlov first conditioned an animal to become afraid by introducing a novel stimulus, one that was initially neutral (such as a tone, or a light). Later he paired this neutral stimulus with an unpleasant (aversive) stimulus, (such as a foot shock or similar unconditioned stimulus). Now, that previously bland tone or light acquired a new meaning: it changed into a conditioned (warning) stimulus. It became a cue that triggered the animal's conditioned response. The animal became conditioned to fear.

Dogs he had earlier conditioned to be fearful could later become deconditioned and less fearful. Pavlov wondered why their fear dwindled. Did such a (temporary) extinction of fear mean that the dogs' newly acquired fear response had been totally erased or passively forgotten? Pavlov thought not. Instead, he hypothesized that extinction was a new dynamic process, one superimposed on the dogs' persistent underlying fear association. He came to view extinction as an *active* form of *new inhibitory learning*. This kind of extinction required work. His bold proposal has since been largely confirmed.[4] To varying degrees, an additional process of erasure may also coincide.[5]

Some Mechanisms of Extinction

The previous chapter discussed the ascending circuits of fear that lead *up* from the amygdala into our inferior and orbitofrontal cortex. Suppose we envisioned one aspect of extinction as a quasi-intelligent process, one that introspective meditators might learn how to turn around, and supervise from the top *down*, both consciously and subconsciously. How can the frontopolar and *medial* prefrontal regions contribute to some of this badly needed practical intelligence?[6]

In fact, preclinical experiments indicate that the medial prefrontal cortex does normally support extinction. How? Glutamate nerve cells in this medial region activate a set of GABA inhibitory circuits down in the *lateral* amygdala. These, in turn, inhibit the *central* nucleus of the amygdala. Subsequent steps go on to enhance both the initial learning of fear extinction *and* to help maintain this ongoing extinction as well.[7] The receptor profiles of neuromessengers in the human amygdala are sufficiently complex to provide the requisite layers of checks and balances [ZB:175–179; ZBR:85–94].

Intriguing clinical studies have been conducted on patients who suffer from posttraumatic stress disorder (PTSD) (chapter 36).[8] Structural MRI scans have suggested that among normal subjects, a thicker ventral medial prefrontal cortex is associated with their retaining a greater capacity to extinguish fearful behavior. Other data suggest that genetic deficits in the way the hippocampus processes cues could also predispose PTSD patients to develop their stress disorder.[9]

Clearly, a complex circuitry is involved in enhancing and suppressing our fears. Simpler practical measures, including mindfulness-based stress reduction

(MBSR) training, and cognitive retraining have much to recommend them as parts of a conservative approach to treating less severe forms of PTSD. The evidence that different subtypes exist among patients who suffer from obsessive-compulsive disorder (OCD) suggests that several different modules in the larger network helps determine which patients are more likely to improve on cognitive behavioral therapy per se[10] [ZBR:84].

Extinguishing the Fear of Death

Sooner or later, each Self must directly confront its ultimate fear. Widely represented learning processes contribute to the extinction of our fear of death, and they are important to define [ZBR:85–137]. The acute, temporary, total loss of fear that occurs during kensho recommends it as one model state in which to study several converging mechanisms (chapters 19, 42). The presence of GABA inhibitory circuits in the amygdala that respond to discharges from frontal lobe pathways suggests only a quasi-intelligent top-down mechanism. Other candidate mechanisms operate at deeper levels. The long-term meditative path itself provides models for several kinds of adaptive "far death attitudes" that can evolve incrementally [ZB:448–452; ZBR:116–120].

54

Anatomical Asymmetries: Autonomic, Emotional, and Temperamental Implications

> [A hypothetical model:] the left forebrain is associated predominantly with parasympathetic activity, and thus with nourishment, safety, positive affect, approach (appetitive) behavior, and group-oriented (affiliative) emotions. The right forebrain is associated predominantly with sympathetic activity, and thus with arousal, danger, negative affect, withdrawal (aversive) behavior and individual-oriented (survival) emotions.
>
> A. Craig[1]

Chapters 36 and 51 called attention to slender sensory fibers. They supply our brain with afferent information ascending via autonomic fibers from our heart, lungs, and other visceral organs. After these interoceptive messages relay up through the ventral medial nucleus of the thalamus, many are represented at the next cortical level in the insula [ZBR:95–99]. The anterior insula on the left side is activated predominantly by sensations, like taste, that we associate with parasympathetic functions. Over on the right side, the anterior insula tends to be activated by sensory messages, like pain, that are associated more with sympathetic functions (see also the updated section on the insula in part VII).

These anatomical and physiological asymmetries begin in the incoming sensory domain, and have outgoing motor parallels. Stimulating the left insula in humans produces chiefly parasympathetic effects: slowing the heart rate and reducing blood pressure. In contrast, stimulation of the right insula is associated with sympathetic effects: increasing the heart rate and raising blood pressure.

Speculations on this hypothetical model seem likely to be tested for decades to come. Currently, they have led to the soft generalizations that the emotional feelings and behaviors lateralized more to the left hemisphere tend to be directed more toward an enrichment of our physical and mental energies, whereas those of the right hemisphere tend to be directed more toward our avoiding potential threats [ZB:358–367; ZBR:213–214, 245–247].

Personality Traits: Structural MRI Correlates of Extroversion and Neuroticism

One approach to a model of human psychology views our normal personality traits as varying along five dimensions. They are extroversion, neuroticism, conscientiousness, agreeableness, and openness to experience.[2] Three dimensions of such a model warrant brief comments. For example, introversion occupies the opposite pole from extroversion. Emotional stability is the polar opposite of neuroticism. Notably, emotional stability is also a key attribute of the sage wisdom that evolves into the advanced stage of ongoing enlightened traits [ZB:641–645].

We observe extroverts manifesting a positive affect, and see them actively engaging in approach behaviors during social interactions. In general, such positive (outgoing) behavior correlates with tendencies toward greater *left* anterior brain activities [ZBR:163–164]. In contrast, other children and adults are obviously more introverted, appear to be more inhibited during unfamiliar situations, and show relatively greater *right* frontal activities.

Wright and colleagues used structural MRI to study 28 right-handed normal subjects of both sexes.[3] The subjects were screened to exclude gross psychological disorders, and averaged 24 years of age. Correlated with greater degrees of extroversion was a thinner right inferior frontal gyrus (BA 45) and a thinner right anterior fusiform cortex (BA 20). Greater degrees of neuroticism, on the other hand, correlated with a thinner *left* anterior orbitofrontal cortex (BA 10, 11). Notably, neither personality dimension correlated with the volume of the amygdala. It will take many multidisciplinary studies to clarify how such gross measurements of thickness might relate to the microstructure and physiological interactions of these cortical regions.

Impulsive behaviors can be studied, using game-playing tasks that offer players the potential opportunity to divide money. Prior damage to the ventral medial prefrontal cortex interferes with the patients' ability to modulate emotional reactions, and correlates with their more impulsive, irrational financial decisions.[4]

Openness to Experience

In order to begin a spiritual quest, and to continue to survive its many vicissitudes, meditators must maintain a variety of open-minded attitudes. One such attitude supports creative activities in general. Sternberg and Lubart defined it this way, in the context of creative insight: "This attitude is one of searching for the unexpected, the novel, and even for what others might label as bizarre."[5] To remain open and to be interested in new experiences are two of the personality traits found in some long-term meditators that correlate with their unusually enhanced capacity to recognize the microemotions expressed on other persons' faces [ZBR:242].

We turn next to consider why one index that an adult has arrived at a less Self-centered level of emotional maturity is described in these terms: "to have ceased growing vertically, but not horizontally."[6]

55

The Cognitive and Emotional Origins of Maturity

> At 30, I planted my feet firm upon the ground. At 40, I no longer suffered from being perplexed. At 50, I knew the entreaties of heaven. At 60, I heard and obeyed them with a docile ear. At 70, I could follow the dictates of my own heart; because what I now desired no longer overstepped the boundaries of what was right.
>
> Confucius (551–479 B.C.E.)

> It is high time for me to depart, because at my age I now begin to see things as they really are.
>
> Bernard DeFontenelle (1657–1757) (at the age of 100)

You don't have to be a DeFontenelle on your deathbed to realize that your views about reality have evolved. Looking back, it's easy to see how we've entertained wildly different views about what "reality" is at different ages. Our emotions also mature at highly individual rates. Only during the later years do some astringent aspects of our personalities become mellower, like those of a slowly ripening persimmon.

Networks Mature as We Grow Up

Parents soon discover how emotionally labile and impulsive their children are. We forget that many of these same problem impulses still lurk in our own adult psyche. What natural developmental changes helped us survive adolescence, reshaping the physiological responses of our own brains?

Our growing mental competence at solving basic problems was crucial, and it remains essential. This current, competitive, multitasking adult environment prompts endless emotional frustrations if general performance skills are not at a high level. Recently, the research team at Washington University in St. Louis asked: how does the maturation profile of fMRI responses evolve in relation to childhood, adolescent, and adult levels of performance skills?[1] Table 16 summarizes the results.

Two very large networks confer these general problem-solving skills. Note how they gradually separate from each other and become activated indepen-

Table 16
Two Macronetworks Involved in General Problem-Solving Tasks and the Ways They Mature with Age

	The Frontoparietal Network	The Cingulo-Opercular Network
Anatomy	Dorsolateral prefrontal cortex; intraparietal sulcus; inferior parietal lobule; precuneus; dorsofrontal; midcingulate gyrus	Dorsal anterior cingulate/medial superior frontal cortex; bilateral anterior insula/frontal operculum, anterior prefrontal cortex, thalamus
Basic function	These separate modules interact to enhance the rapid top-down feedback aspects that *adjust* task performance	These separate modules interact to enhance the top-down *stability* that sustains task performance
Functional differences	Activated by attention to the starting cues that initiate tasks, by the need to detect subsequent errors, and to adjust performance instantly	Activated throughout the long course of more sustained task performance
Pattern in childhood (7–9 years)	The two macronetworks function more as one unit led by the frontoparietal network	
Pattern in adolescence (10–15 years)	The two networks patterns become more segregated, and their disengagement is intermediate between the childhood and adult profiles	
Pattern in adult life (21–31 years)	The two macronetworks are now activated independently; during maturation, their individual modules develop more long-range connections and fewer short-range connections (e.g., long-range connections develop with the cerebellum and also link the posterior cingulate gyrus with the ventral medial prefrontal cortex)	

Adapted from D. Fair, N. Dosenbach, J. Church, et al. Development of distinct control networks through segregation and integration. *Proceedings of the National Academy of Sciences U.S.A.* 2007;104:13507–13512.

dently. This development enables adults to deliberate before acting, to deploy nuances of top-down attention with sufficient flexibility to solve short-term situations, and to sustain mental sets that focus on solving longer-term problems. It will not escape the attentive reader's notice that von Economo nerve cells are in a position to service and sustain the needs of the cingulo-opercular network (chapter 28), and that the frontoparietal network overlaps with many of the attributes of the dorsal attention system (chapter 7).

Suppose we view as affirmative the new perspectives that develop during the decades-long process of normal healthy aging. Could long-term meditative training help to reinforce and enhance this normal developmental trend outlined in table 16?

This is not a new idea. Master Chinul (1158–1212) was the major founder of Korean Zen.[2] Ordained at 15, his first awakening occurred at age 30 when he was reading the liberating words of the sixth Chinese patriarch. Thereafter, Chinul came to view Buddhist training in alertness and calmness as an incremental process comparable with human maturation. This long developmental path resembled his own. It was one of "sudden enlightenment followed by gradual cultivation." Its momentum surged during these early sudden glimpses into the inherent nature of reality. Thereafter, one refined this enlightened perspective in the course of skillfully applying all of one's discriminative faculties and wisdom to meet the needs of daily life practice.

Correlations between Kensho Experiences and Psychological Maturity

MacPhillamy conducted an early longitudinal psychological study of 31 male and female monastic trainees in the Soto Zen tradition.[3] Seven of the monks had experienced kensho during their 5-year period of residence. During this time, they and their cohorts had completed a series of psychological tests using the Minnesota Multiphasic Personality Inventory. The serial MMPI data suggested the possibility that these seven trainees' brief enlightenment experiences had enabled them to mature more rapidly than their cohorts in the direction of becoming more integrated and well-adjusted individuals.

Emotional Clarity in Long-Term Meditators

Nielson and Kaszniak studied 16 meditators representing different Buddhist traditions.[4] Those who had meditated for durations of more than 10 years appeared less focused on physical symptoms and reported greater degrees of "emotional clarity." This capacity of clarity was defined as "the ability to accurately discriminate among, and label, one's feeling states." This kind of clarity correlated with lower arousal ratings, lower skin conductance responses, and with the meditators' greater skills at discerning the emotional valence of masked pictures selected from the International Affective Picture System.

Suppose that long range meditative training does help to nurture and sustain some *basic* developmental processes involved in problem solving, emotional regulation, and personality development. By what physiological mechanisms could it encourage such skills to emerge? [ZBR:399–401].

The Normal Maturation of Emotional Regulation

The subtle physiological processes postulated clearly overlap with the way general cognitive skills mature, as summarized in table 16. Recent experiments suggest how we might loosely describe one such process of maturation. It resembles a tilt in the balance away from the person's old, selfish *I-Me-Mine* kinds of fearful behavior, toward more *You-Us-Ours* modes of allocentric identification.

As noted earlier, fear poses direct threats to all domains of the *I-Me-Mine* and corrupts all our native virtues. Seniors who are more mellow tend to minimize the importance of negative events that in earlier decades they might have overreacted to with emotions of fear or anger. Consider the study of younger and older adults by Mather and Carstensen.[5] They found that older adults, when exposed to stimuli of various kinds, remembered more of the positive items than did younger adults. Moreover, older adults processed their positive memories more elaborately than they processed their negative memories.[6]

On the other hand, older adults tend to become distractible. Suppose the distractions intrude when they first encode events into the early sequences of memory. These older subjects no longer favor positive over negative pictures when their memory recall is tested subsequently. Let us render a charitable interpretation of this result. It suggests that during the *initial* steps of such short-term processing, older adults might have access to, and *use*, some salutary cognitive resources to shape their emotional goals (in a positive direction). (Younger adults did not seem to be using similar cognitive controls to help *them* render their memories more positive.) So, which potential resources might older brains normally be using to help them "accentuate the positive?" Could they improve such functions by further training? If so, could such an approach help seniors tap into resources that are not yet as well-developed in younger brains? Parts I through V have prepared us to consider a variety of potential attentional skills and optional possibilities.

In this regard, Williams and colleagues at the University of Sydney, Australia studied many normal subjects, both male (122) and female (120).[7] Their ages ranged from 12 to 79 years. All subjects viewed standard pictures of facial expressions that varied in emotional valence. Their twofold task was to identify which emotion was imaged, and to rank the intensity of this emotion. fMRI and event-related potentials (ERPs) monitored their responses. Notably, the results described below were paralleled by the scores on their psychological questionnaire. These scores established an important trend: the older subjects were more emotionally stable.

The first group of younger subjects varied from 12 to 19 years of age. Fearful facial expressions generated only slight fMRI responses from their medial prefrontal regions. However, during successive decades (20–29, 30–49, 50–79), this *medial prefrontal* signal activity increased substantially on both sides. Moreover, the ERP responses paralleled this gradual increase in *medial* prefrontal fMRI signals, especially the later ERP potentials that arose *after* 200 ms (chapter 4). This evidence was interpreted as favoring a more reflective variety of subconscious responses during the later decades.

One point of interest: the *orbital* prefrontal cortex did *not* share in these increased signal responses with age. This departure from the medial frontal findings is intriguing. It leads to a plausible hypothesis: As the brain gradually matures, it can draw increasingly on the subconscious resources of the *medial* prefrontal lobe. These medial contributions help contain the way our orbitofrontal region responds when it receives fear-producing stimuli relayed from the amygdala.

Connections in Circuits Involving the Amygdala

Could selective pruning or other atrophic changes inside an aging amygdala per se cause it to respond less to fear-producing stimuli? Structural MRI studies revealed no excessive degree of shrinkage of the subjects' amygdala, only the usual shrinkage expected as the whole brain undergoes normal aging. So, if a normal-sized amygdala still remains as the gateway to our fears [ZBR:85–94], then could aging be associated with a reduction in the *functions* of those particular circuits that project *to* the amygdala? As we grow older, could the earlier *subcortical* flow of impulses change—at conscious and/or subconscious levels—in ways that protect us from being overcome by our fears? (chapter 52).

To answer this crucial question, Williams and colleagues turned to the refined fMRI techniques now aided by functional connectivity analysis.[8] We observed in chapter 22 that connectivity analyses suggest which brain regions in a network are functionally linked during a particular constellation of timed, reported, mental activities. Timing becomes crucial in the interpretation of the next results. Indeed, by the time the subjects *first became conscious* that a face had made them afraid, two mechanisms had already come into play. Each could serve to *reduce* the influence of the amygdala: (1) functional connections were reduced that linked the amygdala with the cortex; (2) functional connections were also diminished along the early subcortical pathways leading *to* the amygdala.

These observations are preliminary, but important. The first provides a hint (as discussed in chapter 6) that *reentrant* feedback (both positive and negative) plays a crucial role in determining whether a stimulus event gains enough momentum to actually pierce our threshold of conscious awareness. The second suggests a compensatory mechanism, one that could cut off some fear responses by disconnecting the earlier fear-generating circuits leading *into* the amygdala [ZB:608–609].

Subliminal Responses to Fearful Stimuli

At an even earlier stage in this study, *before* the subjects had become consciously aware of their own (subconscious) fear responses, what did fMRI monitoring reveal? At this point, the connectivity data suggested that lower subcortical pathways were still connected with the amygdala (mechanism 2). However, these automatic responses to fearful stimuli had not yet been relayed beyond the amygdala to reach the cortex. The limited resolution of current fMRI images does not permit a more detailed conclusion.

An important challenge for future research is to accurately measure and interpret our responses of fear and other emotions. Table 15 suggests why MEG can play a key role in helping to define these critical issues. Using MEG, the longitudinal multidisciplinary research goals will be to measure the physiological responses during life of those rare, enlightened, mature sages whose exemplary lives and psychological profiles have been thoroughly documented. One important target of these studies will be to define accurately the status during life of each major excitatory and inhibitory circuit that governs the responses leading into and out from the amygdala. These studies become the prelude to a detailed postmortem analysis of the paths from both colliculi through the pulvinar to the amygdala and beyond, focusing on the entire circuitry of the limbic and paralimbic systems in particular (chapter 19) [ZB:653–659].

Responses to Happy Faces at Different Ages

The psychological questionnaire showed that emotional *stability* increased over the decades in all of the Australian subjects. Happy facial expressions generated fMRI and ERP responses that contrasted with those to fear. However, the fMRI signals in the medial prefrontal cortex of younger subjects responded much more to happy faces than did the signals of the older subjects. Therefore, much of this age-related difference occurred in younger subjects who were also the most emotionally *labile*. Notably, this gradual decrease in the responsivity to happy faces during successive decades also correlated with a corresponding *decrease* in these subjects' initial ERP responses during the first 150 ms. How are such findings to be interpreted?

Perhaps, as the authors suggest, when adults become less labile emotionally, the need to superimpose as much medial prefrontal "executive control" no longer arises when a happy face signals that an event is a positive one. Accordingly, the decreases with age in the initial ERP responses are consistent with such reduced "requirements" for mature executive control. Whether such a "ho-hum" interpretation is explanatory or descriptive, it is supported by other data. The results indicate that responses do change as we become more mature. Activation can increase *selectively* in those brain areas critical for task performance, whereas noncritical areas become simultaneously less activated.[9]

The Aging Frontal Lobe and its Connections

The structural MRI data on 20 experienced practitioners of insight meditation reported by Sara Lazar and colleagues suggested that "regular meditation practice may slow age-related thinning of the frontal cortex."[10] This relative preservation of brain structure was more evident in the region of the right middle and superior frontal sulci (BA 9, 10). Recent structural MRI studies of 13 Zen meditators indicate that their regular meditative practices correlate with the preservation of their sustained attentive skills, and with the sparing of their left putamen from the age-related shrinkage found in matched controls.[11]

Some of the evidence cited might be consistent with the observed tendencies for a few older meditators to settle down into simpler lifestyles, to show greater emotional stability than their nonmeditating cohorts, and to maintain relatively well-preserved levels of motor skills.

When the normal subjects studied by Urry and colleagues decreased their negative affect, it was the older individuals (in their sixties) who both increased fMRI signals in their ventral medial prefrontal cortex, reduced the activation of their amygdala, and showed steep declines in their saliva cortisol levels.[12]

However, between the ages of 60 and 93, substantial age-dependent disruptions weaken the functional connections that normally link fMRI signals in the medial prefrontal cortex with their partners back in the posterior cingulate/retrosplenial cortex region.[13] These disconnections correlate with a reduced integrity of the white matter tracts that would normally connect the two regions. It is noteworthy that such age-dependent disconnections chiefly impair communications within the more Self-referential and top-down dorsal attention system (table 5). While this loss of connections has obvious disadvantages, it could also contribute to some age-related dissolutions of one's overburdened *I-Me-Mine* and help tilt the balance toward other-referential functions that are more adaptive.

Considered elsewhere are how other aspects of long-term meditative training both contribute to the stability and simplicity implicit in "sage wisdom" [ZB:637–695] and cultivate the kind of selflessness that translates into a larger sense of self-in-the-World [ZBR:346–357]. It remains for future researchers to conduct the rigorously controlled, longitudinal studies that test how long-term meditative training influences the plasticity of each subject's brain during its natural developmental profile in ways relevant to this particular individual's maturing expressions of mental and physical competence.

56

Brain Peptides Help Decode Subtle Facial Emotions

The face is a mirror of the mind, and eyes without speaking confess the secrets of the heart.

St. Jerome (c. 342–420)

Oxytocin

Oxytocin is a peptide composed of nine amino acids. After nerve cells in the hypothalamus release it, oxytocin influences our so-called affiliative interpersonal behaviors. Included in this responsive network are such cortical sites as the fusiform face area (FFA), the superior temporal sulcus (STS), and the amygdala, among the other limbic regions. Women who report that they engage in more hugs with their husbands or partners have higher blood levels of oxytocin and lower baseline levels of blood pressure and heart rate.[1]

How does such a small protein molecule enhance social affiliative responses? [ZBR:120–123, 242, 245–247]. In a recent clinical study, 24 units of oxytocin, or placebo, were administered into the nasal passages of the subjects 45 minutes before their visual responses were tested.[2] The researchers' working hypothesis was simple: After their subjects had absorbed this oxytocin into the basal regions of their brain, its messages would enhance the way the subjects perceived and responded to other persons' faces. Their subjects, all male, then viewed 36 pictures—limited to the eye regions—of different persons' faces. Their task was to select among four options what that person might be thinking or feeling. Oxytocin turned out to help two thirds of the men detect the most subtle social cues by some 3% when contrasted with its placebo.

Normally, intranasal oxytocin inhibits the hypothalamic-pituitary-adrenal axis. This step leads finally to a decrease in the release of cortisol from the adrenal gland. The oxytocin receptor–induced decrease in serum cortisol serves as an indirect test of the functional integrity of this neuroendocrine system. In separate studies, it was observed that children who lose a parent early because of divorce or separation run an increased risk of being depressed when they are adults. To explore the basis for this association, the cortisol responses to intranasal oxytocin were tested in nine healthy men in their twenties. (Each one had experienced such a parental loss before they reached the age of 13 years.) The results were contrasted with ten matched controls.[3] The test subjects showed significantly weakened cortisol responses. These preliminary results suggest that their diminished responses were either (1) genetically determined, or (2) mediated by mechanisms (worthy of further study) that were linked to the various psychosocially adverse circumstances related to their having been deprived of their parent.

Intranasal oxytocin has been shown to generate a substantial increase in interpersonal trust when tested in a model situation involving financial transactions.[4] Even without oxytocin being added, the recipients' perception that a donor is trusting him, and the donor's perception that he himself is being trusted, both correlate with higher blood levels of endogenous oxytocin.[5]

Vasopressin

A similar working hypothesis served as the basis for studying vasopressin, a closely related peptide.[6] Prior research had shown that when vasopressin is given transnasally, it is detectable in spinal fluid ten minutes later and remains elevated for at least 80 minutes. In this study, the subjects looked at pictures of models of the same sex whose facial expressions showed various emotions. Facial EMG, heart rate, and skin conduction responses monitored the subjects' reactions.

Among the women subjects, vasopressin prompted friendly (affiliative) responses toward the faces of the other women pictured. However, when the men viewed the other male faces in the pictures, vasopressin decreased the way they rated the friendliness and approachability of these unfamiliar male faces, *even* when these faces wore expressions that were obviously happy and friendly. An intriguing corollary finding: men who have longstanding aggressive personality disorders have higher vasopressin levels in their spinal fluid.

In sum, the response patterns to vasopressin in women were in the general direction toward "tend and befriend." Among men, the responses were in the opposite direction toward "fight or flight." Men often behave as though they *are* from Mars.

A Testable Hypothesis

Long-term meditative training could increase the endogenous levels of oxytocin but reduce those of vasopressin in spinal fluid. Could meditative training further influence the meditators' responses to the nasal delivery of exogenous oxytocin and vasopressin? The findings of Thompson et al. suggest that such an experiment is feasible, but that the data would need to be interpreted in relation to gender.

57

Did You Really "Have a Good Day?"

> During the day, the optimal point is around noontime as all negative emotions are reduced and all positive emotions are increased well above other points of the working day.
>
> A. Stone and colleagues[1]

Kobori-Roshi introduced me to the way some people in Japan ask their friends: "How is your inner weather?" In fact, this inner weather of our emotions changes substantially during a workday. Stone and colleagues discovered this when they questioned 909 working women about how their hourly emotions varied throughout the period from 7:00 A.M. to 9:00 P.M. The questionnaire listed 12 emotional adjectives. Only three were positive: happy, warm, and enjoy.[2] Most other adjectives described a negative affect. These negative emotions ran the gamut from impatient through frustrated, depressed, hassled, angry, worried, criticized, tired, and depressed.

A glance at the diagrammed swings of their emotions illustrates that a major sharp peak for "impatient" occurs at 4:00 P.M. The lesser peak occurs around 10:00 A.M. "Frustrated" exhibits a similar biphasic pattern, but this emotion is lower in amplitude, and has a slightly higher peak around 10:00 A.M.

These self-rated emotional profiles were different in the younger and older women. The data compared the profiles of women 30 years and under with the profiles of those 50 years and older. For the three positive emotions, the older subjects began their day on a positive note. After the morning hours, they maintained this positive trend with relatively little variation. In contrast, the younger subjects started out lowest in the morning. They didn't reach their first peak until around the noon meal. Then, after the usual 2:00 P.M. postprandial dip, their ratings rose gradually toward higher positive levels in the early evening hours.

The younger subjects tended to be "worrywarts." Their maximum ratings for feeling worried came around 8:00 A.M., but they reported being less worried thereafter. In contrast, the older subjects were less worried in the morning, and didn't reach their worry peak until around 5:00 P.M.

Comment

When you observe your emotions mindfully, you see their amplitudes wax and wane. For meditators, this fact becomes a practical lesson in impermanence, reinforced during a retreat. For investigators, the wide swings in certain emotions during an ordinary day raise a separate practical issue: during longitudinal studies, it can be important to conduct cognitive and emotional tasks at approximately the same hour.

58

Sixth Mondo

The Buddhist Way, the training in Buddhism consists mainly of breaking up I into its component parts and reassembling them in a manner that comes closer to what is truly human.

Myokyo-ni (1921–2007)

You seem to be saying that important but complicated relationships exist between the vagus nerve, the autonomic nervous system, our emotions, and the way we breathe.

Yes. Much more well-controlled research is essential. Stay tuned.

Why can't a person just suppress unwanted emotions?

Top-down willful intentions go only part way. Long-term meditative training helps to sponsor the requisite introspections and deconditionings at deep levels. These support more enduring transformations of consciousness.

What is different about these deep deconditionings?

Brief episodes of selfless insight arrive when the brain shifts into an allocentric mode of processing and engages its receptive, preattentive pathways in other-referential processing.

What's the point in studying how children, adolescents, and adults respond to faces that show emotions, or to tasks in general?

The research suggests potential ways that long-term meditative training could influence brain plasticity and reinforce the trainees' inherent maturational patterns of brain development.

How do current research findings of brain plasticity relate to Siddhartha's legendary enlightenment under the Bodhi tree?

They suggest that many attentive powers of this 35-year-old "Sage of the Sakya clan" had already been highly trained during his rigorous six-year prior meditative quest. At this point, he could have been exceptionally receptive when a bright planet in the pre-dawn sky captured his attention.

Surely, there's more to this story.

Yes, another formative interval of teaching and practice during the next 45 years. After this major episode under the Bodhi tree had further transformed his unusually mature traits of character, it is plausible to consider that his capacities for further realizations of insight-wisdom continued to develop. Indeed, as he related to daily-life events during these next decades, he would then become known as Sakyamuni Buddha.

So, is enlightenment something I can attain?

No. It is a word. It points to the character traits of simplicity and stability that evolve when you keep dropping off your selfish *I-Me-Mine* preoccupations and live a compassionate life with increasing clarity.

Part VII

Updating Selected Research

The art of progress is to preserve order amid change and to preserve change amid order.

Alfred North Whitehead (1861–1947)

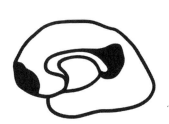

Selected Topics of Current Interest: A Sample

> Science, like life, feeds on its own decay. New facts burst old rules; then newly divined conceptions bind old and new together into a reconciling law.
>
> William James (1842–1910)

Change is in the air. Each month, the swarm of new facts bursts old rules, opening up unexpected vistas. The previous book in this series was published early in 2006, having surveyed the vast Zen-brain literature through the early months of 2005. The pace of research quickened during the following three years. The next pages select three areas of investigation to review and update. For the reader's convenience, the topics follow the general sequence used in the two earlier books, namely: (1) gross functional anatomy, (2) psychophysiology of larger networks, and (3) controversial topics. I apologize to those whose work is not cited here either for lack of space or because it escaped my notice.

Gross Functional Anatomy
The Amygdala

The amygdala is the gateway to our fears [ZBR:85–94]. A fearful amygdala fires faster. Larson and colleagues monitored the fMRI responses of subjects who were afraid of spiders.[1] Their 13 spider-phobic subjects responded faster to phobia-related pictures than did the controls. The data suggested that their amygdala was responding vigorously but briefly to fear-producing stimuli.

Cahill's review documents how diverse are the influences of gender on the amygdala in particular, and on brain function in general.[2] In women, emotionally based visual images preferentially evoke acute responses from the left amygdala; in men, from the right amygdala. As an example, in women the left amygdala is more responsive to happy faces, whereas in men the right amygdala is more responsive to happy faces. Women and men show similar lateralized trends when they actively retrieve emotional material from memory. It seems possible that a careful correlation of first person reports with objective data in the future would disclose that men and women experience kensho differently.

Relevant to meditation are the results of PET scans performed while meditators were simply resting with their eyes closed. In women, the left amygdala tends to covary along with the activity of other brain regions. In men, it is the right amygdala. Cahill suggests that similar trends in laterality—"women left, men right"—reflect asymmetries in their general physiological baseline under resting conditions. Reports in the next section often confirm such a trend.

Nerve cells in the amygdala make a peptide hormone that mediates fear and anxiety behaviors. This corticotrophin-releasing factor (CRF) excites the locus ceruleus down in the brainstem [ZBR.116–120]. The two nuclei are mutually stimulating, because norepinephrine pathways also ascend from the locus ceruleus to excite the amygdala [ZB:201–205]. In female rats, CRF is a stimulus up to 30 times more potent in activating the locus ceruleus than it is in males.[3] In human beings, differences in behavior between men and women might ultimately correlate with similar observations relating both to neuromessengers and to their receptor systems at the cellular level.

The Precuneus and its Potential Functions

The precuneus is the medial extension of the parietal association cortex (shown in figure 2, and again near the top edge of the posterior "hot spot" in figure 5). Currently, the precuneus plays a lesser role in our discussion of Self/other relationships than do the functions of its two close neighbors, the nerve cells in the posterior cingulate and retrosplenial cortex [ZBR:204–205] (chapters 13, 15, 19, 21).

Though the precuneus myelinates late, it goes on to develop the well-differentiated columns and layers of an isocortical structure. Back in 1988, while the writer was engaged in a long interval of quiet, receptive meditation, PET scans of that era showed that the right precuneus was a region of high "resting" metabolism. Research since then—depending on the task—has associated precuneus activities with a wide variety of mental processing at the interface between Self-referential and other-referential functions.[4]

For example, some evidence suggests that the anterior precuneus participates more actively during tasks that engage our capacities to synthesize visuospatial imagery. The (smaller) nerve cells of the posterior precuneus may contribute more to our efforts to retrieve personalized events from memory stores.

Yet, *other*-centered styles of processing tend also to enlist activities represented in the precuneus, including those that arise when visual attention is being diffused in a more global manner.[5] Moreover, the higher resolutions of fMRI show that when we normally localize sounds in external auditory space, we include the right precuneus in the networks that we are using to redirect global auditory attention.[6] A point of related interest is the recent finding that adults who have attention-deficit hyperactivity disorder (ADHD) are deficient in the functional connections that would normally link the precuneus with each end of their cingulate gyrus and their medial prefrontal cortex[7] (chapters 4, 7).

The Insula

The insula is a mound of hidden cortex. It is buried deep in the lateral sylvian fissure, covered over by folds from the frontal and parietal cortex. (In figure 1, it hides deep and posterior to BA 44.) The insula responds during our emotions of disgust, empathy, and love, as well as to interoceptive signals that convey vestibular and other messages from our internal organs. Densely supplied by NMDA glutamate receptors, the insula can act quickly on messages that reach it, even though some had begun slowly in the visceral autonomic pathways far below [ZBR:95–99]. Down in the thalamus, the reticular nucleus is positioned to prevent ascending signals from reaching the insula as they emerge from the ventral medial nucleus.

Some normal people are sensitive to the beating of their own hearts. This heightened visceral sensitivity is termed "interoceptive awareness." The auditory tones from a metronome provide the sounds used to test for this sensitivity. The subject is asked to make a subtle judgement: are these sounds synchronous with the timing of your own silent heartbeats, or not? Source analysis techniques show that during such interoceptive awareness, resources in the subject's right insula are joined by those of the anterior cingulate and prefrontal cortex. Interoceptive awareness can be associated with psychological tendencies to experience emotions more intensely. Supporting this observation, ERP studies indicate that the more sensitive subjects also enhance their P300 amplitudes when they respond to the pleasant *or* unpleasant scenes of emotionally valenced pictures.[8]

The question arises: What happens if the subjects receive *false* feedback information via earphones about the pace of their own heartbeats?[9] The false feedback of an increased heart rate enhanced the salient intensity of neutral faces (but not that of happy or angry faces). At the same time, it also increased fMRI signals in the right anterior insula. One way to interpret these findings is to propose that the insula provides a "comparator" function. When this function detects a mismatch involving the person's own heartbeat, perhaps it regards this as a dissonant event, and joins other regions in an attempt to sharpen the person's attention on what kind of face stimulus is occurring.

This interpretation views the anterior insula as part of the first-order system representing and governing our bodily arousal; it regards the amygdala as encoding the valence of emotionally salient events; and it assigns to the superior temporal gyrus and the lateral temporal cortex the roles of providing second-order layers of interpretation and higher cognitive appraisal.

During studies of human conditioning, fMRI signals indicate that the anterior insula and the orbitofrontal cortex register the coded *valence* of all stimuli, whether the stimuli are appetitive (+) or aversive (−).[10] The anterior insula responds, as does the overlying fold of frontal operculum that covers it, not only to disgusting tastes and smells but also to tastes that are pleasant, unpleasant, or neutral.[11] In addition, when subjects consider themselves as having greater degrees of (self-reported) empathy, they tend to increase fMRI signals in their own insula while they witness *other* persons' pleased or disgusted facial expressions to food.

These new findings extend the empathic functions of our anterior insula and nearby frontal operculum in a positive direction, showing that our response patterns are not limited to other persons' negative expressions of disgust or pain. Indeed, recent fMRI research suggests that the anterior insula shares in the general "sense of fairness or unfairness" that develops when subjects play experimental games with monetary rewards.[12] Chapter 54 suggests anatomical reasons why the right anterior insula is a region prominent among the brain's emotional asymmetries. Chapter 55 indicates that the frontal operculum and insula are also components of a much larger network that helps sustain task performance in general and develops greater independence in adult life (table 16).

Interoceptive sensations threaten certain anxiety-prone individuals. One explanation for this may lie in a neural circuit that includes the anterior insula.[13] Stein and colleagues selected an anxiety-prone group of 16 college students and compared their responses with those of 16 other students whose trait anxiety scores fell in the normal range.[14] Both groups were then monitored with fMRI while they viewed faces that showed different emotions. The anxiety-prone students developed more fMRI signals in their amygdala and insula on both sides. Activations in their amygdala (L) and in their anterior insula (R, L) were associated with psychological tests showing greater degrees of anxiety.

Sarinopoulos and colleagues were concerned about how the power of a prior belief influences test results, and posed a different question.[15] Suppose we first mislead our subjects, allowing them to believe that a forthcoming taste will be only slightly aversive. Does the power inherent in this suggested belief exert a subsequent placebo-like dampening effect on the way their taste circuitry responds in the insula and elsewhere? [ZBR:128–135]. It turned out that the researchers' positive reassuring suggestion that the next taste would be only slightly bad *did* correlate with *decreased* responses in the insula and amygdala when their subjects actually received a much more aversive taste stimulus.

What influenced the *degree* to which the subjects reported that this (bad) taste seemed only mildly aversive? This subjective report correlated with how much their orbital frontal and rostral anterior cingulate gyrus had been activated earlier, at the time when they had first received their reassuring (but misleading) suggestion. The studies point to a "belief" network that becomes active during the placebo effect. With respect to taste, the power of positive thinking taps into this belief circuitry. It includes the functions of the insula, the orbitofrontal cortex, and the anterior cingulate region [ZBR:269–270].

Subliminally, we're constantly informed that we possess a physical body by sensory messages reaching our somatosensory cortex and superior parietal lobule. The insula contributes subtle integrative functions to this subconscious sense that our own soma is the agent responsible for an action.[16] Tsarikiris and colleagues in London used the "rubber hand illusion" to study how normal subjects respond when they misperceive that a fake hand is an integral part of their own body.[17] During PET scanning, the subjects saw that either a right rubber hand or a left rubber hand was being touched. At the same instant, *their own* right hand (masked from sight) might also be touched. During the rubber hand illusion, subjects sense that their own hand shifts toward the position of the fake hand. PET activity increases in their right *posterior* insula and right frontal operculum during this projected illusion of "body ownership" In contrast, even when the subjects' own hand is *not* being touched at the same time, PET activity increases in the appropriate hand region of their somatosensory cortex in the opposite parietal lobe.

The insula enters into longings in subtle ways, participating in sensual, tactile sensations of a sexual nature. When these are delivered to the erect male penis, PET signals increase throughout the *posterior* insula and the nearby secondary somatosensory cortex.[18]

In 29 healthy women, behavioral studies indicated that the closer they felt emotionally to their partner, the more they reported being satisfied with the orgasm they received from their partner.[19] No correlation was found between the intensity of this love relationship and the frequency of these orgasms. Next the subjects were monitored with fMRI while they were receiving, subconsciously, subliminal presentations of their partner's name. Increased signals in their left anterior insula correlated with the prior reports of frequency and the qualitative satisfaction of their orgasms. On the other hand, the intensity with which they had reported being in love was associated with a network involving the angular gyrus [ZBR:255–259].

The anterior insula seems to be one part of a circuit that supports the craving for cigarettes [ZBR:84]. Patients who suffer brain damage to their insula are more likely to abandon easily their habitual addiction to cigarette smoking, and to have fewer relapses than do smokers who sustain damage to regions elsewhere in the brain.[20]

Structural MRI studies on 20 Vipassana meditators who each had practiced on average over 6000 hours each showed that the gray matter concentration was greater in their right insula than in that of the matched controls.[21] This supports the earlier finding by Lazar and colleagues that the right anterior insula was significantly thicker in long-experienced, regular meditators than in controls.[22]

Structural MRI studies contrasted the gray matter volumes of 12 adolescent male patients from an "aggression clinic" in Germany with 12 age and intelligence-matched normal controls. The patients had been diagnosed as having a conduct disorder.[23] Their gray matter volumes were significantly reduced in the anterior insula (R, L) and in the left amygdala. The localized reductions in these patients correlated with their lower psychometric evaluations for empathy, as well as with increased responses consistent with impulsiveness and venture-someness.

The Ventral Medial and Orbitofrontal Cortex

The frontal lobes provide us with a seemingly endless portfolio of practical, "intel-ligent," higher-order associative functions [ZBR:158–167]. Patients who have ventral medial prefrontal damage show significantly impaired judgment prefer-ences.[24] In male patients, damage to this ventral medial prefrontal cortex on the *right* side causes severe defects in their social/emotional and decision-making functions. In women, comparable defects are more marked after damage occurs to the left side.[25]

What does the orbitofrontal cortex contribute? (chapters 4 and 52). Simpli-fied explanations suggest that it helps derive a relative value signal that enters into the decision of how rewarding ($+$) or threatening ($-$) is a given stimulus.[26] Thereafter, once this orbital value signal is held in working memory, (a) the dor-solateral frontal cortex helps plan and supervise ongoing behavior, and (b) the medial prefrontal cortex helps evaluate how much effort is required to meet the desired goal.

Positive social attachment responses correlate with increased fMRI signals in the *medial* orbitofrontal cortex and in nearby portions of the ventral cingulate cor-tex (BA 25) and septal region.[27] In contrast, *lateral* orbitofrontal activity is associ-ated with negative decisions that oppose societal causes. Costly decisions (either to donate or to oppose) generate more signals from the frontal-polar cortex (BA 10) and medial prefrontal gyrus. Looping circuits link the orbital cortex into be-havioral networks that include the ventral candate, globus pallidus and thalamus.

Several lines of evidence indicate that major bidirectional pathways from the amygdala to the orbitofrontal region provide the negative feedback that serves as a normal brake to inhibit behavior [ZBR:160–162]. PET scans monitored the sex-ual climax of 12 normal women during four different conditions. These included sexual arousal, clitoral stimulation, clitorally induced orgasm, or imitation of or-gasm (the last served as the control for motor output).[28] The left lateral orbitofron-tal cortex showed the most *de*activation during orgasm when compared with the ordinary resting state. This decrease in activation was interpreted as evidence consistent with the subject's release from prior behavioral inhibition. Lesser deac-tivations developed in the left inferior temporal gyrus and the anterior temporal pole. In men, PET scan studies confirmed that their *de*activations occurred throughout the prefrontal cortex during ejaculation, in addition to the other wide-spread activations within motor regions.[29]

Psychophysiological Responses in Larger Networks
Relationships between Brain Waves and Higher Networking Functions

How does the brain blend its networks' widely different oscillating frequencies into our coherent conscious and subconscious functions? This continues to be a fertile ground for speculation.[1] A close look at any network within either the physical sciences or the life sciences shows that it manifests two general properties: (1) It coalesces into small, dense clusters. (2) Its connections extend out into intervening space, enabling these local clusters to engage in long-distance global interactions.[2]

Viewed from this larger perspective, our higher mental functions also exhibit two general properties:

- Functional *segregation* enables us rapidly to extract highly selected bytes of information from our external and internal environment.

- Functional *integration* enables us to integrate such discrete information into more coherent, overarching brain states.

Our brains' distributed networks exemplify the same general organizing principle (chapter 55) [ZBR:40–53]. Bassett and colleagues recorded MEG signals from 275 points over the scalp of 22 normal subjects.[3] *At rest*, their activities were distributed throughout the range between slow delta and slow gamma (from 1.1 to 37 cps) in a manner that was both highly clustered *and* highly integrated. Next, their subjects performed a simple *active* task: finger tapping in response to a visual cue. While the subjects' basic MEG patterns remained similar to those at rest, they now showed long-range connectivities within the gamma and *beta* bands. The authors suggest that when we transfer messages from site to site, we use time-related (*temporal*) binding to distribute them within circuits that transmit in particular frequencies. Further phasic modulations are superimposed. In this respect, the dynamic, up-and-down fluctuations in the synchrony of gamma waves could provide different networks with the basic mechanism they need to reconfigure their long-distance connections in *spatial* terms. For example, frontal networks could use such spatial reconfigurations of gamma waves to help modulate distant cortical and subcortical functions.

When Mantini and colleagues recently identified six different intrinsic resting state networks (RSNs), their "RSN 1" cluster tended to correspond with the posterior medial and lateral parietal regions that some researchers refer to with the term "default network."[4] Its EEG signature correlated positively with alpha (8 to 13 cps) and beta (13 to 30 cps) EEG rhythms. In contrast, their "RSN 2" cluster corresponded closely with the dorsal attention system (table 4). Its EEG activities were negatively correlated with alpha and beta rhythms. They related the "RSN 6" cluster to "self-referential" mental activity. This network included the ventral-medial prefrontal cortex and the nearby anterior cingulate region. Its EEG signature correlated with gamma activities (30 to 50 cps). In contrast, the dedicated visual regions were associated with slower rhythms in the delta (1 to 4 cps) and theta (4 to 8 cps) range.

When Kounios and colleagues recently monitored 26 young adults, those who later went on to solve word anagram problems with insight strategies already showed distinctive EEG profiles *at rest*[5] (chapter 34). In their occipital regions at rest, they showed lesser degrees of slow alpha activity (8 to 9.75 cps). This was interpreted as consistent with a generally more active, more open (and less prematurely focused) style of visual receptivity. Such an attitude could allow more creative individuals the chance to sample "a greater range of environmental stimuli." In addition, this group who typically used insight strategies already showed at rest a *right*-sided predominance of beta-2 power (at 18 to 24.75 cps) over their inferior frontal and anterior temporal leads.

Linguistic Implications of Monkeying with Tools

In the laboratory, Iriki's team helped adult monkeys learn how to use a long-handled rake [ZBR:150–152]. Gradually, their educated monkeys extend this rake to retrieve an apple slice that lies beyond their grasp. On their own, no monkeys in the wild develop this skill spontaneously. Training enables the monkeys to enlarge their bimodal somatosensory and visual fields, make their expanding "hand image" actionable, and extend their body schema in an imaginative manner to "assimilate" the tool.[6] Histological studies confirm that monkeys forge novel brain connections after having been trained for only two weeks in this novel use of the rake. Notably, these new connections link their intraparietal sulcus (iPSUL) with their temporoparietal junction (TPJ) (figure 1). This remarkable demonstration of plasticity in the brain of a primate relative is highly relevant to meditative training. It suggests that when parietal nerve cells that are involved in attention learn how to fire together, they can also *wire together* [ZBR:140–141].

That's not all. The results have now evolved in a way that invites a further stretch of the imagination on the part of the monkey and the reader. The monkey's acquired skill goes on to *generalize*. Only those monkeys who were first trained to use tools can develop a new, second, socially useful skill: they start to make voluntary, arbitrary vocalizations. These sounds enable them to report specific objects and particular events. No wild monkeys exhibit this sophisticated form of specialized "speech."

The preliminary step is a trained monkey who, having become aware of its hand and arm, is using these extremities in novel ways that render them equivalent to an external tool. Iriki hypothesizes that training the monkey to develop such an explicit awareness of its own body parts enables the brain's latent capacities to emerge. This boost in the innate capacity of a primate relative suggests the kinds of potential avenues during hominid evolution that might slowly have linked tool usage with the emergence of socially specialized speech.

When meditators practice similarly explicit mindfulness skills, they can also begin with a body scan that focuses attention on particular parts of their bodies and on other stimulus events. Tables 1 and 5 indicate that receptive modes of meditative attention can supervene. Research is gradually documenting the ways that this subsequent processing influences the plasticity and the structure of the brain and enables other subtle long-term latent capacities to emerge.

Getting Personally Located and Navigating Inside Space

We move around a lot in our environment. How does the brain keep track of where our head is pointing in space, so that it "heads" in the direction we want to go? [ZBR:106–108, 153, 172–174, 201–203]. Head direction cells encode how an animal perceives the direction it is heading in with reference to its environment.[7] From the anterior nucleus of the thalamus, many messages about heading relay to the dorsal subiculum, then flow into the entorhinal cortex in the front of the long parahippocampal gyrus [ZB:183–189].

This entorhinal cortex is an intriguing terminus for head direction signals. Here, researchers recently discovered an overlapping, hexagonal latticework of "grid cells." This cellular architecture provides the framework enabling an elementary mapping system to feed precise data on for further processing by the "place" cells of the hippocampal formation [ZBR:100–102]. The roles the human hippocampus plays in allocentric processing and navigation are still being discussed.[8]

Navigation requires sophisticated forms of topographical processing. We have two ways to navigate. We can use our own actual on-the-spot skills (called route skills), or we can refer to a 2-D map and interpret what we see. When we acquire fresh, on-the-spot knowledge about a route, we first use two successive landmarks, then correlate these separate viewpoints with the direction and distance our body has moved in the interim.[9] Subjects can be monitored with fMRI while such complex navigation skills are being tested in a "virtual reality" environment. Note that during their encoding phase, signals increase in the medial frontal gyrus, retrosplenial cortex, and posterioinferior parietal cortex. However, as the subjects later become more skillful, signals increase only in the pootcroinferior parietal regions. This evidence confirms the dynamic parietal contribution to selfothering operations when we engage in first-hand on-the-spot navigation.

Survey learning is different because it is based on navigation skills acquired while reading maps. Map-reading expertise correlates with increased fMRI signals in the retrosplenial cortex on both sides.[10] The posterior parahippocampal gyrus participates in the initial encoding phase, both when we associate an object with a given location, and when a location is associated with a given object. In contrast, signals increase in the left anterior parahippocampal gyrus and in the right anterior medial temporal lobe when we retrieve memories that accurately relate a particular object to a given location.[11]

The Remarkable Properties of Nitric Oxide

We include nitric oxide in this discussion because it exerts a pervasive influence on all networks. Nitric oxide (NO·) is a gas that acts as a highly reactive free radical [ZBR:279–288]. Early research suggested that NO· caused a major increase in the second messenger, cGMP (cyclic guanosine monophosphate). Subsequent studies revealed that NO· has multiple versatile properties. These are potentially important both to the Path of Zen and to brain functions in general [ZB:412–413; ZBR:407–410, 414–432].

Edwards and Rickard begin their recent review with data showing that NO· has an essential role in consolidating memories.[12] For example, in the hippocampus, NO· plays a key role in long-term potentiation and in long-term depression. Here, two different forms of the enzyme synthesize NO·. One form resides inside nerve cells. It generates phasic NO· signals. In contrast, the other synthase occurs in smaller hippocampal blood vessels. Its NO· is the source for the tonic ongoing signals required for the long-term potentiation of memories.[13]

After normal nerve impulses begin in one hemisphere of the brain, they can cross over the corpus callosum to generate local field potentials on the opposite side. Researchers can measure the neuronal "traffic" on this transcallosal system. Some results show that the local field potentials are not decreased even after NO· has been inhibited, and after local blood flow has been reduced by 50%.[14] In other tests of this same transcallosal system, glutamate receptors of the AMPA type *do* help couple cerebral blood flow with the local field potentials. However, tests using a different (somatosensory) system in rat brain have employed the same chemical inhibitor to stop neuronal NO· production. In one report, this inhibitor blocked both the cerebral blood flow response and the fMRI signal, yet it did not cause much change in the sensory evoked potentials themselves.[15] A recent report supports the critical role of neuronally produced NO· in enhancing blood flow, BOLD responses and somatosensory evoked responses.[16] It is essential to reconcile such disparate findings. Vitally important to the ways NO· enters into our understanding of Zen and the brain is how and where its signals influence the brain's blood flow, the fast responses and slow rhythms of its fMRI signals, and its actual neuronal discharges, both locally and at a distance [ZBR:281–282].

In these pages, we refer metaphorically to a bodhisattva (Manjusuri) who "wields the flashing sword of insight-wisdom." Based on its neurochemical properties, NO· is a *two-edged* sword. In in vitro slice preparations, NO· increases the frequency of inhibitory discharges in the lateral geniculate and ventral basal nuclei of the thalamus in a manner consistent with the increased release of GABA from terminals of the reticular nucleus.[17] This suggests an additional source for reinforcing the inhibitory functions of the reticular nucleus (chapter 19). NO· also inhibits cellular respiration in mitochondria secondary to its inhibition of cytochrome-oxidase.[18] (On the other hand, melatonin down-regulates NO· synthase in a manner that reduces some of the harmful effects of its toxic NO· byproduct, peroxynitrite.[19])

NO· has multiple actions, both beneficial and harmful. These actions render it a plausible candidate for some mechanisms intrinsic both to the flash of kensho—to its sword-like cut through the psychic layers of the overconditioned Self—and to a variety of its transforming aftereffects. Serving as a potential example is the latest molecule that mimics nitric oxide: it stimulates the cGMP signal transduction system, *and* reverses the spatial learning deficits caused by acetycholine depletion.[20] This result in an experimental model serves as a reminder that messenger molecules can have beneficial consequences on cognition. These can be both immediate and delayed [ZB:223–225, 659, 794].

With regard to an earlier suggestion that 3-nitrotyrosine could be a useful chemical fingerprint for NO· [ZBR:285], such acute changes after kensho clearly must be distinguished from similar findings in the inferior parietal lobule and hippocampus reported in association with mild cognitive impairment.[21] At present, the wealth of preliminary evidence from *pre*clinical studies suggests that it will take decades to specify with precision what all the cause-and-effect clinical implications of NO· will be for human subjects.[22]

Dusek and colleagues conducted preliminary studies of NO· in the air exhaled by meditators who were enrolled in an eight-weeks' audiotaped relaxation response (RR) course.[23] Interested readers are referred to the authors' discussion and to their accompanying list of 100 relevant references for an appreciation of how difficult it is now to distinguish changes in NO· and its byproducts in the body as a whole from dynamic psychophysiological events that originate within the central nervous system itself.

Successive waves of excitation, inhibition, and disinhibition sculpture the contours of each alternate state of consciousness, enabling the sequence of its phenomena to evolve from start to finish. For example, when a state of internal absorption begins with a visual hallucination, this epiphenomenon serves as a point of distinction from the late visual illusions at the offset of kensho [ZBR:451; table 12].

Fox and colleagues studied the general nature of onset and offset phenomena.[24] They monitored subjects with fMRI during four separate blocks of tasks: working memory, an eyes-open condition, reading, and the analysis of a scene. Signals increased abruptly at the transition intervals between these simple tasks. In each instance, at the moment when attention shifted, large signals arose from three now-familiar sites: the right temporoparietal junction (TPJ), the right precuneus, and the posterior cingulate gyrus. The right TPJ was the most responsive region.

Separate ERP studies confirm that this TPJ makes a major contribution to the prominent P300 potential that develops at the instant we shift mental sets. Moreover, certain transitions give rise to unique response profiles. This observation suggests that a transition is a dynamic interim phase, one that has the potential to yield unique mental phenomena. Instabilities are inherent when existing brain functions are undergoing such rapid reorganizations. Rapid changes invite substates first to dissociate, then to coalesce in novel alternate forms of consciousness.[25] Zen traditions emphasize that triggering stimuli have the potential to shift attention, enabling alternate states to arise (chapter 23) (figure 7).

Controversial Topics
A Sense of "Presence"

Impartial observers recognize that authentic teachers like the Dalai Lama and Thich Nhat Hanh have an *ongoing* quality of character. Their followers describe it as a kind of "presence," a genuine manifestation of compound character traits distinguishable from charisma. The same word, "presence," is used in different ways in relation to mystical experiences, some of which have attracted controversial interpretations [ZBR:157, 191–192].

In the Persinger laboratory in Ontario, Canada, more than 400 subjects have been exposed to transcranial weak, complex magnetic fields during the past two decades. Some subjects report "sensing a presence." The Canadian authors state that the reason Granqvist et al. did not confirm their results was that the subjects in Sweden had "never received an effective field configuration."[1] A subsequent report suggested that the results in one subgroup of 39 Canadian subjects could even have received a subtle boost from the local (Ontario) increase in the Earth's geomagnetic activity (magnetometer-measured) during the particular three-hour period in which the experiences had been induced.[2]

The reply from Sweden seems limited to one analysis of the psychological data on their original subjects.[3] This analysis relied on two definitions. The authors defined an "explicit religious interpretation" as one in which a given subject might say: "I had an experience in which ultimate reality was revealed to me." In contrast, the alternate definition—that of a mystical experience *without* an "explicit religious interpretation"—was one in which the subject might say: "I had an experience in which I realized the oneness of myself with all things."

This follow-up article suggested that the religious individuals in the Swedish study were *not* more suggestible than were the other participants who evidenced a lesser degree of religiousness. Indeed, their psychological analyses suggested that, when religiousness was thus defined, it was not a quality related to aspects of suggestibility, or associated with the traits of absorption, or with "new age characteristics." The authors concluded that their religious Swedish participants (thus defined) were not necessarily prone to have mystical experiences, but simply went on to *interpret*, in religious terms, "the same-level experiences that non-religious participants had."

Adding to the current asymmetry of the exchange between the two groups is the array of evidence St.-Pierre and Persinger marshaled recently in support of their claim that "the sensed presence" of a "Sentient Being" is an experience that is "reliably evoked by very specific temporal patterns of weak (less than 1 microtesla) transcerebral magnetic fields applied across the temporoparietal region of the two hemispheres."[4] Their subsequent experiments indicate that the subjects' prior beliefs can be correlated with the parameters of stimulation, the particular side of the brain that happens to be stimulated, and with the hemisphere to which the stimulation is maximized. Their subjects are said typically to develop "intense, very emotional presences" at times when they generate more alpha rhythms over the temporal lobes (relative to the occipital lobes), and when the complex burst-firing magnetic fields are applied bilaterally.

Although their blindfolded subjects are enclosed in a quiet chamber with a device that has been called "the God machine,"[5] or the "God helmet," the authors concluded that, "Suggestibility was not responsible for the magnetic field effects." Preferential right hemispheric stimulation for 30 minutes within a frequency-modulated field resulted (in more than 80% of the cases) with the sensed presence being felt along the left side. A sense of "evil" arose more often in association with the left-sided experiences, and "marked personal pleasantness" was more often associated with right-sided presences.

Commentary

The temporal lobe has well-known vulnerabilities to déjà vu phenomena. The lateral temporoparietal regions have long been associated with a variety of impressionable experiences [ZBR:414–425]. A recent article in the *New England Journal of Medicine* linked direct stimulation of the right posterior part of the superior temporal gyrus with repeated out-of-body experiences.[6] Psychophysiogical thresholds for responding vary from person to person. This physiological variability must be taken into account during the interpretation of experimental data, and also when evaluating the descriptions that meditation trainees report to their teachers [ZBR:455–457]. The time-honored meditative path is oriented toward incremental, long-term character change. This change evolves as the result of the subject's various internalized practices of attentional training and internal transformations. Artificial experiences induced by electrical currents or drugs are foreign to the Way of Zen.

What Is the Relationship between Seizures and Mystical Experience?

Some patients with epilepsy report unusual "mystical" symptoms only *during* their seizures. Other patients who have epilepsy show unusual behavioral abnormalities during the long intervals *between* their overt seizures. What is an authentic religious experience, and how do seizures relate to it? The whole area remains controversial [ZB:405–407, 349]. Only rarely during a focal temporal lobe seizure does a neurological patient experience some "positive" symptoms consistent with the distinctive psychic state we associate with an authentic "religious" experience. A careful history distinguishes such a rare episode from the fully developed extraordinary alternate states of kensho-satori [ZBR:154–157, 423–424].

   The rarity of the former "religious/seizure" condition is illustrated by a report from an outpatient seizure clinic in Japan.[7] Symptoms regarded as "religious, and related to isolated seizures" occurred in only 3 of 234 patients. Each patient was unusual. Episodes of *psychosis* followed some of their seizures. Moreover, during the intervals between seizures, the patients often showed exaggerated religious preoccupations and behaviors (hyperreligiosity). Electroencephalograms in all three cases showed spike discharges in the anterior temporal region. In two of these, the EEG discharge arose on the left side. The side was not specified in the third patient.

   One other patient, a 35-year old man, had partial complex seizures, and showed evidence of right temporal lobe atrophy on his MRI scan.[8] Between seizures, he exhibited hyperreligiosity together with hyposexuality and humorlessness. On the other hand, no "religious" symptoms occurred during his overt seizures. His sophisticated drawings and paintings of many buildings and houses suggested that he had hypergraphic tendencies.

Some patients who have temporal lobe seizures have silent, recurrent focal temporal lobe spike discharges in their EEG, yet their clinical behavior at these moments does not change.[9] Recently, fMRI has monitored these *sub*clinical EEG discharges. During the spike discharges, fMRI signals are simultaneously reduced in the precuneus, medial prefrontal (BA 8/9), and supramarginal gyrus on the same side.[10] During these distant, local deactivations, hippocampal fMRI signals show transient increases on the same side. However, no hippocampal signals correlate with any particular local anatomical *site* of the EEG spike discharge within the rest of that same temporal lobe. What specific mechanisms relate these clinically silent EEG spikes to reduced fMRI signals both in the precuneus and medial prefrontal area? Would more incisive questioning and testing reveal that some patients manifest a corresponding diminution of Self-relational mentation at these times? Further study is essential.[11]

Does Meditation Increase the Frequency of Seizures?

Some claim that meditation could increase a person's susceptibility to epilepsy.[12] Others reply that meditators who practice the TM technique may show decreased symptoms of epilepsy.[13] An intermediate point of view is also available.[14]

Sleep loss is a very important precipitating cause of seizures. Hyperventilation and low blood sugar also precipitate seizures. A person already susceptible to having seizures should avoid losing sleep, hyperventilating, fasting, and exposure to unusual degrees of physical or mental stress [ZB:235–240]. Rarely does a patient who has temporal lobe seizures manifest a full-fledged hyperreligious personality. If these few patients might later choose to meditate, they could attract unusual attention.

On the other hand, most other people who follow a conservative meditative program can experience some of its positive long-range benefits on various aspects of their mental and physical hygiene (chapter 2). For example, 13 experienced Zen practitioners (each having a minimum of 1000 hours of practice) breathed more slowly, had a higher baseline threshold for pain, and experienced less pain while attending mindfully than did their controls.[15] Greater degrees of practice experience correlated with greater reduction in their experience of pain. Transcendental meditation is reported to reduce the responses to experimental pain at the thalamic level.[16] During Yoga meditation, a Yoga master has shown decreased MEG responses in the primary and secondary somatosensory cortex to noxious laser pain stimulation.[17] fMRI signals were also reduced in the thalamus, the insula, and the cingulate cortex.

In summary, any patient already susceptible to seizures is advised to avoid the kinds of excessive stress-producing events that can occur during rigorous retreats. Yet some patients who have an established seizure disorder could benefit substantially from long-term *conservative* meditative practices. Clearly, individual patients should seek a physician's advice about the best course of action. Zen meditation isn't for everyone, nor is meditation a panacea for all persons who happen to have a tendency toward excessive neuronal discharges.

Semantic Problems in Reconciling Neuroimaging Data with Psychological Terminology

PET scans over a decade ago showed that a large cluster of regions was unusually active at rest. Surprisingly, these regions *reduced their activity* during so-called "goal-oriented tasks" (chapter 13). These brisk task-induced *deactivations* led to this cluster becoming referred to—in shorthand—as "the default network."

Notably, this same cluster of so-called "task-negative" regions also: (a) became *more* activated during various Self-referential functions, (b) was quickly *de*activated whenever attention served its implicit pointing function at the tip of our externally oriented goal-directed behaviors, (c) was hardly ever empty of thoughts. Instead, it was usually preoccupied, at a descriptive phenomenological level, in countless discursive, Self-driven thoughts, even during passive resting conditions in the neuroimaging laboratory.

Substantial semantic issues would complicate the notion that some ultimate baseline, one-level, "default" state might have been reached that has an accurately-matched psychological equivalent in a "baseline" state of consciousness, at least in the neuroimaging literature reported thus far. In principle, we believe in baseline estimations [ZBR:193–199]. However, it has been suggested elsewhere that our ordinary states of consciousness include at least three different categories, that kensho and satori represent a different level, and that ultimate Being might represent an even more extraordinary "basal baseline" state on the endless meditative path [ZB:298–305].

Does Functional Connectivity fMRI Yield "Real" Data?

One could question the validity of the connectivity data in the pioneering fMRI articles (chapter 22). Doubts hinged on the possibility that the slow intrinsic fluctuations were mostly artifacts secondary to subtle cardiac or respiratory (CO_2) changes. Other concerns related to the several seconds' lag time between actual nerve cell discharges and an fMRI signal that reflects subtle differences in magnetic properties between oxygen-rich and oxygen-depleted blood [ZBR:188–189].

Yet other data soon weighed against such doubts. The spontaneous fluctuations in fMRI signals were coherent within networks that were well-defined anatomically and physiologically. In actual practice, a passive rest condition could be used as a quasi-baseline control period, and so-called seed regions could serve as anatomical sites of reference. Soon, the new data analysis technique of independent component analysis confirmed that the fluctuations were reproducible.

Two intriguing reports from the St. Louis group correlated these spontaneous slow fluctuations with significant degrees of variability in subjects' voluntary task performance. The first task seemed simple: watch a movie passively that showed a person performing ordinary domestic chores; then watch it later with a specific active goal in mind.[18] During this later viewing, the subjects pressed a button with their right index finger each time they discerned a clear transition between the major events in the movie. Their event-related fMRI responses turned out to vary from trial to trial in a manner suggesting that the spontaneous fluctuations were almost linearly superimposed on the varying signals of the task-related activities.

The authors recently confirmed these results, monitoring subjects who were looking at a white crosshair centered in a black screen.[19] At rest, the fMRI signals of the one subject shown fluctuated 1.5 times a minute. Later, the task for all subjects was to voluntarily sharpen their attention and then press a response button with their right index finger whenever they saw this crosshair fade from white to dark gray. The force of this button pressing varied. Some 74% of this spontaneous variability in performance correlated with their intrinsic fluctuations in fMRI signal activity.

The 161 references in the latest review by Fox and Raichle confirm that functional connectivity fMRI (fcMRI) is a useful, vital, dynamic index of the brain's spontaneous intrinsic activity.[20] Future studies need to clarify precisely how and when the rhythms of particular intrinsic fluctuating shifts are to be correlated with events all along the Path of Zen.

A Return of the "Magic Mushroom?"

A classic study of psilocybin was conducted on Good Friday in a positive religious setting four and a half decades ago [ZB:436–439, 441–443]. Recently, Griffiths and colleagues at Johns Hopkins contrasted the responses to psilocybin and methylphenidate (Ritalin) in an elegantly designed, triple-blind, crossover study. Their 36 carefully screened mature volunteers averaged 46 years of age.[21] The subjects were monitored individually, wore a mask that covered their eyes, and listened to classical music through headphones while they lay on a couch in an "aesthetic living room-like" setting.

On psilocybin, 22 subjects fulfilled the earlier criteria for having "a complete mystical experience." After methylphenidate, only four did so. During the first seven hours, seven subjects experienced significant episodes of fear, and six had transient ideas of reference/paranoia. Two months later, follow-up telephone interviews of three outside observers verified that, in the interim, their individual subjects had undergone a positive attitudinal and behavioral experience.

From the layered perspectives of the Food and Drug Administration, the Drug Enforcement Agency, the Johns Hopkins Institutional Review Board, and its Department of Psychiatry and Behavioral Sciences, this study was believed to have worthwhile objectives that could justify the minimal risks it posed to its many mature spiritual seekers, 20 of whom had postgraduate degrees.

We live in a drugged culture. Illegal drugs are out there already causing major disruptions in the social fabric [ZB:440–443; ZBR:291–302]. One never knows how many disadvantageous long-term unintended results will be encouraged in the public at large by the fallout from such a "magic mushroom" experiment, given how readily psychedelic drugs tend to fall into less scrupulous hands.

From the age-old perspective of Zen Buddhism, the orthodox Path of moderation begins with ethical layers of Self-disciplined renunciations. (Skt: *shila*) Self-indulgent behavior of every kind is viewed as the legitimate target for training one's traits of character. How is the use of drugs to pursue a "spiritual" journey seen from this perspective? As one more attachment of the pejorative Self, one more "need," one more yielding to the deluded notion that a quick fix could be an acceptable shortcut toward authentic selflessness.

Do Current Quantum Theories Explain Certain Paranormal Phenomena?

How could events that influence one group of isolated nerve cells produce coherent changes in a separate group of distant, shielded nerve cells?[22] [ZBR:192–193]. Theories that relate spontaneous coherence among human brains to a kind of "universal field"[23] remain controversial when they try to explain precisely how energy changes might be transmitted that modify the function of a distant nervous system.[24]

In Closing

What we do know is the greatest hindrance to our learning what we don't know.

Claude Bernard (1813–1878)

The Zen way is a demanding way, but it leads to the depths, to the light of clearly seeing what is when the veil is rent, and to the warmth of heart that touches and engenders growth.

Myokyo-ni[1]

Little insights come as grace notes, usually when one is in solitude. Lighting up our ordinary lives, insights arrive more often after the meditative Path has incubated difficult questions for a long time and begun to ripen into open moments of no-thought clarity.

Meanwhile, regular daily life practice and meditative retreats have continued to hone a variety of subtle top-down and bottom-up skills, both attentive and intuitive. First, the mental landscape is quickened by small surges, then opened partially by the absorptions, and finally turned inside out by kensho's seismic transformations. Only in that rare, deep selfless state does our generic process of intuition unveil its innate other-relational mode of operation. This underlying version of consciousness, shorn of Self-centered intrusions, finally sees into all things as *THEY* really are.

The meditative neurosciences are just beginning to study these Self/other issues. Some newer psychophysiological techniques detect subtle changes in waveforms during the early milliseconds of the brain's responses (ERP, EEG, and MEG). Others reflect changes during the first seconds of the brain's activity as indexed by the varying degrees of oxygenation of its local blood supply (fMRI) or metabolism (PET). The Zen Way looks far beyond the initial results of these first milliseconds, seconds, and early months. It asks, what influence will they have on the lifelong commitment to practice a living Zen?

A few current theories, plausible today, address Self/other issues in ways that clarify how meditation can gradually transform one's consciousness during the daily life practice of mindful attention and the rare moments of insightful illumination.

Now the reader is invited to let go of all such intellectual concepts. Instead, let your footsteps lead you toward that more open awareness first awaiting you on the cushion and the mat. Remember, Zen isn't what you think *it* is. It's more about what is revealed when you let go of your thinking Self.

Glossary

Talking about Zen all the time is like looking for fish tracks in a dry riverbed.

Master Wuzu Fayan (d. 1104)[1]

As soon as you rationalize, Zen becomes hard to understand. Stop rationalizing. Then you'll get it.

Master Foyan Quingyuan (1067–1120)

achronia   Consciousness lacking a sense of time. A zero state of time.

agnosia   A failure to recognize what is clearly perceived. Visual agnosia implies that an object, though seen, is not consciously recognized. But note that some other sensory avenue, such as touch, might still permit the person to identify this object.

amygdala   The complex of nuclei, concentrated near the inner tip of each temporal lobe, which helps generate fear and other emotions.

basal ganglia   The paired deep nuclei on either side of the brain which integrate patterns of motor responses. They include the caudate, putamen, globus pallidus, and substantia nigra.

blindsight   Responding to visual stimuli without being consciously able to "see" them, by using the second visual system which projects through the superior colliculus and the pulvinar.

brainstem   The enlarged stalk which lies between the large forebrain and the long spinal cord. It consists of medulla, pons, and midbrain.

cerebrum   The major, forebrain enlargement of the central nervous system. It lies above the midbrain, and contains the outer layer of cortex, as well as deeper structures such as the basal ganglia, thalamus, and limbic system.

cognition   Our process of knowing in the broadest sense.

coherence   A technical term indicating that the profile of EEG waves in one region resembles that in another. It suggests that both regions are yoked at deeper subcortical or transcortical levels.

conditioned reflex   A basic reflex which has been so modified by past experience that it can now be prompted by a new, conditioned stimulus.

disinhibition   The release of a previously inhibited cell into increased firing, or a release of behavior. In either instance, a prior inhibitory brake is removed.

electroencephalogram (EEG)   The recording of the brain's waves of electrical activity. Electrodes are placed on the scalp, in the cortex (electrocorticogram), or even deeper in the brain (depth electrodes).

enlightenment   Awakening to the reality of the unity of all things. In Zen, it also refers to the temporary states of kensho or satori.

evoked potential   The amplified sum of local brain electrical activity. It is prompted by repeatedly delivering a stimulus at some distance away from the recording site.

experiant   The one experiencing, even though no sense of personal Self remains at that moment. A term used here, not found in dictionaries.

hippocampus   A small region deep in each temporal lobe. It plays a major early role in laying down memory traces, including those that register a sense of "place."

hypothalamus   The small, complex, centrally located region lying below the thalamus and above the pituitary gland. It integrates many vital brain and body functions crucial to survival: eating, drinking, blood pressure, etc.

insight   The sudden act of seeing clearly and comprehensively—without intervening thought—into problem situations or into our own inner nature.

insight-wisdom   The major profound, insightful, comprehension of the existential essence of things, conferred by prajna.

intuition   Our generic faculty of direct knowing. It usually refers to the ordinary, brief intuitive understanding that proceeds quickly without obvious rational thought processes.

kensho   Seeing into the essence of things, insight-wisdom (Chin. *Chien-hsing*). It is regarded as the beginning of true training, a prelude to the depths of satori.

koan   An enigmatic statement serving as a concentration device. Insight resolves it, not logical thought.

limbic system   A series of structures next to the midline on both sides of the brain linked by circuits which generate affective and instinctual responses. It includes the hypothalamus, hippocampus, cingulate gyrus, amygdala, and septal region. Allied regions now tend to be called "paralimbic."

limbic thalamus   A term applied to three thalamic nuclei that have intimate connections with both the limbic system and the cortex: the medial dorsal, anterior, and lateral dorsal nuclei.

meaning The quality conveyed when the brain links the raw perception of an item to its many related associations. Only certain meanings go on to assume major experiential import (salience).

medulla The lower part of the brainstem lying above the spinal cord. It mediates respiratory, cardiovascular, and other vital functions.

paralimbic regions Those with strong affective responses and major connections with the limbic system. The term includes the insula, the orbitofrontal cortex, and sometimes the superior temporal gyrus.

prajna (Skt.; J. *hannya*) The flashing insight-wisdom of enlightenment.

reticular nucleus The thin outer layer of GABA nerve cells capping the thalamus. It plays a pivotal inhibitory role in thalamic functions and in thalamocortical interactions.

roshi Venerable teacher; the Japanese pronunciation (roshi) of the name of the venerated Chinese teacher, Lao-tzu. Usually capitalized when it refers to a particular Zen teacher.

salience The leaping forth into meaning of the special quality which confers significant import.

satori The term frequently reserved for a deeper, more advanced state of insight-wisdom.

sesshin An intensive Zen meditative retreat lasting several days; literally, "to collect the mind."

state A temporary condition involving mentation, emotion, or behavior.

striatum Several nuclei of the basal ganglia which mediate motor functions. The caudate and putamen compose the dorsal striatum. The ventral striatum includes the nucleus accumbens.

synchronization The process of bringing together regions of the cerebrum into regular, rhythmical patterns of firing activity. In the past, it has usually been associated with slower waveforms in the EEG, with drowsiness and slow wave sleep (S sleep). More recently, however, fast activity has been recognized as also rhythmical and synchronized, as, for example, in gamma waves.

trait A distinctive ongoing quality of attitude, character, or behavior. Traits are not usually thought of as subject to change. However, they can be transformed by a series of extraordinary, insightful alternate states superimposed on long-term meditative training.

zazen Zen meditation in the sitting posture; from the Chinese, *tso-ch'an*.

Zen A form of Mahayana Buddhism which emphasizes a systematic approach to meditative training and spiritual growth. Its two major schools, Rinzai and Soto, were imported from China and developed in Japan during the twelfth and thirteenth centuries.

References and Notes

Preface

1. I. Schloegl. *The Zen Way*. London, Sheldon Press, 1977, 92.

By Way of Introduction

1. Cf. T. Cleary. *Zen Essence, The Science of Freedom*. Boston, Shambhala, 1989, 14.

Chapter 1   Training Attention

1. Cf. P. Kapleau. *The Three Pillars of Zen*. Boston, Beacon Press, 1967, 10–11. Ikkyu Sojun was an eccentric Zen master. Fortunately for those who trained later at Daitoku-ji, his efforts succeeded in rebuilding it after it was destroyed by war in the fifteenth century.
2. B. Wallace. *The Attention Revolution. Unlocking the Power of the Focused Mind*. Boston, Wisdom, 2006. The current "Shamatha Project" represents a milestone in comprehensive research on the meditative training of attention during a closely monitored 3-months' retreat. The immediate and follow-up results are awaited with great interest.
3. Sheng-yen and D. Stevenson. *Hoofprint of the Ox. Principles of the Chan Buddhist Path as Taught by a Modern Chinese Master*. New York, Oxford University Press, 2001, 147.
4. A. Lutz, J. Dunne, and R. Davidson. Meditation and the neuroscience of consciousness: An introduction, in P. Zelazio, M. Moscovitch, and E. Thompson, eds., *Cambridge Handbook of Consciousness*. Cambridge, UK, Cambridge University Press, 2008.
5. Two elastic Sanskrit terms are encountered along the path of concentrative meditation. One of them, *samadhi*, can often be translated as absorption (ZB:473–478, 530–534). The other, *shamatha*, can cause confusion, as reference 4 observes. Sometimes it is used to refer to the (nine) successive levels on the path of training attention, and sometimes only to the culminating stage of an attention so refined that it can be effortlessly sustained for many hours (see references 2 and 4 above.) Some Sanskrit translations suggest that the old term *shamatha* meant, literally, "dwelling in tranquility." In Tibetan traditions, the term *shamatha* has also come to refer to the tranquility that one first develops during preliminary practices which then goes on subsequently to be highly refined in association with "special insight." (See *The Encyclopedia of Eastern Philosophy and Religion*. Boston, Shambhala, 1994, 314.) In this context, (and still referring to this further refinement of the word) the encyclopedia cites an image suggesting that *shamatha* practice later becomes increasingly complex. Thus, the actual ongoing dwelling in advanced tranquility is now referred to as comparable to that of a calm, clear lake in which now *plays* the "fish of special insight." For teaching purposes, I prefer the more traditional Zen view: absorptions represent preliminary states distinct from the other more advanced states of kensho-satori, during which enlightened awakenings strike in the form of insight-wisdom (*prajna*) [ZB:589–592, 617]. For a recent comprehensive discussion of Zen meditation, the reader is referred to reference 3.
6. The reader interested in the absorptions is referred to Wallace's recent review and its tabulation of the nine successive stages in attentional training emphasized in earlier Indo-Tibetan Buddhist traditions. *The Attention Revolution*, (Wallace. 174–175.) In brief, the first four of these stages involve paying close attention to one's breathing. The next three involve settling the mind, in the course of which visualized objects begin to appear more vividly. The last two describe a single-pointedness of attention followed by greater degrees of attentional balance, each representing a sustained degree of absorption. Thus, step 8 reaches a

single-pointed degree of sustained attention. During this, no thoughts occur. The advanced meditator experiences this field of absorption as the uninterrupted *stillness* of a deep waveless ocean. During step 9, only the highly skilled meditator reaches that degree of attentional balance which enables absorption to be effortlessly sustained at a level of "flawless perfection" for up to 4 hours or so. Clearly, in order to arrive at such advanced levels of concentrated meditative absorption, the person must make a major commitment to daily meditative training and to intensive retreats, usually in some monastic-like context.

7. B. Wallace and S. Shapiro. Mental balance and well-being: Building bridges between Buddhism and Western psychology. *American Psychologist* 2006; 61:690–701.

8. Western dictionary definitions suggest that this term, *tranquility*, implies a state that is steady and stable, and one that is free from any disturbance of thoughts or emotions.

9. H. Guogu. Hongzhi Zhengjue on silent illumination Ch'an. *Ch'an Magazine* 2007; 27:14–17. This master (a.k.a Hung-Chih) was the author of the *Book of Serenity*, a collection of 100 koans used by the Caodong (J. Soto) Zen school.

10. Wallace. *The Attention Revolution*. Such states of "meditative quiescence" may illustrate the paradox just described: extraordinarily high levels of one-pointed, stable attention that become coupled with deep silent relaxation.

11. J. Kornfield. This fantastic unfolding experiment. *Buddhadharma* 2007; 5:32–39.

12. O. Carter, D. Presti, C. Callistemon, et al. Meditation alters perceptual rivalry in Tibetan Buddhist monks. *Current Biology* 2005; 11:R412–R413. The research was conducted at or near the places where the monks had been in an isolated mountain retreat. The parallel lines (gratings) were green. The compassion meditation was described as a nonreferential contemplation of suffering within the world, one which included emanations of loving kindness.

13. H. Slagter, A. Lutz, L. Greischar, et al. Mental training affects distribution of limited brain resources. *Public Library of Science Biology* 2007; 5(6):e138.doi:10. The Vipassana training at the Insight Meditation Society cultivates both concentration and bare attention. It also includes loving-kindness and compassion meditation. The 23 matched controls were subjects "interested in learning about meditation" who meditated for twenty minutes daily, for 1 week before each recording session. The task consisted of a few numbers embedded in a rapid stream of many distractor letters. The pertinent event-related potential (ERP) is the so-called P3b. It is detected in the mid–parieto-occipital region during the time window of 350 to 650 ms.

14. J. Galvin, H. Benson, G. Deckro, et al. The relaxation response: Reducing stress and improving cognition in healthy aging adults. *Complementary Therapy in Clinical Practice* 2006; 12:186–191.

15. M. Thimm, G. Fink, J. Kust, et al. Impact of alertness training on spatial neglect: A behavioral and fMRI study. *Neuropsychologia* 2006; 47:1230–1246.

Chapter 2   Meditating Mindfully at the Dawn of a New Millennium

1. J. Kabat-Zinn. Mindfulness-based stress reduction (MBSR). *Constructivism in the Human Sciences* 2003; 8:73–107. My apologies to the author for condensing into one sentence the gist of a long introductory paragraph in his original version. Soko-Roshi's six words remain intact.

2. J. Kabat-Zinn. Lecture at the Mind and Life Summer Research Institute, June 2006, Garrison, NY.

3. R. Baer, G. Smith, J. Hopkins, et al. Using self-report assessment methods to explore facets of mindfulness. *Assessment* 2006; 13:27–45. This is a cross-sectional study, not a longitudinal study.

4. J. Creswell, B. Way, N. Eisenberger, et al. Neural correlates of dispositional mindfulness during affect labeling. *Psychosomatic Medicine* 2007; 69:560–565.

5. S. Jain, S. Shapiro, S. Swanick, et al. A randomized controlled trial of mindfulness meditation versus relaxation training: Effects on distress, positive states of mind, rumination, and distraction. *Annals of Behavioral Medicine* 2007; 33:11–21.

6. J. Kristeller. Mindfulness meditation, in P. Lehrer, W. Sime, and R. Woolfolk, eds., *Principles and Practice of Stress Management*. 3rd ed. New York, Guilford Press, 2007.

7. D. MacCoon, A. Lutz, M. Rosenkranz, et al. Lessons from an active control condition: "McMindfulness," shams, and the one-fold path. Poster presentation. Mind and Life Summer Research Institute. June 22–27, 2007, Garrison, NY.

8. D. Siegel. *The Mindful Brain: Reflection and Attunement in the Cultivation of Well-being*. New York, Norton, 2007.

9. R. Walsh and S. Shapiro. Meditation and Western psychology. *American Psychologist* 2006; 61:227–239.

10. R. Aitken. *The Dragon Who Never Sleeps*. Berkeley, CA, Parallax Press, 1992.

11. J. Ford. *Zen Master Who? A Guide to the People and Stories of Zen*. Boston, Wisdom, 2006.

12. M. Kwee. Neo Zen: A "structing" psychology into non-self and beyond. *Constructivism in the Human Sciences* 2003; 8:181–202.

13. M. Kwee, K. Gergen, F. Koshikawa, eds. *Horizons in Buddhist Psychology. Practice, Research, and Theory*. Chagrin Falls, OH, Taos Institute, 2006.

Chapter 3   Meditation: "JUST THIS"

1. A. Olendzki. Back to the beginning. *Tricycle 13*, Winter 2003, p 47 (an interview conducted by Helen Tworkov).

2. H. Roth. *Original Tao, Inward Training and the Foundations of Taoist Mysticism*. New York, Columbia University Press, 1999, 66–67. Harold Roth's translation of this ancient text illustrates that China had already in place a substantial foundation of Taoist mysticism centuries before Indian Buddhist influences arrived.

3. Christian "centering prayer" begins with a simple, silent word. It implies that you consent to your intentions to listen—in quiet and with eyes closed—to the truth of who you are. The explicit question "Who?" remains a simplified capping phrase for a Zen koan [ZBR:61–64].

4. A. Ferguson. *Zen's Chinese Heritage. The Masters and Their Teachings*. Boston, Wisdom, 2000, 153. This master is Tianhuang Daowu.

5. I am indebted to Robert Aitken-Roshi in his letter of March 20, 2007. In response to my earlier inquiry, he points me toward these other two Ch'an masters who also used an equivalent of this phrase. He refers Yunyan's version of "JUST THIS!" to case 49 in the *Book of Serenity*, and Yantou's statement both to the *Book of Serenity* case 50, and to the *Blue Cliff Record*, case 51. These two masters were in the lineage of Master Shih-T'ou (700–790) [ZBR:330–333].

6. S. Morinaga. *Novice to Master; An Ongoing Lesson in the Extent of My Own Stupidity*. Boston, Wisdom, 2004; 108:154. Sir William Osler (1849–1919), the distinguished Canadian-born physician, recommended this *aequanimitas* to health professionals in a classic address.

7. B. Cahn and J. Polich. Meditation states and traits: EEG, ERP, and neuroimaging studies. *Psychological Bulletin* 2006; 132:180–211. The nine pages of reference citations review a variety of research reports up to 2005.

8. M. Ospina, K. Bond, M. Karkhaneh, et al. Meditation practices for health: State of the research. *Evidentiary Report of Technological Assessments* 2007; 155:1–263. Health-related outcomes were the focus of this extensive review.

Chapter 4   Neurologizing about Attention

1. For example, as Moore notes, attention can be voluntary (top-down, goal-directed) or involuntary (bottom-up, stimulus-driven); spatial (directed toward a location in space) or object-based (focused on some feature of an object); overt or covert. T. Moore. The neurobiology of visual attention: Finding sources. *Current Opinion in Neurobiology* 2006; 16:159–165. Knudson observes that our voluntary control of attention involves the following ongoing steps: access to working memory, a top-down sensitivity control, and a selection among several competing targets. E. Knudson. Fundamental components of attention. *Annual Reviews in Neuroscience* 2007; 30:57–78.

2. A. Raz and J. Buhle. Typologies of attentional networks. *Neuroscience* 2006; 7:367–379.

3. M. Koivisto, M. Lähteenmäki, T. Sørensen, et al. The earliest electrophysiological correlate of visual awareness? *Brain and Cognition* 2008; 66:91–103.

4. M. Overgaard, M. Koivisto, T Sorensen, et al. The electrophysiology of introspection. *Consciousness and Cognition* 2006; 15:662–672.

5. D. Lenz, J. Schadow, S. Thaerig, et al. What's that sound? Matches with auditory long-term memory induced gamma activity in human EEG. *International Journal of Psychophysiology* 2007; 64:31–38. Gamma frequencies differ from person to person. Sensitive magnetoencephalogram (MEG) techniques detect these induced gamma oscillations sooner than do the standard EEG methods, and show that they also last longer. For example, some recent MEG research detects the slower gamma oscillations (those at 44–66 cps) when we focus top-down attention more *deliberately* on a visual task. These occur down in the lateral parieto-occipital region. In contrast, the faster gamma oscillations (at 70 to 120 cps) arise when we respond more reflexly to external stimuli with the aid of *bottom-up* processing. See J. Vidal, M. Chaumon, J. O'Regan, et al. Visual grouping and the focusing of attention induce gamma-band oscillations at different frequencies in human magnetoencephalogram signals. *Journal of Cognitive Neuroscience* 2006; 18:1850–1862.

6. T. Demiralp, Z. Bayraktaroglu, D. Lenz, et al. Gamma amplitudes are coupled to theta phase in human EEG during visual perception. *International Journal of Psychophysiology* 2007; 64:24–30. How gamma and theta coupling (or nesting) occurs, and what it means remains speculative [ZBR:44–47].

7. T. Grent-'t-Jong and M. Woldorff. Timing and sequence of brain activity in top-down control of visual-spatial attention. *Public Library of Science Biology* 2007; 5e12.

8. C. Ruff, F. Blankenburg, O. Bjoertomt, et al. Concurrent TMS-fMRI and psychophysics reveal frontal influences on human retinotopic visual cortex. *Current Biology* 2006; 16:1479–1488.

9. A. Hampshire and A. Owen. Fractionating attentional control using event-related fMRI. *Cerebral Cortex* 2006; 16:1679–1689.

10. S. Gilbert, S. Spengler, J. Simons, et al. Differential functions of lateral and medial rostral prefrontal cortex (area 10) revealed by brain-behavior associations. *Cerebral Cortex* 2006; 16:1783–1789.

11. M. Bar, K. Kassam, A. Ghuman, et al. Top-down facilitation of visual recognition. *Proceedings of the National Academy of Sciences U.S.A.* 2006; 103:449–454. A pathway from the medial pulvinar to the orbital cortex is of interest in this regard [ZBR:175–176]. This study combined MEG and fMRI monitoring of the behavioral task. A later review summarizes the evidence that the early recognition of a low spatial frequency image up in the orbitofrontal cortex helps facilitate the subsequent integration of visual responses back in the fusiform gyrus and inferior temporal cortex. See K. Kveraga, A. Ghuman, and M. Bar. Top-down predictions in the cognitive brain. *Brain and Cognition* 2007; 65:145–168.

12. T. Wager, J. Jonides, E. Smith, et al. Toward a taxonomy of attention shifting: Individual differences in fMRI during multiple shift types. *Cognitive Affective and Behavioral Neuroscience* 2005; 5:127–143. In contrast, other sites are activated when shifts of attention are accompanied by poorer task performance. These other sites are linked with the kinds of executive control that wrestle with the overall demands of the task. They include the dorsolateral, medial prefrontal, and parietal cortex. Most Zen meditation is oriented toward a nonstriving approach. During the openly receptive meditation of shikantanza, "letting go" is an underlying operational principle.

13. R. Mitchell. Anterior cingulate activity and level of cognitive conflict: Explicit comparisons. *Behavioral Neuroscience* 2006; 120:1395–1401.

14. B. Haas, K. Omura, R. Constable, et al. Interference produced by emotional conflict associated with anterior cingulate activation. *Cognitive Affective and Behavioral Neuroscience* 2006; 6:152–156.

15. C. Wu, D. Weissman, K. Roberts, et al. The neural circuitry underlying the executive control of auditory spatial attention. *Brain Research* 2007; 1134:187–198.

16. A. Barrett, R. Schwartz, G. Crucian, et al. Attentional grasp in far extrapersonal space after thalamic infarction. *Neuropsychologia* 2000; 38:778–784. The mechanisms governing this patient's strong, right-sided attentional bias in far space could be sensory-attentional, motor-attentional, or both. Normally, the firing of head direction cells in the anterior thalamus anticipates the next head direction [ZBR:172–174].

Chapter 5   On Remaining Attentive while We Meditate

1. D. Weissman, K. Roberts, K. Visscher, et al. The neural bases of momentary lapses in attention. *Nature Neuroscience* 2006; 9:971–978.

2. The term *temporoparietal junction* (TPJ) could refer to a relatively long interface leading toward the supramarginal gyrus. It dates from an earlier era when a clot in the middle cerebral artery or its branches could infarct relatively large areas of cortex on both sides of this general region and damage several kinds of attentive functions.

3. G. Schulman, S. Astafiev, M. McAvoy, et al. Right TPJ deactivation during visual search: Functional significance and support for a filter hypothesis. *Cerebral Cortex* 2007; 17:2625–2633. TPJ activations are behaviorally relevant, suggesting that messages reaching it have first been filtered to remove the irrelevant information.

4. D. Chan and M. Woollacott. Effects of level of meditation experience on attentional focus: Is the efficiency of executive or orientation networks improved? *Journal of Alternative Complementary Medicine* 2007; 13:651–658. The data from 20 subjects who practiced forms of concentrative meditation, and 30 subjects who practiced forms of "opening up" meditation were compared with data from 10 nonmeditating controls of comparable age.

Chapter 6   Perceiving Clearly

1. I. Schloegl. *The Zen Way.* London, Sheldon Press, 1977, 114. Irmgard Schloegl's Buddhist name is Myokyo-ni.

2. M. Christensen, T. Ramsoy, T. Lund, et al. An fMRI study of the neural correlates of graded visual perception. *Neuroimage* 2006; 31:1711–1725. The circle, triangle, and square rendered here are a pale contemporary version, not Sengai's originals.

3. S. Dehaene, J.-P. Changeux, L. Naccache, et al. Conscious, preconscious, and subliminal processing: A testable taxonomy. *Trends in Cognitive Sciences* 2006; 10:204–211.

4. C. Koch and N. Tsuchiya. Attention and consciousness: Two distinct brain processes. *Trends in Cognitive Sciences* 2006; 11:16–22.

5. R. Szczepanowski and L. Pessoa. Fear perception: Can objective and subjective awareness measures be dissociated? *Journal of Vision* 2007; 7:1–17.

Chapter 7 Network Systems Serving Different Forms of Attention

1. M. Fox, M. Corbetta, A. Snyder, et al. Spontaneous neuronal activity distinguishes human dorsal and ventral attention systems. *Proceedings of the National Academy of Sciences U.S.A.* 2006; 103:10046–10051.
2. S. Astafiev, G. Schulman, and M. Corbetta. Visuospatial reorienting signals in the human temporo-parietal junction are independent of response selection. *European Journal of Neuroscience* 2006; 23:591–596.
3. J. Serences and S. Yantis. Selective visual attention and perceptual coherence. *Trends in Cognitive Sciences* 2006; 10:41–45. In itself, this region, localized using fMRI, appears too small to account for the entire large area of the P3b waveform that is revealed using ERP. However, its nearness to the somatosensory association cortex suggests that reduced "wiring costs" are associated with its instant contributions to egocentric processing.
4. Y. Golland, S. Bentin, H. Gelbard, et al. Extrinsic and intrinsic systems in the posterior cortex of the human brain revealed during natural sensory stimulation. *Cerebral Cortex* 2007; 17:766–777.

Chapter 8 The Implications of Training More Efficient Attentional Processing

1. S. Shipp. The brain circuitry of attention. *Trends in Cognitive Sciences* 2004; 8:223–230.
2. J. Hopf, C. Boehler, S. Luck, et al. Direct neurophysiological evidence for spatial suppression surrounding the focus of attention in vision. *Proceedings of the National Academy of Sciences U.S.A.* 2006; 103:1053–158.
3. S. Adler and J. Orprecio. The eyes have it: Visual pop-out in infants and adults. *Developmental Science* 2006; 2:189–206. Note that the path through the inferior colliculus and the pulvinar provides for comparable auditory stimuli to serve as a trigger for kensho (chapter 23).
4. Shipp, The brain circuitry.
5. Q. Luo, T. Holroyd, M. Jones, et al. Neural dynamics for facial threat processing as revealed by gamma band synchronization using MEG. *Neuroimage* 2007; 34:839–847. See table 15. Pop-out functions can be enhanced by spatial priming cues involving the left FEF. See J. O'Shea, N. Muggleton, A. Cowey, et al. Human frontal eye fields and spatial priming of pop-out. *Journal of Cognitive Neuroscience* 2007; 19:1140–1151.
6. H. Slagter, A. Lutz, L. Greischar, et al. Mental training affects distribution of limited brain resources. *Public Library of Sciences Biology* 2007; 5(6):e138.doi:10. One hopes researchers will use a similar approach to study the auditory blink phenomenon in well-trained meditators.
7. J. Brefczynski-Lewis, A. Lutz, H. Schaefer, et al. Neural correlates of attentional expertise in long-term meditation practitioners. *Proceedings of the National Academy of Sciences U.S.A.* 2007; 104:11483–11488. The authors matched the expert groups in terms of their ethnic origins. Notably, when compared with novices, the experts showed *reduced* fMRI responses in the amygdala and posterior cingulate regions. However, their left insula and subthalamic responses were enhanced. See also the discussion in the next chapter.

Chapter 9 Studying Meditators' Brains

1. B. Hölzel, U. Ott, H. Hempel, et al. Differential engagement of anterior cingulate and adjacent medial frontal cortex in adept meditators and non-meditators. *Neuroscience Letters* 2007; 421:16–21.

2. A. Jha, J. Krompinger, and M. Baime. Mindfulness training modifies subsystems of attention. *Cognitive, Affective, and Behavioral Neuroscience* 2007; 7:109–119. A reduction in conflict monitoring means that the flanker arrows are less distracting.

3. J. Brefczynski-Lewis, A. Lutz, H. Schaefer, et al. Neural correlates of attentional expertise in long-term meditation practitioners. *Proceedings of the National Academy of Sciences U.S.A.* 2007; 104:11483–11488. See the additional discussion in part V.

4. A. Lutz, J. Dunne, R. Davidson. Meditation and the neuroscience of consciousness: An introduction, in P. Zelazo, M. Moscovitch, and E. Thompson, eds., *The Cambridge Handbook of Consciousness.* Cambridge, UK, Cambridge University Press. 2008.

5. A. Lutz, J. Brefczynski-Lewis, T. Johnstone, et al. Regulation of the neural circuitry of emotion by compassion meditation: effects of meditative expertise. *Public Library of Science. ONE.* 2008 March 26; 3(3): 1897. The experts were selected from either Asian or European origins. The novices were recruited from the local Wisconsin community and had practiced this compassion style of meditation and two other varieties for one week.

6. Hölzel et al., Differential engagement. Long practice, in itself, provides no absolute barrier to the "demand characteristics" that enter into an experiment. Conscientious subjects can experience mental dissonance if they feel unusual task demands are being imposed, or if their own self-imposed pressures remain unusually high.

7. Y. Tang, T. Ma, J. Wang, et al. Short-term meditation training improves attention and self-regulation. *Proceedings of the National Academy of Sciences U.S.A.* 2007; 104:17152–17156.

8. Substantial semantic and theoretical issues complicate the motion that one single "default-like" state, prone to be Self-preoccupied at the phenomenological level with a stream of thoughts, has connectivities that fluctuate several times a minute between introspective and extrospective modes (chapter 22).

Chapter 10   Inward Turned Attention: Induced Experiences

1. M. Beauregard and V. Paquette. Neural correlates of a mystical experience in Carmelite nuns. *Neuroscience Letters* 2006; 405:186–190.

2. The nuns had only five minutes during which to develop and intensify their induced absorption, with the aid of the reverberations that normally link the lateral posterior nucleus of the thalamus with this superior cortex (figure 6). Induced absorptions that are sustained for a much longer period could activate a secondary, inhibitory response from the reticular nucleus of the thalamus. This could later "cap" these induced oscillations and *decrease* the previous activitation of the superior parietal lobule [ZBR:219–223].

3. N. Azari, J. Nickel, G. Wunderlich, et al. Short communication: Neural correlates of religious experience. *European Journal of Neuroscience* 2001; 13:1649–1652. During the resting period, the eyes were covered. The control conditions included reading or reciting a nursery rhyme or instructions for using a telephone. A trend toward a decrease in negative affect was measured using the Affect Scale (PANAS), and it was apparent only during the religious condition. Less consistent activations occurred in the left dorsolateral prefrontal and right medial precuneus regions. Further details about a subjects "conversion experience" could help interpret whether it could be categorized as an absorption, or as a deeper state of awakening comparable with insight-wisdom.

Chapter 11   First Mondo

1. S. Heine and D. Wright, eds. *Zen Classics: Formative Texts in the History of Zen Buddhism.* Oxford, Oxford University Press, 2006, 6.

Chapter 12   You Are the "Person of the Year"

1. Epictetus was a Stoic philospher who lived in Phrygia and proclaimed the brotherhood of man. Greek legends associate this ancient region (now in central Turkey) with two local kingdoms, one of Gordius (he of the knot) and the other of Midas (who knew the curse of gold).

2. The *Atlantic* has risen to defend Facebook, concluding that it has surpassed the other "social media" sites, brought order to the web, and could become as important as Google. See M. Hirschorn. "About Facebook," *Atlantic*, October 2007, 148–155.

3. This author-researcher does not question the absolute right of any other person to Self-expression as a liberal art form. Nor does he devalue the Internet as a positive resource for free communication throughout the world. In the context of this book on Zen, the sole issue to be raised on the downside is the sheer volume, variable quality, and time diverted into unrestrained, Self-indulgent electronic expression. When the term, I-Generation was first introduced, the *I* stood for Internet. Now it can also represent the excesses of the I-Me-Mine.

Chapter 13   On the Nature and Origins of the Self

1. M. Nardini, N. Burgess, K. Breckenridge, et al. Differential developmental trajectories for egocentric, environmental and intrinsic frames of reference in spatial memory. *Cognition* 2006; 101:153-172.

2. Of course, it is our own brain that processes the coding of stimuli that mediate this object-centered mode of perception; the apple always remains a passive object. The old term, *ap-perception*, applies to the egocentric process that relates each new event and sensation to one's personal emotions and memories of previous experiences. Meanwhile, and only to illustrate the converse, it might help envision what "object-centered" perception implies if you were to "let go" sufficiently to imagine that an apple might possess a nose. Then, as the apple "faces" back toward you, its *own* two halves are positioned on either side of this midline.

3. "Positive prejudice. Really loving your neighbor," *Economist* 2007, March 17, 66.

4. S. Neggers, R. Van der Lubbe, N. Ramsey, et al. Interactions between ego- and allocentric neuronal representations of space. *NeuroImage* 2006; 31:320–331. See also the EEG study by K. Gramann, H. Muller, B. Schonebeck, et al. The neural basis of ego- and allocentric reference frames in spatial navigation: Evidence from spatio-temporal coupled current density reconstruction. *Brain Research* 2006; 1118:116–129. These findings confirm that the egocentric reference frame is represented along an extensive network in the posterior parietal-premotor-frontal regions. Its initial path is distinct from the occipito-temporal representation of the allocentric reference frame.

5. E. Rolls. Neurophysiological and computational analyses of the primate presubiculum, subiculum and related areas. *Behavioral Brain Research* 2006; 174:289–303. For a model of how the compass-like coding functions of head-direction cells participate in dynamic shifts between Self-centered and other-centered processing, see P. Byrne, S. Becker, and N. Burgess. Remembering the past and imagining the future: A neural model of spatial memory and imagery. *Psychological Review* 2007; 114:340–375.

6. Rolls, ibid.

Chapter 14   Selective Deficits of Egocentric or Allocentric Processing in Neurological Patients

1. H. Ota, T. Fujii, K. Suzuki, et al. Dissociation of body-centered and stimulus-centered representations in unilateral neglect. *Neurology* 2001; 57:2064–2069. When smart people get into

big controversies in the neurosciences, there's usually some merit to each side, and perhaps some higher level of meaning.

2. A. Hillis, M. Newhart, J. Heidler, et al. Anatomy of spatial attention: Insights from perfusion imaging and hemispatial neglect in acute stroke. *Journal of Neuroscience* 2005; 25:3161–3167. As part I explains, the right side of our brain plays the predominant role in attentive functions. The clinical defects after right-sided parietal damage become most obvious within the patient's left field of space. The clinical defects of right-sided temporal damage become most obvious when they interfere with the way the patient attends to and processes that other side of an *object* wherever it is out there. The authors' previous studies indicated that underperfused cortex is the cause of the visuospatial neglect rather than the small subcortical infarct. At this writing, it is plausible to consider that some anterosuperior temporal gyrus deficits could represent an allocentric disorder at some higher level of disintegration and misinterpretation than do those deficits that are referable to local damage far down in area 37 of the fusiform gyrus. However, the precise nature(s) of such higher-level functions remain to be described in detail and translated into the specific visual tests that could help characterize the differences between normal and patient populations.

3. J. Vincent, A. Snyder, M. Fox, et al. Coherent spontaneous activity identifies a hippocampal-parietal memory network. *Journal of Neurophysiology* 2006; 96:3517–3531.

4. J. Kleinman, M. Newhart, C. Davis, et al. Right hemispatial neglect: Frequency and characterization following acute left hemisphere stroke. *Brain and Cognition* 2007; 64:50–59. Right superior temporal lesions are not represented. Future acute studies are awaited that distinguish in greater detail among the discrete neuropsychological deficits referable to the superior temporal, supramarginal, and angular gyrus on each side, and between homologous sites on the two sides. The authors' attribution to the left hemisphere of a more general role in allocentric processing (table 8) raises an intriguing possibility for the future to test. If some episodes of kensho-satori were to be accompanied by a more asymmetrical inhibition of right hemispheric functions (absolute or relative), then would both the dissolution of the Self and the predominance of the OTHER each be experienced to a greater degree?

Chapter 15   The Brain's Active Metabolism during Resting Conditions

1. D. Gusnard, and M. Raichle. Searching for a baseline: Functional imaging and the resting human brain. *Nature Reviews Neuroscience* 2001; 2:685–694. In this article, their figure 1a emphasizes the substantial *decreases* in PET scan activities that occur during a variety of "active goal-directed behaviors." Part I of this book has emphasized that attention can be conceptualized as the sharp point at the leading edge of such external goal-driven behaviors. Figure 7 in this book depicts the de-activation of Self-referential processing that occurs as a reaction to a major triggering stimulus in the external environment.

2. A prolific novelist like Joyce Carol Oates draws on similar resources for enough material to invent countless semifictional characters each fleshed out with a different lifetime narrative. Klein cites case studies relevant to a theory that we normally develop a "trait summary database." Then, to address the specific needs for pertinent self-knowledge that a particular situation requires, we quickly blend its coarse abstractions with fine-tuned, highly selected episodic memories. See S. Klein. The cognitive neuroscience of knowing one's self, in M. Gazzainga, ed., *The Cognitive Neurosciences*, 3rd ed. Cambridge, MA, MIT Press, 2004, 1077–1089.

3. R. Rosenbaum, M. Ziegler, G. Winocur, et al. "I have often walked down this street before:" fMRI studies on the hippocampus and other structures during mental navigation of an old environment. *Hippocampus* 2004; 14:826–835.

4. L. Frings, K. Wagner, A. Quiske, et al. Precuneus is involved in allocentric spatial location encoding and recognition. *Experimental Brain Research* 2006; 173:661–672.

5. G. Committeri, G. Galati, A.-L. Paradis, et al. Reference frames for spatial cognition: Different brain areas are involved in viewer-, object-, and landmark-centered judgements about object location. *Journal of Cognitive Neuroscience* 2004; 16:1517–1535.

6. T. Zaehle, K. Jordan, T. Wüstenberg, et al. The neural basis of the egocentric and allocentric spatial frame of reference. *Brain Research* 2007; 1137:92–103. A specific example of the two word tasks is instructive. Allocentric description: "The blue triangle is to the left of the green square. The green square is above the yellow triangle. The yellow triangle is to the right of the red circle." Question: "Is the blue triangle above the red circle?" Correct answer: "Yes." Egocentric word task description: "The blue circle is in front of you. The yellow circle is to your right. The yellow square is to the right of the yellow circle." Question: "Is the yellow square to your right?" Correct answer: "Yes."

7. J. Pfeifer, M. Lieberman, and M. Dapretto. "I know you are but what am I?!": Neural bases of self- and social knowledge retrieval in children and adults. *Journal of Cognitive Neuroscience* 2007; 8:1323–1337.

8. D. Amodio, and C. Frith, Meeting of minds: The medial frontal cortex and social cognition. *Nature Reviews Neuroscience* 2006; 7:268–277.

9. J.-D. Haynes, K. Sakai, G. Rees, et al. Reading hidden intentions in the human brain. *Current Biology* 2007; 17:323–328.

10. L. Zhang, T. Zhou, J. Zhang. In search of the Chinese self: An fMRI study. *Science in China, Series C: Life Sciences* 2006; 49:89–96. This study, using trait objectives, explores the very close identification between Self and mother in Chinese culture, and notes how close together their representations were in the medial prefrontal cortex.

11. R. Saxe. Uniquely human social cognition. *Current Opinion in Neurobiology* 2006; 16:235–239.

12. J. Beer. The default self: Feeling good or being right? *Trends in Cognitive Sciences* 2007; 11:187–189.

13. Gusnard and Raichle. Searching for a baseline.

Chapter 16   Internal "Mirrors" Facing Outward

1. V. Gazzola, G. Rizzolatti, B. Wicker, et al. The mirror neuron system responds to human and robotic actions. *Neuroimage* 2007; 35:1674–1684.

2. V. Gallese. Embodied simulation: From mirror neuron systems to interpersonal relations. *Novartis Foundation Symposium* 2007; 278:3–12.

3. Gazzola, et al. The mirror neuron system. Subjects who observe a novel behavior can develop increased fMRI signals in mirror neuron regions, even though they do not understand the *intention* underlying this particular behavior. See J. Kilner, C. Frith. Action observation: Inferring intentions without mirror neurons. *Current Biology* 2008; 18:R32–33.

4. V. Gazzola, L. Aziz-Zadeh, and C. Keysers. Empathy and the somatotopic auditory mirror system in humans. *Current Biology* 2006; 16:1824–1829.

5. Almost as if in fulfilment of some expectations of an animated, empathetic, ethnic stereotype, it happens that many pioneering researchers contributing to this field bear names of Italian origin. The dorsolateral prefrontal cortex serves to inhibit the expression of such politically incorrect ethnic stereotypes. See K. Knutson, L. Mah, C. Manly, et al. Neural correlates of automatic beliefs about gender and race. *Human Brain Mapping* 2007; 28:915–930.

6. M. Iacoboni and M. Dapretto. The mirror neuron system and the consequences of its dysfunction. *Nature Reviews Neuroscience* 2006; 7:942–951. Cortical thinning occurs in adult, high-functioning patients who have autism. These local decreases of cortical gray matter

are not restricted to regions corresponding to the often elastic boundaries of the classical "mirror neuron system" (said here to include the opercular portion of the inferior frontal gyrus [BA 44], the angular gyrus (BA 39), and the superior temporal sulcus [BA 22]). Thinning also occurs in other areas involved in social cognition and in the recognition of emotion. See N. Hadjikhani, R. Joseph, J. Snyder, et al. Anatomical differences in the mirror neuron system and social cognition network in autism. *Cerebral Cortex* 2006; 16:1276–1282.

7. In category III, the impression of oneness is speculated to occur in a state also regarded as being internally empty of Self. Yet the mental field could become sufficiently inclusive to embrace some subtle manifestations consistent with functions attributable to the *psyche*. Will current limits placed on any such conceptual projections of a "mirror" system stretch to accommodate this variety of oneness in the decades to come? Future studies may clarify this issue.

8. L. Uddin, M. Iacoboni, C. Lange, et al. The self and social cognition: The role of cortical midline structures and mirror neurons. *Trends in Cognitive Sciences* 2007; 11:153–157.

9. B. Leggenhager, S. Smith, and O. Blanke. Functional and neural mechanisms of embodiment: Importance of the vestibular system and the temporal parietal junction. *Reviews in Neuroscience* 2006; 17:643–657.

10. C. Devue, F. Collette, E. Balteau, et al. Here I am: The cortical correlates of visual self-recognition. *Brain Research* 2007; 1143:169–182.

11. M. Tsakiris, M. Hesse, C. Boy, et al. Neural signatures of body ownership: A sensory network for bodily self-consciousness. *Cerebral Cortex* 2007; 17:2235–2244.

12. S. Arzy, G. Thut, C. Mohr, et al. Neural basis of embodiment: Distinct contributions of temporoparietal junction and extrastriate body area. *Journal of Neuroscience* 2006; 26:8074–8081.

Chapter 17   Subcortical Contributions to Self/Other Distinctions

1. N. Kobori. The ripening persimmon: An interview with Kobori Nanrei Roshi. *Parabola* 1985; 10:72–79.

2. How much of our brain's activities are *sub*conscious? Freud guessed about six sevenths. On one occasion, he compared the human mind with an iceberg that floated "with only one-seventh of its bulk above water." After the *Titanic* sank in 1912, iceberg metaphors captured the imagination, and eight ninths or nine tenths were common estimates.

3. The earlier PET scan data condensed in figures 4 and 5 show that the medial temporal lobe can be partially deactivated during a variety of "active goal-directed behaviors" (which necessarily involve attention). These medial deactivations are referable to the region around the hippocampus and parahippocampus, not included in figure 5 for purposes of visual clarity.

4. D. Hassabis, D. Kumaran, S. Vann, et al. Patients with hippocampal amnesia cannot imagine new experiences. *Proceedings of the National Academy of Sciences U.S.A.* 2007; 104:1726–1731.

5. B. Zikopoulous and H. Barbas. Prefrontal projections to the thalamic reticular nucleus form a unique circuit for attentional mechanisms. *Journal of Neuroscience* 2006; 26:7358–7361.

6. I. Schloegl. *The Zen Way*. London, Sheldon Press, 1977, 15.

Chapter 19   Seeing Selflessly in a New Dimension

1. M. Buchsbaum, B. Buchsbaum, S. Chokron, et al. Thalamocortical circuits: fMRI assessment of the pulvinar and medial dorsal nucleus in normal volunteers. *Neuroscience Letters* 2006; 404:282–287.

2. K. Young, L. Holcomb, W. Bonkale, et al. 5HTTLPR polymorphism and enlargement of the pulvinar: Unlocking the backdoor to the limbic system. *Biological Psychiatry* 2007; 61:813–818.

3. S. Shipp. The functional logic of cortico-pulvinar connections. *Philosophical Transactions of the Royal Society of London. Part B* 2003; 358:1605–1624. Two of the visual domains in the ventral pulvinar (termed VP1 and VP2) have cortical counterparts within the ventral, object-centered visual stream. Auditory domains have yet to be studied in this detail. In general, the tendency is for top-down indirect circuits (those from cortex → pulvinar → cortex) to mimic the direct transcortical circuits.

4. The older literature had implied that connections were relatively less well-developed between the thalamus and the temporal lobe cortex. Sometimes the word, "athalamic" was used to describe the temporal lobe [ZB:763; ZBR:169].

5. J. Kaas and D. Lyon. Pulvinar contributions to the dorsal and ventral streams of visual processing in primates. *Brain Research Reviews* 2007; 55:285–296. The nearby ventrolateral nucleus of the lateral pulvinar also connects with the ventral stream, whereas the medial nuclei of the inferior pulvinar connect chiefly with the dorsal stream.

6. The gap junctions in the reticular nucleus augment its already powerful inhibitory effects. Nuclei of the dorsal thalamus also contain their own small *intrinsic*, local circuit GABA nerve cells. They exert localized inhibitory effects. These too can be inhibited by the reticular nucleus, adding to the organizational complexities that underlie thalamocortical oscillations. See M. Steriade, E. Jones, and D. McCormick. *Thalamus. Vol. 1. Organization and Function.* Oxford, Elsevier, 1997, 491–513.

7. In vitro intracellular recordings in brain slices from young rats show that neurons in the ventral part of the reticular nucleus have more obvious burst firing properties than do those in the dorsal part. With respect to the absorptions and kensho, it will be important to discover how these burst-firing functions translate into the dynamic aspects of in vivo information processing and reshape adult thalamocortical patterns of oscillation. See S. Lee, G. Fovindaiah, and C. Cox. Heterogeneity of firing properties among rat thalamic reticular nucleus neurons. *Journal of Physiology* 2007; 582:195–208.

8. The distinction between kensho and internal absorption becomes clear at this thalamic level. The GABA cap in internal absorption inhibits transmissions lower down, at the level of the sensory relay nuclei. In kensho, the GABA cap tightens on these five adjacent nuclei of the dorsal thalamus. Some of the resulting effects could be attributable to inhibiting the anterior thalamic nucleus and its path to the anterior cingulate gyrus. Adding to the phenomena of kensho, such inhibitions could help render its emptiness ineffable, help dissolve that sense of "heading" involved in approach behavior, and contribute to kensho's impression of having entered that deepest level of peace that "passeth all understanding." The fact that the normal olfactory pathway runs directly to our cortex, bypassing the thalamus, offers a potential way to gather sensory information from a meditator immediately after kensho. Theoretically, if GABA inhibition is limited to the reticular nucleus and its cap is restricted solely to the thalamus, one might expect that the early steps in the transmission of unthreatening odors would be relatively spared (at least when compared with data for smell thresholds obtained during earlier baseline control periods).

9. *Udana* 2:1 (Pali Canon).

Chapter 20   On the Long Path toward Selflessness

1. Cf. T. Cleary. *Zen Essence, The Science of Freedom.* Boston, Shambhala, 1989, 11.

2. A prior event and some sense of novelty may have contributed to that episode: I woke up an hour earlier than usual in order to take a rare trip to Cambridge University.

3. A. Gunji, R. Ishii, W. Chau, et al. Rhythmic brain activities related to singing in humans. *NeuroImage* 2007; 34:426–434.

4. ZBR: Table 11, page 415 summarizes kensho's measurable succession of earlier and late visual phenomena, including both the initial preservation of color, its later disappearance, and its final recovery of color. For visual clarity, figure 5 in chapter 13 of the present book chose not to show two hippocampal pathways in its summary of PET scan data.

5. D. Simonton. Foresight in insight? A Darwinian answer. In R. Sternberg and J. Davidson, eds., *The Nature of Insight*. Cambridge, UK. Cambridge University Press, 1995, 465–494.

6. The explanations proposed are plausible, and await confirmation. The pivotal roles of the ego/allo cycle involving the thalamus and its reticular nucleus in the taste of kensho are summarized in J. Austin. Selfless insight-wisdom: A thalamic gateway, in *Measuring the Immeasurable*. Louisville, CO, Sounds True, 2008, 211–230, 480.

Chapter 21   Neuroimaging during Tasks That Shift the Brain from Self-Referential to Other-Referential Modes of Attention

1. M. Raichle and M. Mintun. Brain work and brain imaging. *Annual Review of Neuroscience* 2006; 29:449–476. See a recent review which also emphasizes the cortical midline regions: G. Northoff, A. Heinzel, M. de Greck, et al. Self-referential processing in our brain—a meta-analysis of imaging studies on the self. *NeuroImage* 2006; 31:440–457. It is clear that a resting "baseline" represents a temporary abstraction of convenience, the more so when many research reports now appreciate that it is also an active mental interval during which their subjects experience a swarm of mind-wandering thoughts. An increase in fMRI signals during mind-wandering epochs is also reported in other lateral satellite regions, not just in the angular gyrus. These regions can include the insula (BA 13) and the left (BA 22) and right (BA 41) superior temporal gyrus.

2. Unless such a shift remains object-centered and other-referential, it would be a misnomer to describe it as allocentric attention.

3. Resource management is crucial. When a stimulus event occurs, how can a brain shift *efficiently* into the most appropriate practical response? It needs (a) to highlight only the relevant information stored in its vast memory networks, and (b) to impose simultaneously just a brief, *selective, partial restriction of access* on all the other irrelevant historical baggage previously stored in these same networks. In fact, this is what the PET and fMRI data reveal: only very slight deactivations do occur in certain brain regions. In fMRI, the decreases prompted during attentive processing are usually only in the range of 1% or 2% or less. These partial attenuations speak volumes. They tell us normal mechanisms exist that accomplish a discrete process of data *disengagement*. These minimal deactivations suggest that we do not respond to a new event by losing *all* our Self/other memory data permanently. Instead, the neuroimaging evidence confirms that we pinpoint—with astonishing precision—*only what needs to be recalled*, while *selectively detaching access* to the huge bulk of other irrelevant details. This neat trick would seem to create working room in which immediate memory functions can operate freely. Detached where? Perhaps nearest whatever served as the point of access for the process of attention that had originally focused on such details; nearest whatever functions had then been engaged at that site and were then used to index them for future reference.

4. Meditators are uniquely qualified to appreciate the nature of the journal entries. Not until one begins to meditate, and then encounters all the random channel-surfings of one's usual stream of consciousness/unconsciousness, does one begin to appreciate how vast are the resources of trivia maintained in this personal journal, and how Self-preoccupied we are in our efforts to plan future scenarios that add even more trivia.

5. M. Mason, M. Norton, J. Van Horn, et al. Wandering minds: The default network and stimulus-independent thought. *Science* 2007; 315:393–395.

Chapter 22   Slow Fluctuations, Revealing How Networks Shift Spontaneously

1. M. Fox, A. Snyder, J. Vincent, et al. The human brain is intrinsically organized into dynamic, anticorrelated functional networks. *Proceedings of the National Academy of Sciences U.S.A.* 2005; 102:9673–9678. The pattern in figure 3 of this article shows lateral activities that are relatively symmetrical. Those attention systems discussed in chapter 7 in this book are more right-sided (figure 3). Gross estimates suggest one reciprocal cycle of fluctuations every 21 seconds or so.

2. P. Fransson. Spontaneous low frequency BOLD signal fluctuations: An fMRI investigation of the resting-state default mode of brain function hypothesis. *Human Brain Mapping* 2005; 26:15–29. This study was based on 13 subjects, both male and female. Scanning at two different rates produced "virtually identical results," suggesting that cardiac "noise" did not play a significant role. Gross estimates suggest one reciprocal fluctuation every 16 seconds. In a recent confirming study, Fransson processed new data using the mathematical technique called independent component analysis (ICA). He found that a strenuous, sustained working memory task did not extinguish, but only attenuated, the intrinsic spontaneous activity in the several medial parietal and angular gyrus regions representing the Self-referential network. Notably, this rigorous mental task did *not* decrease signals in the medial prefrontal cortex. This result suggested that one role of this medial region might be to participate more autonomously in the particular kinds of Self-awareness functions that can proceed further removed from memory. Not surprisingly, task-*un*related thoughts decreased during all the distractions that were caused by this added rigorous task. See P. Fransson. How default is the default mode of brain function? Further evidence from intrinsic BOLD signal fluctuations. *Neuropsychologia* 2006; 44:2836–2845.

3. R. Wise, K. Ide, M. Poulin, et al. Resting fluctuations in arterial carbon dioxide induce significant low frequency variations in BOLD signal. *NeuroImage* 2004; 21:1652–1664.

4. M. DeLuca, C. Beckmann, N. De Stefano, et al. fMRI resting state networks define distinct modes of long-distance interactions in the human brain. *NeuroImage* 2006; 29:1359–1367. The authors used "probabilistic independent component analysis" (PICA), showing that the slow fluctuations occurred in clusters bilaterally and varied in space and time.

5. Ibid.

6. One inference is that the brain develops individual well-connected networks poised to support its multiple, alternative modes of operation. The hypothesis is testable that certain individual clusters could be found to assume patterns that would correspond with the several phenomena distinctive of alternate states of consciousness [ZBR:297–298]. The figures and table 1 in reference 4 show that their second resting state network (termed "RSN2") corresponds with what the St. Louis team had originally called the "default" network. It includes the hippocampus on both sides. It also includes a bilateral posterolateral temporal lobe contribution (not specifically identified as area MT). Its midline thalamic component is consistent with the medial dorsal nucleus of the thalamus, using criteria suggested by the authors' other diffusion tensor imaging studies.

In reference 4, the large visual brain is well represented (even though the subjects' eyes were closed while they relaxed). This "RSN1" network occupies both the right and left occipital and inferior temporal regions. "RSN4" corresponds with the usual dorsolateral parietal and frontal pathways (of the "where?" type), those that mediate our immediate visual preparations for action. "RSN5" corresponds with only some parts of the ventral ("what?")

pathway. Their "RSN3" network is a large cluster of six subregions. It includes the sensori-motor cortex and allied thalamic nuclei. The current consensus is that multiple intrinsic networks engage in slow rhythms of functional connectivity in the resting state. Figure 7 in the next chapter emphasizes that our Self-referential networks deactivate quickly whenever attention is captured and activated (including at the initiation of goal-directed tasks).

7. J. Vincent, A. Snyder, M. Fox, et al. Coherent spontaneous activity identifies a hippocampal-parietal memory network. *Journal of Neurophysiology* 2006; 96:3517–3531. The activity links that extend to include the hippocampal formation (in the medial temporal lobe), and which occurred spontaneously at rest, were spatially similar to those links that also developed when the subjects engaged in deliberate attempts to recall information from memory. However, they appeared distinct from those other correlations associated with area MT in the lateral temporal lobe that are cited in note 6 above.

8. Perhaps in the future, implicit association tests (IATs) could be used to assess the discrete timing of any subtle subconscious biases.

9. C. Landisman and B. Connors. Long-term modulation of electrical synapses in the mammalian thalamus. *Science* 2005; 310:1809–1813. Gap junctions interconnect nerve cells of the reticular nucleus. This electrical coupling synchronizes, and strengthens, many of the inhibitory capacities of this nucleus. These dual attributes enable the reticular nucleus to exert a major inhibitory influence on thalamo ↔ cortical oscillations.

10. The glutamate-calcium-nitric oxide-cyclic GMP cascade offers one neurochemical avenue to explore, in view of its cyclic electrophysiological, metabolic, and blood flow correlates [ZBR:279–288].

11. S. Horovitz, M. Fukunaga, J. de Zwart, et al. Low frequency BOLD fluctuations during resting wakefulness and light sleep: A simultaneous EEG-fMRI study. *Human Brain Mapping* 2008; 6:671–682.

12. J. Vincent, G. Patel, M. Fox, et al. Intrinsic functional architecture in the anaesthetized monkey brain. *Nature* 2007; 447:83–86.

Chapter 23   The Balance of Opposing Functions: Age-Old Perspectives and the Destablizing Effect of Triggers

1. Much later on, suppose that certain skilled meditators did in fact develop such attributes as more efficient attentive and intuitive skills, greater degrees of clear "ever-present awareness," and faster behavioral responses that were more selfless and altruistic. The questions would then arise: which of these perceptual, attitudinal, and behavioral changes correlate with greater degrees, or kinds, of difference in the several parameters of the fMRI shifts discussed above? To begin to answer such questions, it could help to plot on graphs the baseline data both from *adequate* genuine, no-thought resting states and from *well-designed* tasks. Then, the amplitude, frequency, and durations of the responses in the activated networks would need to be plotted separately from those responses cycling simultaneously in their opposing, deactivated counterparts. (Figure 7 is illustrative.)

2. The spontaneous shifts that occur at intervals of around 16 to 24 seconds are estimates based on only two human subjects. In large populations, the rhythms and amplitudes of the normal fluctuations under discussion could vary substantially. The questions to be studied are straightforward: Do the innate anatomical and physiological patterns of such intrinsic fluctuations correlate with any particular psychological profiles? Do any of these patterns evolve, over long periods of time, in persons who engage in a regular program of meditative training? How do these patterns change during alternate states of consciousness?

3. S. Horovitz, M. Fukunaga, J. de Zwart, et al. Low frequency BOLD fluctuations during resting wakefulness and light sleep: A simultaneous EEG-fMRI study. *Human Brain Mapping* 2008; 6:671–682. The normal subjects showed fluctuations of fMRI signals in gray matter at rest. These were 1.14% that of the baseline signal intensity, and were comparable to the percent changes in signals during the actual performance of assigned tasks.

4. S. Sdoia, A. Couyoumdjian, and F. Ferlazzo. Opposite visual field asymmetries for egocentric and allocentric spatial judgments. *NeuroReport* 2004; 15:1303–1305. Egocentric processing responses in the lower field are much faster (378 ms) than in the upper field (404 ms). Even so, allocentric processing in the upper field (447 ms) is slightly faster than in the lower field (465 ms). The slight differences were considered significant. Further confirmations are indicated, using techniques (that minimize the motor component) suitably modified with the aid of mirrors, to test the different visual quadrants for such differences in processing efficiency. It might be of interest to test subjects' responses to discrete bird calls located either above or below the acoustic horizon in 3-d space.

5. *Treasures of Dunhuang Grottos*. Hong Kong. Polyspring Co. Ltd. 2002. Revised first edition, plate 220, page 250 (ISBN 962-85787-2-3).

6. Psalm 121, Old Testament. Celestial objects in the sky are but one of countless reminders that we share the same stardust with other beings and things—all gifts from the same universe.

7. M. Ricard. *Tibet. An Inner Journey*. New York. Thames and Hudson, 2006. 195. Shabkar was an ordained itinerant sage in the Dzogchen tradition, renowned for his composing and singing "The Flight of the Garuda." See K. Dowman. *The Flight of the Garuda. The Dzogchen Tradition of Tibetan Buddhism*. Boston, Wisdom, 2003.

8. Tulken Urgen. *Rainbow Painting*. Hong Kong. Rangjung Yeshe Publications. 1995, 63–64. The Tibetan Dzogchen tradition speaks of *rigpa* as the "knowing" of unconstructed space devoid of all concepts, the "unity of emptiness and cognizance" (59–62). This nonduality corresponds with the states of kensho-satori in Zen. See also A. Lutz, J. Dunne, and R. Davidson. Meditation and the Neuroscience of Consciousness: An Introduction, in P. Zelazo, M. Moscovitch and E. Thompson. *Cambridge Handbook of Consciousness*. New York. Cambridge University Press. 2008. This chapter discusses how delicate it is even for an adept to *voluntarily* and *discursively* cultivate such an advanced refinement of open receptivity.

9. We make allowances for artistic license by the unknown artist who portrays this monk as appearing startled and as possessing large earlobes. Large earlobes are among the physical attributes ascribed to the historical Buddha. The strained posture and grasping hand might suggest an artist who had worked previously on fierce temple guardians and was not yet personally familiar with the way kensho releases the psyche from an expression of anxiety.

10. M. Palmer. *The Jesus Sutras*. New York. Ballantine Wellspring, 2001.

11. J. Henderson, C. Larson, and D. Zhu. Cortical activation to indoor versus outdoor scenes: an fMRI study. *Experimental Brain Research* 2007; 179:75–84.

12. F. Previc. The role of extrapersonal brain systems in religious activity. *Consciousness and Cognition* 2006; 15:500–539. With regard to the particular school of Zen Buddhism being discussed in this book, the emphasis places *selfless insight* at the core of the Zen transformation of states and traits. Accordingly, the orientation in these pages is twofold: First, toward the *fast* transmitter systems (both excitatory and inhibitory) that underlie our mechanisms of attention; second, toward the complex thalamocortical interactions that suddenly shift the brain into allocentric processing. This approach minimizes neither the role of biogenic

amines nor that of other messenger molecules [ZB:197–208]. It does reflect a different, more selective multifactorial explanation for the Zen Way than for the spectrum of religiosity in general, given that the term *religion* is often used to include a wide range of beliefs, experiences, and practices.

13. W. Schultz. Multiple dopamine functions at different time courses. *Annual Reviews in Neuroscience* 2007; 30:259–288.

14. R. Ronci. *This Rented Body*, Boston, Pressed Wafer, 2006, 78.

Chapter 24   Third Mondo

1. Jean Francois Fernel was an unusual Renaissance physician. His writings emphasized how organs actually *function*, not just their gross anatomy. Because he introduced the term "physiology," we owe a special debt to Fernel in the context of the functional anatomy reviewed in these pages.

Chapter 25   Intuitions about Insight

1. J. Austin. *Chase, Chance, and Creativity. The Lucky Art of Novelty.* New York, Columbia University Press, 1978. Revised edition Cambridge, MA, MIT Press, 2003; K. Heilman. *Creativity and the Brain.* New York. Psychology Press, 2005.

2. R. Sternberg and J. Davidson, eds. *The Nature of Insight.* Cambridge, MA, MIT Press, 1995.

3. J. Austin. *Zen and the Brain. Toward an Understanding of Meditation and Consciousness.* Cambridge, MA, MIT Press, 1998.

4. J. Austin. Consciousness evolves when the self dissolves. *Journal of Consciousness Studies* 2000; 7:209–230.

5. J. Austin. Your self, your brain, and Zen. *Cerebrum.* The Dana Forum on Brain Science, New York, 2003; 5:47–66.

6. J. Austin. *Zen-Brain Reflections. Reviewing Recent Developments in Meditation and States of Consciousness.* Cambridge, MA, MIT Press, 2006.

7. J. Davidson. The suddenness of insight, in R. Sternberg and J. Davidson, eds., *The Nature of Insight*, Cambridge, MA, MIT Press, 1995, 125–155.

8. U. Wagner, S. Gals, H. Halder, et al. Sleep inspires insight. *Nature* 2004; 427:352–355.

9. J. Ellenbogen, J. Hulbert, R. Stickgold, et al. Interfering with theories of sleep and memory: Sleep, declarative memory, and associative interference. *Current Biology* 2006; 16:R596–R597.

10. J. Ellenbogen, P. Hu, J. Payne, et al. Human relational memory requires time and sleep. *Proceedings of the National Academy of Sciences U.S.A.* 2007; 104:7723–7728. Reverie is a fruitful interval. Its boundaries need to be well-defined so that it can be studied as a distinct phenomenon.

11. Austin. *Chase, Chance, and Creativity*, 162, 184, 188.

12. Rarely, I'm under the impression that some answer might lie vaguely up "there," a foot away from the *right* side of my head, off at a variable angle. However, people reach other insight solutions much more successfully by using one or more of the three special processes cited that suddenly restructure the problem.

13. M. Ippolito and R. Tweney. The inception of insight, in R. Sternberg and J. Davidson, eds., *The Nature of Insight.* Cambridge, MA, MIT Press, 1995, 443–462.

14. M. Glick and R. Lockhart. Cognitive and affective components of insight, in R. Sternberg and J. Davidson, eds., *The Nature of Insight.* Cambridge, MA, MIT Press, 1995, 197–228.

15. Ippolito and Tweney, Cognitive and affective components.

16. www.sciam.com/ontheweb (D. Biello, "Fact or Fiction." *Science News*, December 8, 2006).

Chapter 26   A Lotus Puzzle

1. R. Sternberg and J. Davidson. *The Nature of Insight.* Cambridge, MA, MIT Press, 1995, 315. Adapted from the authors' earlier water lily problem.

Chapter 27   Our Normal Quest for Meaning

1. A. Ferguson. *Zen's Chinese Heritage. The Masters and Their Teachings.* Boston, Wisdom, 2000, 68.

2. A. Ropper and R. Brown, eds. *Adams and Victor's Principles of Neurology*, 8th ed. New York, McGraw-Hill, 2005, 406–408. Pure visual and auditory agnosias are more common after lesions of the dominant hemisphere (usually the left when the patient is right-handed). Anomias (word finding difficulties) are much more common. Normally, we engage and disengage several kinds and degrees of attention in order to grasp different associative threads and to weave them together into a more sustained, meaningful tapistry [ZB:601–603]. Current classifications list a disorder of piecemeal visual perception among the agnosias (and spell it simultanagnosia). However, different case reports suggest several alternative explanations for this uncommon condition. Among them is a basic defect *not* primarily in synthesizing meaning (as in other agnosias) but in *sustaining more global forms of attention* on more than one item in space at a time, or on more than one object at a time.

3. M. Vandenbulcke, R. Peeters, K. Fannes, et al. Knowledge of visual attributes in the right hemisphere. *Nature Neuroscience* 2006; 9:964–968. The patient had a bilateral left upper quadrant visual field defect accompanying the infarct of her right mid- and anterior fusiform gyrus. Her color vision remained essentially intact, but her visual feature matching, facial identification, and object decision task performances were impaired. All 27 normal controls were right-handed.

4. R. Rumiati, P. Weiss, A. Tessari, et al. Common and differential neural mechanisms supporting imitation of meaningful and meaningless actions. *Journal of Cognitive Neuroscience* 2005; 17:1420–1431. Imitation per se showed activation of the primary sensorimotor cortex, the supplementary motor area, and the ventral premotor cortex.

5. D. Kumaran, E. Maguire. Match mismatch processes underlie human hippocampal responses to associative novelty. *Journal of Neuroscience* 2007; 27:8517–8524. In the pages of this book, no brief is being made that déjà vu impressions are 100% accurate, just that they are fast, multifaceted, and widely distributed.

6. K. Watson, B. Matthews, and J. Allman. Brain activation during sight gags and language-dependent humor. *Cerebral Cortex* 2007; 17:314–324. Cartoons were selected from "The Far Side" and from *The New Yorker*. The researchers used language-independent sight gags that often challenged the viewers' first expectation. Other cartoons were language-based, and often contained an incongruity between the visual image and its caption.

7. D. Mobbs, P. Petrovic, J. Marchant, et al. When fear is near: Threat imminence elicits prefrontal-periaqueductal shifts in humans. *Science* 2007; 317:1079–1083. The central gray substance surrounds the core of the aqueduct in the midbrain. It serves as the core of our fearful defense responses.

Chapter 28   Studies of Meaningful Coherence in Visual Images

1. S. Han, Y. Jiang, and L. Mao. Right hemisphere dominance in perceiving coherence of visual events. *Neuroscience Letters* 2006; 398:18–21. The subjects correctly identified the coherent vs. the incoherent epochs.

2. J. Kable, J. Lease-Spellmeyer, and A. Chatterjee. Neural substrates of action event knowledge. *Journal of Cognitive Neuroscience* 2002; 14:795–805.

3. R. Saxe, D.-K. Xiao, G. Kovacs, et al. A region of right posterior superior temporal sulcus responds to observed intentional actions. *Neuropsychologia* 2004; 42:1435–1446.

4. J. Kable and A. Chatterjee. Specificity of action representations in the lateral occipitotemporal cortex. *Journal of Cognitive Neuroscience* 2006; 18:1498–1517. See also the following reaction-time study. It shows that the right lateral occipital complex (LOC) contributes not only to our perception of shapes but also to how we begin to estimate spatial position and distance. A. Ellison and A. Cowley. TMS can reveal contrasting functions of the dorsal and ventral visual processing streams. *Experimental Brain Research* 2006; 175:618–625. (TMS is transcranial magnetic stimulation.)

5. R. Saxe and L. Powell. It's the thought that counts: Specific brain regions for one component of theory of mind. *Psychological Science* 2006; 7:692–699.

6. A. Ciaramidaro, M. Adenzato, I. Enrici, et al. The intentional network: How the brain reads varieties of intentions. *Neuropsychologia* 2007; 45:3105–3115.

7. The sequence in kensho was different. The essentials were grasped as the old barriers collapsed. The incongruities could be discerned only after the "oneness" had arrived and then faded [ZBR:333–342, 361–371].

8. T. Tucker and J. Adler. *Zen Dog*. New York, Clarkson Potter, 2001. See also *The New Yorker Book of Dog Cartoons*. New York, Knopf, 1992. Different jokes wag different folks.

9. K. Watson, B. Matthews, and J. Allman. Brain activation during sight gags and language-dependent humor. *Cerebral Cortex* 2007; 17:314–324. The authors used cartoons both by Gary Larson and from the *New Yorker*. Their figure 2b shows the increases referable to the frontal operculum and the cingulate gyrus. Their figure 3 shows the many other regions that responded. A general "climate of uncertainty," "great doubt," and "not knowing" prevails throughout Zen training. It might be suggested that such uncertainty could subtly enhance the functional activity of von Economo nerve cells in ways that could contribute to several other processing benefits attributed to zazen.

10. K. Watson, T. Jones, and J. Allman. Dendritic architecture of the von Economo neurons. *Neuroscience* 2006; 141:1107–1112. These neurons have recently been found among granular cells in the normal prefrontal cortex of BA 9. See C. Fajardo, M. Escobar, E. Buritica, et al. Von Economo neurons are present in the dorsolateral (dysgranular) prefrontal cortex of humans. *Neuroscience Letters* 2008; 435: 215–218.

11. W. Seeley, D. Carlin, J. Allman, et al. Early frontotemporal dementia targets neurons unique to apes and humans. *Annals of Neurology* 2006; 60:660–667. Represented in the control brains were five cases of Alzheimer's disease and seven age-matched non-neurological diseases.

12. V. Goffaux, A. Mouraux, S. Desmet, et al. Human non–phase-locked gamma oscillations in experience-based perception of visual scenes. *Neuroscience Letters* 2004; 354:14–17.

13. D. Lenz, M. Jeschke, J. Schadow, et al. Human EEG very high frequency oscillations reflect the number of matches with a template in auditory short-term memory. *Brain Research* 2008; 1220:81–92.

Chapter 29   Dynamic Aspects of Truth

1. K. Taylor, H. Moss, E. Stamatakis, et al. Binding crossmodal object features in perirhinal cortex. *Proceedings of the National Academy of Sciences U.S.A.* 2006; 103:8239–8244. This is an fMRI study. The local anatomical details provide informative hints about function. The posterior end of this superior temporal sulcus rises up to enter the angular gyrus. In contrast, the posterior end of the lateral sylvian fissure rises up to enter the supramarginal gyrus (figures 1, 4). This gyrus corresponds with much of the TPJ in the data reported by Fox, Corbetta, and Snyder (chapter 7, reference 1).

2. H. Eichenbaum, A. Yonelinas, and C. Ranganath. The medial temporal lobe and recognition memory. *Annual Reviews in Neuroscience* 2007; 30:123–152.

3. H. Kim and R. Cabeza. Differential contributions of prefrontal, medial temporal, and sensory-perceptual regions to true and false memory formation. *Cerebral Cortex* 2007; 17:2143–2150. We await the detailed study of déjà vu episodes in this context [ZBR:422].

Chapter 30   Value Systems for Truth, Beauty, and Reality

1. Pierce's choice of the real as "the *object*" seems apt. At least, it appears to be in line with the curious proposal in part III that the collective interpretations within the ventral stream during *object-based* processing could contribute to the apparent sense of "reality" during kensho.

2. P. Winkielman, J. Halberstadt, T. Fazendeiro, et al. Prototypes are attractive because they are easy on the mind. *Psychological Science* 2006; 17:799–806. Fluency is definable as fast, efficient categorizing.

3. The facial expressions of bliss that accompany the absorptions would occur much more frequently. Collecting a detailed database on these changes during absorption would be a prerequisite to identifying whatever facial changes occur in kensho-satori and are manifest in an ongoing manner in a sage.

4. R. Zahn, J. Moll, F. Krueger, et al. Social concepts are represented in the superior anterior temporal cortex. *Proceedings of the National Academy of Sciences U.S.A.* 2007; 104:6430–6435. This same anterior superior region of the temporal pole is also involved in the general semantic processing of words (chapter 34).

Chapter 31   The Temporal Lobe: Harmonies of Perception and Interpretation

1. H. Roth. *Original Tao. Inward Training and the Foundations of Taoist Mysticism.* New York, Columbia University Press, 1999, 50–51.

2. L. Stewart, K. von Kriegstein, J. Warren, et al. Music and the brain: Disorders of musical listening. *Brain* 2006; 219:2533–2553.

3. S. Koelsch and W. Siebel. Towards a neural basis of music perception. *Trends in Cognitive Sciences* 2005; 9:578–584.

4. Arthur Sullivan (1842–1900) is also known for "Onward Christian Soldiers" and for his collaborations with William Gilbert in the Gilbert and Sullivan operettas.

5. This outstanding documentary was sponsored by the National Geographic Society and is available in a DVD. It is not to be missed. Ceramic replicas of this Tang dynasty camel are sold at museums in the People's Republic of China.

6. S. Koelsch. Investigating emotion with music: Neuroscientific approaches. *Annals of the New York Academy of Sciences* 2005; 1060:412–418. See also D. Sammler, M. Grigutsch, T. Fritz, et al. Music and emotion: Electrophysical correlates of the processing of pleasant and unpleasant music. *Psychophysiology* 2007; 44:293–304.

7. N. Gosselin, S. Samson, R. Adolphs, et al. Emotional responses to unpleasant music correlate with damage to the parahippocampal cortex. *Brain* 2006; 129:2585–2892.

8. N. Gosselin, I. Peretz, E. Johnsen, et al. Amygdala damage impairs emotion recognition from music. *Neuropsychologia* 2007; 45:236–244.

9. C. Conrad, H. Niess, K. Jauch, et al. Overture for growth hormone: Requiem for interleukin-6? *Critical Care Medicine* 2007; 35:2858–2859. This study was randomized, double-blind, and placebo-controlled. Slow measurements were chosen from various andante and adagio sonatas.

10. L. Patson, I. Kirk, M. Hsin, et al. The unusual symmetry of musicians: Musicians have equilateral interhemispheric transfer for visual information. *Neuropsychologia* 2007; 45:2059–2065. Nonmusicians transfer information faster from right to left, and the left occipital N1 component of their ERP occurs sooner.

11. C. Limb and A. Braun. Neural substrates of spontaneous musical performance: An fMRI study of jazz improvisation. *Public Library of Science ONE.* 2008. February 27; 3(2): e1679.

12. An extraordinary, passionate, all-consuming interest in and over-attachment to music can rarely develop in adults in the context of acquired structural brain disease, often in ways that can influence the temporal lobe. It is not yet clear which precise connections and phenomena (including disinhibition) are responsible for each of the individual case reports. See O. Sachs. *Musicophilia. Tales of Music and the Brain.* New York, Knopf, 2007.

Chapter 32   The Temporal Lobe: Word Thoughts Interfere with No-Thought Processing

1. J. Schooler, S. Ohlsson, and K. Brooks. Thoughts beyond words: When language overshadows insight. *Journal of Experimental Psychology: General* 1993; 122:166–183. Although "thinking aloud" types of verbalizations do interfere with solving problems directly by insight, they help groups solve problems indirectly, by so-called brain-storming approaches.

2. S. Virtue, J. Haberman, Z. Clancey, et al. Neural activity of inferences during story comprehension. *Brain Research* 2006; 1084:104–114.

3. J. Austin. *Chase, Chance, and Creativity: The Lucky Art of Novelty.* Cambridge, MA, MIT Press, 2003, 97–192.

4. J. Loori. *The Zen of Creativity. Cultivating Your Artistic Life.* New York, Ballantine, 2004.

5. J. Taylor. *My Stroke of Insight: A Brain Scientist's Personal Journey.* New York, Viking, 2008.

Chapter 33   The Pregnant Meditative Pause; Introspection; Incubation

1. M. Csikszentmihalyi and K. Sawyer. *Creative Insight: The Social Dimension,* in R. Sternberg and J. Davidson, eds. *The Nature of Insight.* Cambridge, MA, MIT Press, 1995, 329–363. The italics are mine. Most experts, years before they had their major insight, had become sufficiently resourceful to have gleaned essential facts from more than one domain.

2. Ibid.

3. J. Austin. *Chase, Chance and Creativity: The Lucky Art of Novelty.* New York, Columbia University Press, 1978. Revised edition: Cambridge, MA, MIT Press, 2003.

4. The Dalai Lama. *Mind and Life XIII. The Science and Clinical Applications of Meditation.* Washington, DC, November 9, 2005.

5. J. Ford. *Zen Master Who? A Guide to the People and Stories of Zen.* Boston, Wisdom, 2006, 35–43, 50.

6. Austin, *Chase, Chance, and Creativity,* 159–164.

7. A. Dijksterhuis and T. Meurs. Where creativity resides: The generative power of unconscious thought. *Conscious, Consciousness, and Cognition* 2006; 15:135–146.

8. H. Lau and R. Passingham. Unconscious activation of the cognitive control system in the human prefrontal cortex. *Journal of Neuroscience* 2007; 27:580–581. On the other hand, conflict signals from elsewhere can also activate this mid-dorsolateral cortex.

9. V. Sogen-Hori. Zen koan capping phrase books: Literary study and the insight "not founded on words or letters," in S. Heine and T. Wright, eds., *Zen Classics. Formative Texts in the History of Zen Buddhism.* Oxford, England, Oxford University Press, 2006, 171–214.

10. Ibid., 197.

11. Ibid., 173.

12. Ibid., 201.

13. "Contemplative" is a word that has taken on a variety of meanings in the West. Historically, they began with the spiritual practices that one might perform in a temple, including one's prayer and expressions of penance. In some instances, the meaning has expanded to include mystical absorptions. Yet the usual meaning suggests that the person's mental field is occupied by some form of thoughtful ideation. The implicit orientation of formal Zen meditation remains toward intuitions, not thoughts, not words.

14. Cf. T. Cleary. *Zen Essence. The Science of Freedom*. Boston, Shambhala, 1989, 41.

15. I. Schloegl. *The Zen Way*. London, Sheldon Press, 1977, 106.

Chapter 34   Recent, Ongoing Neuroimaging Studies of Ordinary Forms of Insight

1. J. Luo, K. Niki, and S. Phillips. The function of the anterior cingulate cortex (ACC) in the insightful solving of puzzles: The ACC is activated less when the structure of the puzzle is known. *Journal of Psychology in Chinese Societies* 2004; 5:195–213.

2. K. Niki and J. Luo. Letter, November 15, 2004.

3. M. Jung-Beeman, E. Bowden, J. Haberman, et al. Neural activity when people solve verbal problems with insight. *Public Library of Science Biology* 2004; 2:500–510. Interested readers can now access an excellent recent discussion of the rationale behind the various methods this group has used in their pioneering studies on insight in E. Bowden and M. Jung-Beeman. Methods for investigating the neural components of insight. *Methods* 2007; 42:87–99. See chapter 35 for its review of the companion article that was published in this same issue of *Methods*.

4. E. Bowden, M. Jung-Beeman, J. Fleck, et al. New approaches to demystifying insight. *Trends in Cognitive Sciences* 2005; 9:322–328. These word problems are called "compound remote associates" problems. A recent fMRI study of 15 male subjects used a variation of the remote word association task that demanded a snap judgment in only the first 1.5 seconds. The data contrasted the subjects' impressions of coherence with and without their having actually retrieved a solution word during this short interval. Again, the right superior temporal sulcus (STS) stood out in the results. So did the supramarginal gyrus (R > L). See R. Ilg, K. Vogeley, T. Goschke, et al. Neural processes underlying intuitive coherence judgments as revealed by fMRI on a semantic judgment task. *NeuroImage* 2007; 38:228–238.

5. M. Jung-Beeman. Bilateral brain processes for comprehending natural languages. *Trends in Cognitive Sciences* 2005; 9:512–518.

6. A. Revonsuo, M. Wilenius-Emet, J. Kuusela, et al. The neural generation of a unified illusion in human vision. *NeuroReport* 1997; 8:3367–3870. The resulting mental image was called a "stereoscopic Gestalt." It resembles the one you visualize when you see into the 2-D ambiguity of a "Magic Eye" picture and abruptly transform (transfigure) it into a coherent, meaningful stable image in three dimensions. Only minimal beta and alpha activities were seen in the midline occipital regions at the same time that this gamma burst appeared.

7. Y. Nir, L. Fisch, R. Mukamel, et al. Coupling between neuronal firing rate, gamma LFP, and BOLD fMRI is related to interneuronal correlations. *Current Biology* 2007; 17:R768–770.

8. M. Jung-Beeman, E. Bowden, J. Haberman, et al., Neural activity, 2004.

9. G. Knyazev. Motivation, emotion, and their inhibitory control mirrored in brain oscillations. *Neuroscience Biobehavioral Reviews* 2007; 31:377–395.

10. J. Kounios, J. Frymiare, E. Bowden, et al. The prepared mind: Neural activity prior to problem presentation predicts subsequent solution by sudden insight. *Psychological Science* 2006; 17:882–890. For technical reasons, confirmatory gamma EEG activity could not be reliably estimated during this study. The interval selected for fMRI monitoring corresponded (in its timing) with the subjects' next period of rest (rest periods varied from 2 to 8 seconds.) They

rested just *after* they had solved a problem successfully by insight. The duration of the rest periods was varied deliberately. The fact that the subjects could not predict precisely when they would be tested next rendered their preparation potentially more passive. No button press signals were required in the fMRI study, but a bimanual button press was required when the subjects decided that they felt prepared to start the trial. A later button press was required to specify that the verbalized solution had been accompanied by an insight-like experience. The subjects were limited to 30 seconds to solve each set of word problems.

11. C. Babiloni, F. Vecchio, A. Bultrini, et al. Pre- and poststimulus alpha rhythms are related to conscious visual perception: A high-resolution EEG study. *Cerebral Cortex* 2006; 16:1690–1700. An array of 128 EEG electrodes was used. Theta rhythms (between 4 and 6 cps) did not correlate with successful task performance. In these subjects, alpha frequencies were highest between 9 and 11 cps. People differ in the frequencies of their brain waves. This suggests that longitudinal studies could benefit from individualized analyses. Alpha rhythms are traditionally measured at 8 to 12 cps, and theta at 4 to 7 cps. The interval cited in this study (from 6 to 12 cps) is of interest in view of the earlier evidence that it happens to correspond with the increased coherence of waking waveforms found in those long-term meditators who report greater degrees of "ever-present awareness." [ZBR:237–239].

12. J. Lachaux, N. George, C. Talon-Baudry, et al. The many faces of the gamma band response to complex visual stimuli. *NeuroImage* 2005; 30:173–187.

13. J. Lachaux, J. Jung, N. Mainy, et al. Silence is golden: Transient neural deactivation in the prefrontal cortex during attentive reading. *Cerebral Cortex* 2008; 18:443–450. Gamma band synchronous activities appeared elsewhere in the expected network used for reading.

14. A. Brovelli, A. Lachaux, P. Kahane, et al. High gamma frequency oscillatory activity dissociates attention from intention in the human premotor cortex. *NeuroImage* 2005; 28:154–164. Reference 13 in chapter 28 discusses the higher gamma band frequencies that correlate with short-term memory.

15. G. Winterer, F. Carver, F. Musso, et al. Complex relationship between BOLD signal and synchronization/desynchronization of human brain MEG oscillations. *Human Brain Mapping* 2007; 28:805–816.

16. D. Senkowski, S. Molholm, M. Gomex-Ramirez, et al. Oscillatory beta activity predicts response speed during a multisensory audiovisual reaction time task: A high-density electrical mapping study. *Cerebral Cortex* 2006; 16:1556–1565.

17. D. Senkowski, D. Talsma, M. Grigutsch, et al. Good times for multisensory integration: Effects of the precision of temporal synchrony as revealed by gamma-band oscillations. *Neuropsychologia* 2007; 45:561–571.

Chapter 35   Alternative Ways to Study Ordinary Insight Using Neuroimaging Techniques

1. J. Luo, G. Knoblich. Studying insight problem solving with neuroscientific methods. *Methods* 2007; 42:77–86. This journal is to be congratulated for having brought to its pages in one issue the two reviews by each of the major groups studying insight.

Chapter 36   Does Eliminating the Negative Help to Accentuate the Positive?

1. H. Critchley, P. Lewis, M. Orth et al. Vagus nerve stimulation for treatment-resistant depression: Behavioral and neural effects on encoding negative material. *Psychosomatic Medicine* 2007; 69:17–22. FDA approval was for adults only. Vagal stimulation is a very expensive procedure (currently $25,000 to $30,000). As is true for any stimulation of neural systems, the parameters of stimulation are critical. They determine which will occur: physiologically comparable results or "jamming." Human and animal research suggests that

favorable clinical results evolve slowly and involve biochemical mechanisms both in brain and body. Longitudinal data on many patients are awaited.

2. Z. Nahas, C. Teneback, J. Chae, et al. Serial vagus nerve stimulation; Functional MRI in treatment-resistant depression. *Neuropsychopharmacology* 2007; 32:1649–1660. One interpretation of these data is that the ventral medial region would then be "needed" less.

3. T. Johnstone, C. van Reekum, H. Urry, et al. Failure to regulate: Counterproductive recruitment of top-down prefrontal-subcortical circuitry in major depression. *Journal of Neuroscience* 2007; 27:8877–8884. Attention points and notices instantly, whereas *reappraisal* is defined as an active, mindful reinterpretation of the content of a stimulus event that is intended to reduce its affective impact.

4. M. Greicius, B. Flores, V. Menon, et al. Resting-state functional connectivity in major depression: Abnormally increased contributions from subgenual cingulate cortex and thalamus. *Biological Psychiatry* 2007; 62:429–437. Compare these results with those in a meta-analysis: P. Fitzgerald, A. Laird, J. Maller, et al. A meta-analytic study of changes in brain activation in depression. *Human Brain Mapping* 2008; 29:683–695.

5. C. van Reekum, H. Urry, T. Johnstone, et al. Individual differences in amygdala and ventromedial prefrontal cortex activity are associated with evaluation speed and psychological well-being. *Journal of Cognitive Neuroscience* 2007; 19:237–248. The authors include area 24 in the ventral anterior cingulate and ventromedial prefrontal cortex.

6. D. Sharp, S. Scott, M. Mehta, et al. The neural correlates of declining performance with age: Evidence for age-related changes in cognitive control. *Cerebral Cortex* 2006; 16:1739–1749. See also a more intricate set of experiments conducted with fMRI at various ages reported by R. Gould, R. Brown, A. Owen, et al. Task-induced deactivations during successful paired associates learning: An effect of age but not Alzheimer's disease. *NeuroImage* 2006; 31:818–831.

7. A. Etkin, T. Egner, D. Peraza, et al. Resolving emotional conflict: A role for the rostral anterior cingulate cortex in modulating activity in the amygdala. *Neuron* 2006; 51:871–882. When the Stroop Conflict Task is used, conflict is inferred by lesser degrees of interference with the reaction time for an incongruent trial when it is preceded by an incongruent trial. When incongruent trials follow a congruent trial, the inference is that an "anticipatory" mechanism has been activated during the "conflict" generated by a prior incongruent trial, and that this expectation can lead to an improved resolution of the conflict during the next trial. A logical assumption underlies such experiments: A region responsible for conflict *resolution* should be more active during the trials that reflect this reduction in conflict. In contrast, a region implicated in *generating* conflict or in monitoring conflict should be more active when behavioral conflict is increased and when its successful resolution is less likely. The kinds of conflict that subjects experience during a task depend critically on which particular level is the site of the interference: Stimulus encoding, response selection, or the execution of the response. The patterns of fMRI signals vary accordingly. D. Nee, T. Wager, and J. Jonides. Interference resolution: Insights from a meta-analysis of neuroimaging tasks. *Cognitive Affective Behavioral Neuroscience* 2007; 7:1–17.

8. C. Grady, M. Springer, D. Hongwanishkul, et al. Age-related changes in brain activity across the adult lifespan. *Journal of Cognitive Neuroscience* 2006; 18:227–241.

9. T. Kircher, S. Weis, K. Freymann, et al. Hippocampal activation in MCI patients is necessary for successful memory encoding. *Journal of Neurology, Neurosurgery and Psychiatry* 2007; 78:812–818. MCI refers to mild cognitive impairment.

10. D. Margulies, A. Kelly, L. Uddin, et al. Mapping the functional connectivity of anterior cingulate cortex. Neuroimage 2007; 37:579–588.

11. Etkin et al. Resolving emotional content.

Chapter 37   Balancing One's Assets and Liabilities

1. Cf. T. Cleary. *Zen Essence. The Science of Freedom*. Boston, Shambhala, 1989, 58.
2. N. Kapur. Paradoxical functional facilitation in brain-behaviour research: A critical review. *Brain* 1996; 119:1775–1790.
3. B. Miller, J. Cummings, F. Mishkin, et al. Emergence of artistic talent in frontotemporal dementia. *Neurology* 1998; 51:978–982. The progression of the natural disease later eroded all these talents. The patients seem motivated to express in realistic terms what they experience as visual reality. Our current cultural belief system places a higher priority on many of the other ingredients of artistic creativity.
4. C. Hou, B. Miller, J. Cummings, et al. Autistic savants. *Neuropsychiatry and Neuropsychology Behavioral Neurology* 2000; 1:29–38.
5. L. Mottron, M. Dawson, I. Soulieres, et al. Enhanced perceptual functioning in autism: An update, and eight principles of autistic perception. *Journal of Autism and Developmental Disorders* 2006; 36:27–43.
6. With regard to such processing, though blindsighted patients might appear blind when tested conventionally, their second visual system readily detects certain small, low-contrast stimuli that are relayed through the pulvinar [ZBR:242–244]. C. Trevethan, A. Sahraie, and L. Weiskrantz. Can blindsight be superior to "sighted-sight?" *Cognition* 2007; 103:491–501. Subconsciously, the pulvinar processes "happy" body images via the second visual system and refers them up to cortical area MT. See B. de Gelder and N. Hadjikhani. Non-conscious recognition of emotional body language. *NeuroReport* 2006; 17:583–586.
7. J. Luo and G. Knoblich. Studying insight problem solving with neuroscientific methods. *Methods* 2007; 42:77–86.
8. C. Reverberi, A. Toraldo, S. D'Agostini, et al. Better without (lateral) frontal cortex? Insight problems solved by frontal patients. *Brain* 2005; 128:2882–2890. Nineteen of these 35 patients had meningiomas, and were studied between 7 and 150 days after their surgery. The authors provide alternative explanations for their findings.
9. An example of a more difficult task might be to change the matches of a plus sign into an equals sign. For example, when the false equation is VI = VI + VI, the result of moving one matchstick is to transform it into a tautology: VI = VI = VI. (I struck out on that one.) The dorsolateral frontal functions of patients in reference 8 are not strictly comparable to those patients in reference 3.
10. Confirming this major caveat are two other studies showing, for example, that patients with left lateral frontal lobe damage fail on tasks that require them to develop *new* abstract rules on the basis of inductive reasoning. See C. Reverberi, S. D'Agostini, M. Skrap, et al. Generation and recognition of abstract rules in different frontal lobe subgroups. *Neuropsychologia* 2005; 43:1924–1937; C. Reverberi, M. Laiacona, and E. Capitani. Qualitative features of semantic fluency performance in mesial and lateral frontal patients. *Neuropsychologia* 2006; 44:469–478.
11. C. Limb and A. Braun. Neural substrates of spontaneous musical performance: An fMRI study of jazz improvisation. *Public Library of Science ONE*. 2008 February 27; 3(2): e1679.
12. H. Gak (Ed.) *Wanting Enlightenment Is A Big Mistake. Teachings of Zen Master Seung Sahn*. 2006 Boston, Shambhala. 101, 145–146.
13. M. Corbetta, M. Kincade, C. Lewis, et al. Neural basis and recovery of spatial attention deficits in spatial neglect. *Nature Neuroscience* 2005; 8:1603–1610. The putamen was also involved. The contributions by the right temporoparietal junction (TPJ), the right superior temporal sulcus (STS), and of the underlying disconnections in the white matter fasciculi to

such neglect are considered further in the latest 2007 article from this group at Washington University. B. He, A. Snyder, J. Vincent, et al. Breakdown of functional connectivity in frontoparietal networks underlies behavioral deficits in spatial neglect. *Neuron* 2007; 53:905–918. It is not clear the degree to which these patients' clinical neglect was either object-centered, body-centered, or mixed. Some aspects of the patients' neglect were attributed to their problems in disengaging from visual stimuli. A single cause for the imbalance between the right and left intraparietal sulci is not evident. A major question remains: Do patients who have a *different* pattern of selective structural damage, this time involving *only* the cortical networks of the more *dorsal*, *egocentric* system, also show a measurable functional imbalance, and does it then contribute to the measured release of *hyperactive* responses within the *object*-centered network of the *allocentric* temporal lobe system? Multidisciplinary studies can resolve it only by correlating detailed behavioral neurological descriptions with neuroimaging data.

14. V. Goel, M. Tierney, L. Sheesley, et al. Hemispheric specialization in human prefrontal cortex for resolving certain and uncertain inferences. *Cerebral Cortex* 2007; 17:2245–2250. The different subdivisions of the prefrontal cortex play roles in creative problem solving that need to be evaluated separately.

Chapter 39   The Broken Water Bucket

1. J. Schooler, M. Fallshore, S. Fiore. Epilogue: Putting insight into perspective, in R. Sternberg and J. Davidson, eds., *The Nature of Insight*. Cambridge, MA, MIT Press, 1995, 559–587.
2. Cf. T. Cleary. *Classics of Buddhism and Zen*, vol. 4. Boston. Shambala, 2001, 553. This Ch'an master (also known as Hung-Chih Cheng-chueh) was both a poet and eloquent speaker in the Caodong (J. Soto) lineage.
3. Schooler et al., Epilogue.
4. www.google:Mugai-Nyodai In Japan, her Chinese Zen master was known as Bukko [ZB:117, 495].
5. A. Ferguson. *Zen's Chinese Heritage. The Masters and Their Teachings*. Boston, Wisdom, 2000, 364–366.
6. Schooler et al. Epilogue.

Chapter 40   The Construction and Dissolution of Time

1. D. Tranel, R. Jones. Knowing "what" and knowing "when." *Journal of Clinical Experimental Neuropsychology* 2006; 28:43–66.
2. B. Bennett, J. Reynolds, G. Prusky, et al. Cognitive deficits in rats after forebrain cholinergic depletion is reversed by a novel NO mimetic nitrate ester. *Neuropsychopharmacology* 2007; 32:505–513. This new molecule, mimicking nitric oxide, stimulates the cyclic GMP signal transduction system in the brain.
3. J. Okuda, F. Toshikatsu, H. Ohtake, et al. Differential involvement of regions of rostral prefrontal cortex (Brodmann Area 10) in time- and event-based prospective memory. *International Journal of Psychophysiology* 2007; 64:233–246. These are short-term experiments.
4. L. Battelli, A. Pascual-Leone, P. Cavanagh. The "when" pathway of the right parietal lobe. *Trends in Cognitive Sciences* 2007; 11:204–210. It would be of interest to determine if the lower visual fields have some relative and absolute advantage in this timing metric function. In this one respect, the way this right-sided network is responsible for processing the acute timing relationships for *both* sides of the environment resembles the bilateral responsibilities similarly assumed by the ventral attention system, as summarized in table 4. Note the functional distinction: this mostly *right*-sided representation of the so-called when pathway

normally focuses its metrics of attention on the milliseconds of short-term *timing*. In contrast, as discussed in part I, the dorsal path of the "where" pathways employs each intraparietal sulcus (IPS) to focus attention on *spatial discriminations*. Each IPS is chiefly oriented toward the *opposite side* of its environment, not toward *both sides* of the environment.

5. L. Uddin, I. Molnar-Szakacs, E. Zaidel, et al. rTMS to the right inferior parietal lobule disrupts self-other discrimination. *Social, Cognitive, and Affective Neuroscience* 2006; 1:65–71. Further studies are indicated in order to clarify the precise basis for this impairment in higher-level discrimination.

Chapter 42   Cutting into the Layers of Self

1. J. Burgdorf, J. Panksepp. The neurobiology of positive emotions. *Neuroscience Biobehavioral Reviews* 2006; 30:173–187. The sensorimotor sequences of several dopamine options become tricky to interpret in primates. Recent studies suggest that when trained monkeys confront a choice between two options for a potential reward, dopamine neurons tend to fire in accord with their latest snap decision. See Y. Niv, N. Daw, and P. Dayan. Choice values. *Nature Neuroscience* 2006; 9:987–988.

2. C. Martin-Soelch, J. Linthicum, and M. Ernst. Appetitive conditioning: Neural bases and implications for psychopathology. *Neuroscience and Biobehavioral Reviews* 2007; 31:426–440.

Chapter 43   Striking at the Roots of Overconditioned Attitudes

1. A. Ferguson. *Zen's Chinese Heritage: The Masters and Their Teachings.* Boston, Wisdom, 2000, 79–80.

2. S. Morinaga. *Novice to Master. An Ongoing Lesson in the Extent of My Own Stupidity.* Boston, Wisdom, 2004, 142.

3. J. Horgan. *Rational Mysticism. Dispatches from the Border between Science and Spirituality.* Boston, Houghton Mifflin, 2003, 230.

4. "Forum: How Does Karma Really Work?" *Buddhadharma* Spring 2007; 5:48–57.

5. D. Chadwick. *Crooked Cucumber. The Life and Zen Teachings of Shunryu Suzuki.* New York, Broadway, 1999, 345, 384. A similar not-knowing is associated with Bodhidharma and Nagarjuna.

6. T. Kuhn, cited in J. Austin. *Chase, Chance and Creativity. The Lucky Art of Novelty.* Cambridge, MA, MIT Press, 2003, 114–115.

7. D. Scott, M. Heitzeg, R. Koeppe, et al. Variations in the human pain stress experience mediated by ventral and dorsal basal ganglia dopamine activity. *Journal of Neuroscience* 2006; 26:10789–10795.

8. A. Galvan, T. Hare, C. Parra, et al. Earlier development of the accumbens relative to orbitofrontal cortex might underlie risk-taking behavior in adolescents. *Journal of Neuroscience* 2006; 26:6885–6892.

9. S. Floresco, S. Ghods-Sharifi, C. Vexelman, et al. Dissociable roles for the nucleus accumbens core and shell in regulating set shifting. *Journal of Neuroscience* 2006; 26:2449–2457.

10. J. Jensen, A. Smith, M. Willeit, et al. Separate brain regions code for salience vs. valence during reward predictions in humans. *Human Brain Mapping* 2007; 28:294–302. The results imply that the dopamine-accumbens circuit is the hub of a network that is involved in our anticipating an event.

11. A. Hampton, J. O'Doherty. Decoding the neural substrates of reward-related decision making with functional MRI. *Proceedings of the National Academy of Sciences U.S.A.* 2007; 104:1377–1382.

12. Q. Luo, M. Nakic, T. Wheatly, et al. The neural basis of implicit moral attitude—an IAT study using event-related fMRI. *NeuroImage* 2006; 30:1449–1457. (Table 13 in the next chapter summarizes how the subjects responded—with shorter or longer reaction times—to implicit association types of visual images.) The left precuneus and left insula were active participants in the incongruent responses. The superior temporal sulcus was an active participant in the responses to illegal pairings that were inherently immoral. This finding is in keeping with prior reports suggesting that the STS is involved in processing intentionality.

13. U. Herwig, T. Kaffenberger, T. Baumgartner, et al. Neural correlates of a "pessimistic" attitude when anticipating events of unknown emotional valence. *NeuroImage* 2007; 34:848–858.

Chapter 44   Neuroimaging Our Representations of Shoulds and Oughts

1. Q. Luo, M. Nakic, T. Wheatly, et al. The neural basis of implicit moral attitude—an IAT study using event-related fMRI. *NeuroImage* 2006; 30:1449–1457. The experiments covered a full range of options. For example, during the first phase of the study, the subjects recognized *legal* behaviors by pressing a button with their left hand. In contrast, they recognized illegal behaviors by pressing a different button with their right hand. (Subsequently, throughout the whole series of ten phases, they also alternated hands.)

2. K. Knutson, L. Mah, C. Manly, et al. Neural correlates of automatic beliefs about gender and race. *Human Brain Mapping* 2007; 28:915–930.

Chapter 45   Distinctions between Intuitive Mind Reading, Simple Empathy, and Compassion

1. T. Singer. The neuronal basis and ontogeny of empathy and mind reading: Review of literature and implications for future research. *Neuroscience and Biobehavioral Reviews* 2006; 30:855–863.

2. T. Whitford, C. Rennie, S. Grieve, et al. Brain maturation in adolescence: Concurrent changes in neuroanatomy and neurophysiology. *Human Brain Mapping* 2007; 28:228–237. The reductions in EEG power are attributed to the "synaptic pruning" that occurs in healthy adolescents. Parietal white matter volumes increase during these two decades.

3. S. Blakemore, H. den Ouden, S. Choudhury, et al. Adolescent development of the neural circuitry for thinking about intentions. *Social, Cognitive, and Affective Neuroscience* 2007; 2:130–139. The study by Williams et al. included a greater age range (from 12 to 79), and showed that the responses to fearful faces increased more in the medial but not the orbitofrontal cortex. See reference 6, chapter 55.

Chapter 46   Empathy, Forgivability, and the Responses of the Medial Prefrontal Cortex

1. K. Lee, W. Brown, P. Egleston, et al. A functional magnetic resonance imaging study of social cognition in schizophrenia during an acute episode and after recovery. *American Journal of Psychiatry* 2006; 163:1926–1933. All comparisons cited are made with reference to the data obtained during the subjects' baseline social reasoning judgments. All the schizophrenic patients were receiving conventional inpatient treatment and antipsychotic medication. The authors relate some left lateralized findings to the language-based material used throughout their study.

Chapter 47   Rigorous Retreats, and the Supporting Influence of a Friendly Hand

1. S. Ader. *Thoughts without Thinking. A Gathering of Wisdoms That Seeks Nothing and Finds Nothing.* Durham, NC, Acorn Press, 2004, 45.

2. B. Seymour, T. Singer, and R. Dolan. The neurobiology of punishment. *Nature Reviews in Neuroscience* 2007; 8:300–311. Zen masters were not the subject of this article. An ideal Zen

master is supposed to remain so objective that, aside from the actual energy efficiently expended, no personal cost would be incurred.

3. J. Coan, H. Schaefer, and R. Davidson. Lending a hand: Social regulation of the neural response to threat. *Psychological Science* 2006; 17:1032–1039. One wonders: What are the results when the wives provide emotional support for their husbands?

Chapter 48   Show Me

1. Willard Vandiver, a lawyer, registered Democrat, and oft-reelected congressman, was a distinguished public servant. He made his remarks in a playful spirit at a banquet in 1899.

2. A. Ropper, R. Brown. *Adams and Victor's Principles of Neurology*, 8th ed. New York, McGraw-Hill, 2005, 304–306, 359–394. The Greek root of the term might suggest that it was regarded chiefly as a disorder of top-down decision making.

3. M. Habib. Athymhormia and disorders of motivation in basal ganglia disease. *Journal of Neuropsychiatry and Clinical Neurosciences* 2004; 16:509–524. The disorders included under the established terms of *abulia* and *akinetic mutism* are distinct from those causing classic Parkinson's disease. Multiple neuromessengers interconnect these regions [ZBR:75–79].

Chapter 49   Fifth Mondo

1. Cf. T. Cleary. *Zen Essence. The Science of Freedom*. Boston, Shambhala, 1989, 31.

Chapter 51   Modulating the Emotions

1. T. Straube, H. Mentzel, W. Miltner. Waiting for spiders: Brain activation during anticipatory anxiety in spider phobics. *NeuroImage* 2007; 37:1427–1436.

2. N. Harrison, C. Wilson, H. Critchley. Processing of observed pupil size modulates perception of sadness and predicts empathy. *Emotion* 2007; 7:724–729.

3. C. Côté, M. Beauregard, A. Girard, et al. Individual variation in neural correlates of sadness in children: A twin fMRI study. *Human Brain Mapping* 2007; 28:482–487.

4. J. Peper, R. Brouwer, D. Boomsma, et al. Genetic influences on human brain structure: A review of brain imaging studies in twins. *Human Brain Mapping* 2007; 28:464–473.

5. P. Rainville, A. Bechara, N. Naqvi, et al. Basic emotions are associated with distinct patterns of cardiorespiratory activity. *International Journal of Psychophysiology* 2006; 61:5–18. The decrease in heart rate variability during fear appeared to be secondary to a reduction in respiratory sinus arrhythmia. However, the decreases during happiness and sadness were not coupled with these changes linked to respiration. Normally the intervals between heartbeats vary in relation to respiration in the following manner: Slow changes index the heart rate variations *between* respiratory cycles. These "low-frequency" changes recur at a slow rhythm between 3.6 and 6.0 times a minute. Rapid changes index the variations *within* one respiratory cycle. These can recur at a rhythm between 9 and 30 times a minute. See R. Nolan, M. Kamath, J. Floras, et al. Heart rate variability biofeedback as a behavioral neuro-cardiac intervention to enhance vagal heart rate control. *American Heart Journal* 2005; 149:1137.

6. The scope of this book limits our discussion of the technical issues involved. A recent review with three full pages of references is S. Porges. The polyvagal perspective. *Biological Psychology* 2007; 74:116–143. Controversial aspects related to any expansive theory of heart rate variability are aired elsewhere in this February issue of *Biological Psychiatry*.

7. H. Song, P. Lehrer. The effects of specific respiratory rates on heart rate and heart variability. *Applied Psychophysiological Biofeedback* 2003; 28:13–23. The heart rate normally increases during inspiration and decreases during expiration. It is an interesting commentary on the

"gentling" approach recommended for training both meditators and horses that the phenomenon of sinus arrhythmia was first observed in horses in 1733.

8. E. Vaschillo, B. Vaschillo, P. Lehrer. Characteristics of resonance in heart rate variability stimulated by biofeedback. *Applied Psychophysiological Biofeedback* 2006; 31:129–142. The author's caveat: The biofeedback procedure must train the subjects "not to breathe too deeply while they breathe slowly, at the resonant frequency."

9. M. Karavidas, P. Lehrer, E. Vaschillo, et al. Preliminary results of an open label study of heart rate variability biofeedback for the treatment of major depression. *Applied Psychophysiological Biofeedback* 2007; 32:19–30. The study was not placebo-controlled.

10. S. Phongsuphap, Y. Phongsupap, P. Chandanamattha, et al. Changes in heart rate variability during concentration meditation. *International Journal of Cardiology* 2008; in press. Authentic Zen emphasizes meditation. Its age-old path of Self-effacing restraint does not endorse artificial electronic devices. In the long-term approach of living Zen, character traits do not depend on silicon circuits. However, among meditators in this millennium, some beginners might find that a handheld visual device helps them learn how to focus attention on the in-and-out movements of breathing.

11. This discussion is intended solely to reflect the increased public interest in the sensory and motor functions of the vagus nerve (chapter 36) and in the growing preoccupation with electronic biofeedback techniques. Its inclusion here constitutes no endorsement. The discussion relates only tangentially to other important issues on the subject of respiration [ZBR:58–61]. No device is viewed as a substitute for Zen meditation. A controlled study is essential to determine which advanced meditators—those already breathing at slow rates—have arrived at a natural, spontaneous manner of breathing that might have been optimally synchronized with their vagal efferent and afferent rhythms.

12. The reference pages cited by Rainville et al., Nolan et al., and Porges (see references 5 and 6) survey the existing literature, but do not address the separate issue of what happens when *both* the sensory and motor fibers of the left vagus nerve are stimulated electronically (chapter 36).

13. P. Vestergaard-Poulson, M. vanBeek, J. Skewes, et al. Increased brainstem gray matter density in experienced meditators. Submitted for publication, 2008. The ten meditators and ten controls were matched for age (55 to 58), handedness, and gender. The increases in density in the upper medulla and left superior frontal gyrus were not obviously correlated with the subjects' age or their total hours of practice. One wonders whether the increased densities might correlate with their actual proficiency as meditators, with their degree of sinus arrythmia, or with the initial decline in their breathing rate during the first six minutes as they began to meditate (as described by S. Lazar et al. *NeuroReport* 2005; 16:1893–1897). The region of increased density also includes the inferior vestibular nucleus, the inferior olivary complex, and might influence some functions of the ninth (glossopharyngeal) cranial nerve.

14. C. van Reekum, T. Johnstone, H. Urry, et al. Gaze fixations predict brain activation during voluntary regulation of picture-induced negative affect. *NeuroImage* 2007; 36:1041–1055. Gaze can be softened and attention diffused during receptive meditation.

Chapter 52   How Could the Long-Term Meditative Path Modulate the Emotions?

1. Q. Luo, T. Holroyd, M. Jones, et al. Neural dynamics for facial threat processing as revealed by gamma band synchronization using MEG. *NeuroImage* 2007; 34:839–847. These sensitive MEG techniques now detect some fear responses in the hypothalamus and thalamus as early as 15 ms. It is being assumed that transmissions this fast in the thalamus are

being relayed via the colliculo-pulvinar visual system. If the fastest transmission times are referable to substance P fibers, it could be possible to slow them by giving a neurokinin-1 receptor antagonist. Later waves reflect processing in the geniculostriate visual system [ZB:241–244].

2. B. Wallace. A mindful balance. *Tricycle* 2008; 17:60–63, 109–111.

3. R. Kessler, W. Chiu, R. Jin, et al. The epidemiology of panic attacks, panic disorder, and ag-oraphobia in the National Comorbidity Survey Replication. *Archives of General Psychiatry* 2006; 63:415–424. The study was conducted from 2001 to 2003.

4. R. Kessler, E. Coccaro, M. Fava, et al. The prevalence and correlates of DSM-IV intermittent explosive disorder in the National Comorbidity Survey Replication. *Archives of General Psychiatry* 2006; 63:669–678.

5. R. Ward, A. Calder, M. Parker, et al. Emotion recognition following human pulvinar damage. *Neuropsychologia* 2007; 45:1973–1978.

6. B. Depue, T. Curran, M. Banich. Prefrontal regions orchestrate suppression of emotional memories via a two-phase process. *Science* 2007; 317:215–219.

Chapter 53   Newer Views of Extinction

1. M. Barad, P.-W. Gean, and B. Lutz. The role of the amygdala in the extinction of conditioned fear. *Biological Psychiatry* 2006; 60:322–328. The authors' physiological hypothesis is that learned extinction occurs within the lateral amygdala, and is a result of "long-term potentiation of one or both synapses in the feedforward inhibitory circuit."

2. Extinction in neurology is a different phenomenon. It describes a disorder of attentional balance. The patient cannot detect a target on the side opposite the lesion when a competing stimulus also occurs on the same side as the lesion. This disorder of attention often accompanies damage to the temporoparietal junction (TPJ).

3. D. Hermans, M. Craske, S. Mineka, et al. Extinction in human fear conditioning. *Biological Psychiatry* 2006; 60:361–368.

4. G. Quirk, R. Garcia, and F. Gonzalez-Lima. Prefrontal mechanisms in extinction of conditioned fear. *Biological Psychiatry* 2006; 60:337–343. The suggestion is that this medial region and other prefrontal regions go on, in turn, to inhibit regions elsewhere that had been serving to help *express* conditioned fear responses. These fear-generating regions include the ventral midbrain and medial dorsal thalamus, not just the auditory system that first transmits the sensory signals of the warning sound.

5. M. Barad. Is extinction of fear erasure or inhibition? Why both, of course. *Learning and Memory* 2006; 13:108–109. Currently, extinction is regarded as a process of new learning that inhibits previous kinds of learning, including that learned response to a stimulus which had acquired aversive properties.

6. F. Sotres-Bayon, C. Cain, J. LeDoux. Brain mechanisms of fear extinction: Historical perspectives on the contribution of prefrontal cortex. *Biological Psychiatry* 2006; 60:329–336.

7. F. Sotres-Bayon, D. Bush, J. LeDoux. Acquisition of fear extinction requires activation of NR2B-containing NMDA receptors in the lateral amygdala. *Neuropsychopharmacology* 2007; 32:1929–1940. The authors note that the term "medial prefrontal cortex" is often used to cover a wide region that can overlap with portions of the anterior cingulate gyrus and the medial orbital region.

8. S. Rauch, L. Shin, E. Phelps. Neurocircuitry models of post-traumatic stress disorder and extinction: Human neuroimaging research past, present, and future. *Biological Psychiatry* 2006; 60:376–382.

9. M. Gilbertson, S. Williston, L. Paulus, et al. Configural cue performance in identical twins discordant for posttraumatic stress disorder: Theoretical implications for the role of hippocampal function. *Biological Psychiatry* 2007; 62:513–520.

10. A. Brody, S. Saxena, J. Schwartz, et al. FDG-PET predictors of response to behavioral therapy and pharmacotherapy in obsessive compulsive disorder. *Psychiatry Research* 1998; 84:1–6. Zen practice employs mindful introspection and analysis (chapter 33). With regard to this top-down capacity to modulate the emotions, it is important to appreciate how effective a tool cognitive retraining is in defusing the urgency of obsessive and compulsive behaviors in some patients, and in reversing their PET scan abnormalities.

Chapter 54 Anatomical Asymmetries: Autonomic, Emotional, and Temperamental Implications

1. A. Craig. Forebrain emotional asymmetry: A neuroanatomical basis? *Trends in Cognitive Sciences* 2005; 9:566–571.

2. C. Wright, D. Williams, E. Feczko, et al. Neuroanatomical correlates of extraversion and neuroticism. *Cerebral Cortex* 2006; 16:1809–1819. Cortical surface analysis techniques were used.

3. Ibid.

4. M. Koenigs and D. Tranel. Irrational economic decision-making after ventromedial prefrontal damage: Evidence from the Ultimatum Game. *Journal of Neuroscience* 2007; 27:951–956.

5. R. Sternberg, T. Lubart. An investment perspective on insight, in D. Sternberg and J. Davidson, eds., *The Nature of Insight*. Cambridge, MA, MIT Press, 1995, 535, 558.

6. An anonymous saying.

Chapter 55 The Cognitive and Emotional Origins of Maturity

1. D. Fair, N. Dosenbach, J. Church, et al. Development of distinct control networks through segregation and integration. *Proceedings of the National Academy of Sciences U.S.A.* 2007; 104:13507–13512. See also the companion article: N. Dosenbach, D. Fair, F. Miezin, et al. Distinct brain networks for adaptive and stable task control in humans. *Proceedings of the National Academy of Sciences U.S.A.* 2007; 104:11073–11078. Signals shown in one subject fluctuate twice a minute in the right and left anterior insula-fronto-opercular regions. These regions are in the ventrolateral prefrontal cortex cited in table 3 (see chapter 55 and table 16). The frontoparietal component is the larger region. It helps maintain adaptive adjustments during our goal-directed behaviors. The "cingulo-opercular" network helps sustain a more stable task performance. The authors make an important point: the networks engaging in spontaneous fMRI signal fluctuation are, in fact, reflecting "a longstanding history of coactivation." Their connectivities provide a basis for consistently greater "synaptic efficiencies."

2. C. Buswell. *Tracing Back the Radiance. Chinul's Korean Way of Zen*. Honolulu. University of Hawaii Press 1991. 28, 59, 62–63.

3. D. MacPhillamy Some personality effects of long-term Zen monasticism and religious understanding. *Journal for the Scientific Study of Religion* 1986; 26:304–319.

4. L. Nielson, A. Kaszniak. Awareness of subtle emotional feelings: A comparison of long-term meditators and nonmeditators. *Emotion* 2006; 6:392–405.

5. M. Mather, L. Carstensen. Aging and motivated cognition: The positivity effect in attention and memory. *Trends in Cognitive Sciences* 2005; 9:496–502.

6. M. Mather, M. Knight. Goal-directed memory: The role of cognitive control in older adults' emotional memory. *Psychology of Aging* 2005; 20:554–570.

7. L. Williams, K. Brown, D. Palmer, et al. The mellow years?: Neural basis of improving emotional stability over age. *Journal of Neuroscience* 2006; 26:6422–6430. The study does not cite parallel evidence of the heart rate, respiratory rate, and blood pressure responses. This would help establish that the autonomic and respiratory responses of the maturing adults were correspondingly reduced. Cf. reference 3, chapter 45.

8. L. Williams, P. Das, B. Liddell, et al. Mode of functional connectivity in amygdala pathways in dissociated level of awareness signals of fear. *Journal of Neuroscience* 2006; 26:9264–9271. In themselves, connectivity analyses indicate that the two regions are linked, but do not indicate the direction of impulse flow.

9. S. Durston and B. Casey. What have we learned about cognitive development from neuroimaging? *Neuropsychologia* 2006; 44:2149–2157. Note that children become more mature in their abilities to override competing responses at around age 12 or so, whereas seniors become more distractible as their attentional skills wane.

10. S. Lazar, C. Kerr, R. Wasserman, et al. Meditative experience is associated with increased cortical thickness. *NeuroReport* 2005; 16:1893–1897.

11. G. Pagnoni and M. Cekic. Age effects on gray matter volume and attentional performance in Zen meditation. *Neurobiology of Aging* 2007; 10:1623–1627. Rapid visual attention processing was tested using a stream of fast-occurring digits in the center of a computer screen. The task was to detect three specific target sequences. The flexible merger of the cognitive skills inherent in both columns of table 16 would be an advantage in such a task.

12. H. Urry, C. van Reekum, T. Johnstone, et al. Amygdala and ventromedial prefrontal cortex are inversely coupled during regulation of negative affect and predict the diurnal pattern of cortisol secretion among older adults. *Journal of Neuroscience* 2006; 26:4415–4425.

13. J. Andrews-Hanna, A. Snyder, J. Vincent, et al. Disruption of large-scale brain systems in advanced aging. *Neuron* 2007; 56:924–935. Alzheimer changes were excluded as the explanation for the disconnection. The white matter tracts show abnormal degrees of anisotropy when studied with diffusion tensor imaging.

Chapter 56   Brain Peptides Help Decode Subtle Facial Emotions

1. K. Light, K. Grewen, J. Amico. More frequent partner hugs and higher oxytocin levels are linked to lower blood pressure and heart rate in premenopausal women. *Biological Psychology* 2005; 69:5–21.

2. G. Domes, M. Heinrichs, A. Michel, et al. Oxytocin improves "mind-reading" in humans. *Biological Psychiatry* 2007; 61:731–733. The pictures were displayed on a computer screen.

3. G. Meinlschmidt, C. Heim. Sensitivity to intranasal oxytocin in adult men with early parental separation. *Biological Psychiatry* 2007; 61:1109–1111. All studies were conducted at 4:30 P.M. Cortisol levels were determined in saliva.

4. P. Zak, A. Fakhar. Neuroactive hormones and interpersonal trust: International evidence. *Economics and Human Biology* 2006; 4:412–429.

5. It remains to be established how the oxytocin data is to be correlated with other data that links interpersonal trust with fMRI activity in the paracingulate cortex, conditional trust with activity in the ventral tegmental region, and unconditional trust with the septal area and adjoining hypothalamus. F. Krueger, K. McCabe, J. Moll, et al. Neural correlates of interpersonal trust. *Proceedings of the National Academy of Sciences U.S.A.* 2007; 104:20084–20089.

6. R. Thompson, K. George, J. Watson, et al. Sex-specific influences of vasopressin on human social communication. *Proceedings of the National Academy of Sciences U.S.A.* 2006; 103:7889–

7894. The left corrugator muscle above the brow contracts in response to anger and threat. The left zygomatic muscle over the cheek contracts during the kinds of smiling associated with "friendliness" responses. The authors have set a high standard in the design and execution of this study, and in the careful interpretation of the data.

Chapter 57   Did You Really "Have a Good Day?"

1. A. Stone, J. Schwartz, D. Schkade, et al. A population approach to the study of emotion: Diurnal rhythms of a working day examined with the Day Reconstruction Method. *Emotions* 2006; 6:139–149. Figure 3 compared the two age groups.

2. While we have attributed an implicit positive interpretation to competence in problem solving in table 16, the adjective *competent* remained a neutral option for subjects in this study.

Chapter 59   Selected Topics of Current Interest: A Sample
Gross Functional Anatomy
The Amygdala

1. C. Larson, H. Schaefer, G. Siegle, et al. Fear is fast in phobic individuals: Amygdala activation in response to fear-relevant stimuli. *Biological Psychiatry* 2006; 60:410–417.

2. L. Cahill. Why sex matters for neuroscience. *Nature Reviews Neuroscience* 2006; 7:477–484.

3. Ibid.

The Precuneus and Its Functions

4. A. Cavanna, M. Trimble. The precuneus: A review of its functional anatomy and behavioral correlates. *Brain* 2006; 129:564–583. Figures 1 and 2 in this article illustrate anatomical details of the precuneus. Readers should note that at this early moment in the evolving history of the so-called default system, a consensus view about the precuneus awaits the reconciliation of complex semantic and technical issues. Among them: The individual variations among histological boundaries, precise definition of intention vs. each of the two modes of attention, co-registration of earlier PET data with later fMRI data, and the influence of normalizing fMRI signals. A recent detailed review discusses these and other issues: R. Buckner, J. Andrews-Hanna, and D. Shacter. The brain's default network. Anatomy, function and relation to disease. *Annals of the New York Academy of Sciences* 2008; 1124:1–38.

5. W. Sturm, B. Schmenk, B. Fimm, et al. Spatial attention: More than intrinsic alerting? *Experimental Brain Research* 2006; 171:16–25.

6. A. Mayer, D. Harrington, J. Adair, et al. The neural networks underlying endogenous auditory covert orienting and reorienting. *NeuroImage* 2006; 30:938–949.

7. F. Castellanos, D. Margulies, C. Kelly, et al. Cingulate-precuneus interactions: A new locus of dysfunction in adult attention-deficit/hyperactivity disorder. *Biological Psychiatry* 2008; 63:332–337.

The Insula

8. O. Pollatos, K. Gramann, R. Schandry. Neural systems connecting interoceptive awareness and feelings. *Human Brain Mapping* 2007; 28:9–18. For contrast, a study of Tibetan Buddhist and Kundalini meditators indicates that several decades of formal practice did not enhance the accuracy of their heartbeat detection skills. S. Khalsa, D. Rudrauf, A. Damasio, et al. To feel or not to feel: Interoceptive awareness in experienced meditators. Poster: 2007 Mind and Life Summer Research Institute, June 3–9, 2007, Garrison, NY.

9. M. Gray, N. Harrison, S. Wiens, et al. Modulation of emotional appraisal by false psychological feedback during fMRI. *Public Library of Science ONE* 2007; 2:e546. "First-level"

physiological arousal prompted by physical exercise did not influence the data, presumably because the subjects correctly attributed their response to exercise.

10. J. Jensen, A. Smith, M. Willeit, et al. Separate brain regions code for salience vs. valence during reward prediction in humans. *Human Brain Mapping* 2007; 28:294–302.

11. M. Jabbi, M. Swart, and C. Keysers. Empathy for positive and negative emotions in the gustatory cortex. *NeuroImage* 2007; 34:1744–1753.

12. T. Singer. The neuronal basis of empathy and fairness. *Novartis Foundation Symposium* 2007; 278:20–30. Discussions:30–40.

13. M. Paulus and M. Stein. An insular view of anxiety. *Biological Psychiatry* 2006; 60:383–387.

14. M. Stein, A. Simmons, J. Feinstein, et al. Increased amygdala and insula activation during emotion processing in anxiety-prone subjects. *American Journal of Psychiatry* 2007; 164:318–327.

15. I. Sarinopoulos, G. Dixon, S. Short, et al. Brain mechanisms of expectation associated with insula and amygdala response to aversive taste: Implication for placebo. *Brain, Behavior, and Immunology* 2006; 20:120–132.

16. C. Farrer, C. Frith. Experiencing oneself vs. another person as being the cause of an action: The neural correlates of the experience of agency. *NeuroImage* 2002; 15:596–603.

17. M. Tsakiris, M. Hesse, C. Boy, et al. Neural signatures of body ownership: A sensory network for bodily self-consciousness. *Cerebral Cortex* 2007; 17:2235–2244.

18. J. Georgiadis, G. Holstege. Human brain activation during sexual stimulation of the penis. *Journal of Comprehensive Neurology* 2005; 493:33–38.

19. S. Ortigue, S. Grafton, F. Bianchi-Demicheli. Correlation between insula activation and self-reported quality of orgasm. *NeuroImage* 2007; 37:551–560.

20. N. Naqvi, D. Rudrauf, H. Damasio, et al. Damage to the insula disrupts addiction to cigarette smoking. *Science* 2007; 315:531–534.

21. B. Hölzel, U. Ott, T. Gard, et al. Investigation of mindfulness meditation practitioners with voxel-based morphometry. *Social Cognitive and Affective Neuroscience* 2008. In press. Gray matter concentration was also greater in the left inferior temporal gyrus in those who had more meditative training.

22. S. Lazar, C. Kerr, R. Wasserman, et al. Meditation experience is associated with increased cortical thickness. *NeuroReport* 2005; 16:1893–1897. The meditators were typical Western practitioners, not monks, who averaged 9 years of insight meditation experience. Their right middle and superior frontal region was also thicker.

23. P. Sterzer, C. Stadler, F. Poustka, et al. A structural neural deficit in adolescents with conduct disorder and its association with lack of empathy. *NeuroImage* 2007; 37:335–342.

The Ventromedial and Orbitofrontal Cortex

24. L. Fellows, M. Farah. The role of ventromedial prefrontal cortex in decision making: Judgment under uncertainty or judgment per se? *Cerebral Cortex* 2007; 17:2669–2674. The experimental conditions exclude uncertainty and test value judgments per se.

25. D. Tranel, H. Damasio, N. Denburg, et al. Does gender play a role in functional asymmetry of ventromedial prefrontal cortex? *Brain* 2005; 128:2872–2881.

26. J. Wallis. Orbitofrontal cortex and its contributions to decision-making. *Annual Reviews in Neuroscience* 2007; 30:31–56.

27. J. Moll, F. Krueger, R. Zahn, et al. Human fronto-mesolimbic networks guide decisions about charitable donation. *Proceedings of the National Academy of Sciences U.S.A.* 2006; 103:15623–15628.

28. J. Georgiadis, R. Kortekaas, R. Kuipers, et al. Regional cerebral blood flow changes associated with clitorally induced orgasm in healthy women. *European Journal of Neuroscience* 2006; 24:3305–3316.

29. J. Georgiadis, A. Simone Reinders, F. Van der Graaf, et al. Brain activation during human male ejaculation revisited. *NeuroReport* 2007; 18:553–557.

Psychophysiological Responses in Larger Networks
Relationships between Brain Waves and Higher Networking Functions

1. G. Knyazev. Motivation, emotion, and their inhibitory control mirrored in brain oscillations. *Neuroscience and Biobehavioral Reviews* 2007; 31:377–395.

2. O. Sporns, C. Honey. Small worlds inside big brains. *Proceedings of the National Academy of Sciences U.S.A.* 2006; 103:19219–19220.

3. D. Bassett, A. Meyer-Lindenberg, S. Achard, et al. Adaptive reconfiguration of fractal small-world human brain functional networks. *Proceedings of the National Academy of Sciences U.S.A.* 2006; 103:19518–19523.

4. D. Mantini, M. Perrucci, C. Del Gratta, et al. Electrophysiological signatures of resting state networks in the human brain. *Proceedings of the National Academy of Sciences U.S.A.* 2007; 104:13170–13175. The 15 male subjects lay quietly with their eyes closed. Their mental content is not described.

5. J. Kounios, J. Fleck, D. Green, et al. The origins of insight in resting-state brain activity. *Neuropsychologia* 2008; 46:281–291.

Linguistic Implications of Monkeying with Tools

6. A. Iriki. The neural origins and implications of imitation, mirror neurons and tool use. *Current Opinion in Neurobiology* 2006; 16:660–667. Surprisingly, monkeys in the wild tend not to imitate the actions of other monkeys. Chimpanzees are different.

Getting Personally Located and Navigating Inside Space

7. J. Taube. The head direction signal: Origins and sensory-motor integration. *Annual Reviews in Neuroscience* 2007; 30:181–207.

8. See: T. Hartley, C. Bird, D. Chan, et al. The hippocampus is required for short-term topographical memory in humans. *Hippocampus* 2007; 17:34–48; Y. Schager, P. Bayley, B. Bontempi, et al. Spatial memory and the human hippocampus. *Proceedings of the National Academy of Sciences U.S.A.* 2007; 104:2961–2966; H. Spiers, E. Maguire. The neuroscience of remote spatial memory: A tale of two cities. *Neuroscience* 2007; 149:7–27.

9. T. Wolbers, C. Weiller, C. Buchel. Neural foundations of emerging route knowledge in complex spatial environments. *Brain Research and Cognitive Brain Research* 2004; 21:401–411.

10. T. Wolbers, C. Buchel. Dissociable retrosplenial and hippocampal contributions to successful formation of survey representations. *Journal of Neuroscience* 2005; 25:3333–3340.

11. T. Sommer, M. Rose, J. Glascher, et al. Dissociable contributions within the medial temporal lobe to encoding of object-location associations. *Learning and Memory* 2005; 12:343–351.

The Remarkable Properties of Nitric Oxide

12. T. Edwards, N. Rickard. New perspectives on the mechanisms through which nitric oxide may affect learning and memory processes. *Neuroscience and Biobehavioral Reviews* 2007; 31:413–425.

13. R. Hopper, J. Garthwaite. Tonic and phasic nitric oxide signals in hippocampal long-term potentiation. *Journal of Neuroscience* 2006; 26:11513–11521. Note: Elsewhere in the brain, the

endothelial layer of small vessels can release its NO· to act on axons. In this manner, it can generate both tonic and phasic NO· signals. See also G. Garthwaite, K. Bartus, D. Malcolm, et al. Signaling from blood vessels to CNS axons through nitric oxide. *Journal of Neuroscience* 2006; 26:7730–7740. These endothelial sources of NO· also provide a mechanism for increasing stem cell proliferation within the hippocampus after exercise. See M. Moon, Y. Huh, C. Park. L-Nitroimidazole ornithine limits exercise-induced increases in cell proliferation in the hippocampus of adult mice. *NeuroReport* 2006; 17:1121–1125. Moreover, the dilation of smaller blood vessels caused by flavanols appears to be related to the release of NO· N. Fisher, F. Sarond, N. Hollenberg. Cocoa flavanols and brain perfusion. *Journal of Cardiovascular Pharmacology* 2006; 47:210–214.

14. H. Hoffmeyer, P. Enager, K. Thomsen, et al. Nonlinear neurovascular coupling in rat sensory cortex by activation of transcallosal fibers. *Journal of Cerebral Blood Flow Metabolism* 2007; 27:575–587.

15. M. Burke, C. Buhrle. BOLD response during uncoupling of neuronal activity and CBF. *NeuroImage* 2006; 32:1–8. The inhibitor was 7-nitroindazole.

16. B. Stepanovic, W. Schwindt, M. Hoehn, et al. Functional uncoupling of hemodynamic from neuronal response by inhibition of neuronal nitric oxide synthase. *Journal of Cerebral Blood Flow and Metabolism* 2007; 27:741–754.

17. S. Yang, C. Cox. Modulation of inhibitory activity by nitric oxide in the thalamus. *Journal of Neurophysiology* 2007; 97:3386–3395.

18. S. Moncada, J. Bolanos. Nitric oxide, cell bioenergetics and neurodegeneration. *Journal of Neurochemistry* 2006; 97:1676–1689.

19. R. Reiter, D.-X. Tan, M. Terron, et al. Melatonin and its metabolites: New findings regarding their production and their radical scavenging actions. *Acta Biochimica Polonica* 2007; 54:1–9.

20. B. Bennett, J. Reynolds, G. Prusky, et al. Cognitive deficits in rats after forebrain cholinergic depletion are reversed by a novel NO mimetic nitrate ester. *Neuropsychopharmacology* 2007; 32:505–513.

21. D. Butterfield, T. Reed, M. Perluigi, et al. Elevated levels of 3-nitrotyrosine in brain from subjects with amnestic mild cognitive impairment: Implications for the role of nitration in the progression of Alzheimer's disease. *Brain Research* 2007; 1148:243–248.

22. J. Jeong, C. Kum, H. Choi, et al. Extremely low frequency magnetic field induces hyperalgesia in mice modulated by nitric oxide synthesis. *Life Sciences* 2006; 78:1407–1412; A. Jelenkovic, B. Janac, V. Pesic, et al. Effects of extremely low-frequency magnetic field in the brain of rats. *Brain Research Bulletin* 2006; 68:355–360; S. Lores-Arnaiz, J. Bustamante, M. Arismendi, et al. Extensive enriched environments protect old rats from the aging dependent impairment of spatial cognition, synaptic plasticity and nitric oxide production. *Behavioral Brain Research* 2006; 169:294–302; J. Calka. The role of nitric oxide in the hypothalamic control of LHRH and oxytocin release, sexual behavior and aging of the LHRH and oxytocin neurons. *Folia Histochemica et Cytobiology* 2006; 44:3–12; D. Emmanouil, A. Dickens, R. Heckert, et al. Nitrous oxide–antinociception is mediated by opioid receptors and nitric oxide in the periaqueductal gray region of the midbrain. *European Neuropsychopharmacology Journal* 2008; 18:194–199.

23. J. Dusek, B.-H. Chang, J. Zaki, et al. Association between oxygen consumption and nitric oxide production during the relaxation response. *Medical Science Monitor* 2006; 12:CR1–CR10.

Transition Phenomena at the Boundary between States of Consciousness

24. M. Fox, A. Snyder, D. Barch, et al. Transient BOLD responses at block transitions. *NeuroImage* 2005; 28:956–966.

25. J. Austin. Consciousness evolves when the self dissolves. *Journal of Conscious Studies* 2000; 7:209–230.

Controversial Topics
A Sense of "Presence"

1. M. Persinger and S. Koren. A response to Granqvist et al. "Sensed presence and mystical experiences are predicted by suggestibility, not by the application of transcranial weak magnetic fields. *Neuroscience Letters* 2005; 380:346–347.

2. J. Booth, S. Koren, and M. Persinger. Increased feelings of the sensed presence and increased geomagnetic activity at the time of the experience during exposures to transcerebral weak complex magnetic fields. *International Journal of Neuroscience* 2005; 115:1053–1079. The subjects reported "sensing a presence or Sentient Being" while being exposed to the weak, complex magnetic fields over their right hemisphere.

3. P. Granqvist and M. Larsson. Contribution of religiousness in the prediction and interpretation of mystical experiences in a sensory deprivation context: Activation of religious schemas. *Journal of Psychology* 2006; 140:319–327. The reader will note that the term "religion" is being used in a context that is culture-bound. The complex culture-bound concepts of "Oneness" are discussed elsewhere [ZBR:333–357].

4. L. St.-Pierre and M. Persinger. Experimental facilitation of the sensed presence is predicted by the specific patterns of the applied magnetic fields, not by suggestibility: re-analyses of 19 experiments. *International Journal of Neuroscience* 2006; 116:1079–1096. The wording suggests that the subjects' parietal *and* temporal lobes were both exposed to the magnetic fields. The authors recently reported that adult rats develop increased ambulation behavior after a 15-minute exposure to weak, complex magnetic fields (0.5 to 1.0 µT). L. St.-Pierre, S. Koren, M. Persinger. Ambulatory effects of brief exposures to magnetic fields changing orthogonally in space over time. *International Journal of Neuroscience* 2007; 117:417–420.

5. J. Horgan, *Rational Mysticism: Dispatches from the Border between Science and Spirituality.* Boston, Houghton-Mifflin 2003, 91–105.

6. D. DeRidder, K. VanLaere, P. Dupont, et al. Visualizing out-of-body experience in the brain. *New England Journal of Medicine* 2007; 357:1829–1833. PET scans showed activations in and around the right TPJ, right precuneus, and posterior thalamus.

What Is the Relationship between Seizures and Mystical Experience?

7. A. Ogata, T. Miyakawa. Religious experiences in epileptic patients with a focus on ictus-related episodes. *Psychiatry and Clinical Neurosciences* 1998; 52:321–325. These three patients (two women and one man) were in that subgroup of 137 patients who had temporal lobe epilepsy, an incidence of 2.7%.

8. P. Trevisol-Bittencourt, A. Troiano. Interictal personality syndrome in non-dominant temporal lobe epilepsy: Case report [in Portugese]. *Arquives de Neuropsiquiatry* 2000; 58:548–555.

9. M. LeVan-Quyen, I. Khalilov, Y. Ben-Ari. The dark side of high-frequency oscillations in the developing brain. *Trends in Neuroscience* 2006; 29:419–427.

10. H. Laufs, K. Hamandi, A. Salek-Haddadi, et al. Temporal lobe interictal epileptic discharges affect cerebral activity in "default mode" brain regions. *Human Brain Mapping* 2007; 28:1023–1032.

11. The data suggest that an excessive degree of excitation spreads within the temporal lobe and then secondarily inhibits the precuneus, medial prefrontal, and supramarginal gyrus on that same side. Alternatively, does some primary, unilateral subcortical process excite the hippocampus *and* inhibit these other key regions? The answers have an important bearing on the Self/other issues raised in these pages.

Does Meditation Increase the Frequency of Seizures?

12. Jaseja H. Meditation and epilepsy: The ongoing debate. *Medical Hypotheses* 2007; 68:916–917.
13. D. Orme-Johnson. Evidence that the transcendental meditation program prevents or decreases diseases of the nervous system and is specifically beneficial for epilepsy. *Medical Hypotheses* 2006; 67:240–246.
14. E. Lansky and E. St. Louis. Transcendental meditation: A double-edged sword in epilepsy? *Epilepsy and Behavior* 2006; 9:394–400.
15. J. Grant, P. Rainville. Effects of Zen meditation and mindful states on pain sensitivity. *Psychosomatic Medicine* 2008. Submitted.
16. D. Orme-Johnson, R. Schneider, Y. Son, et al. Neuroimaging of meditation's effect on brain reactivity to pain. *NeuroReport* 2006; 17:1359–1363.
17. R. Kakigi, H. Nakata, K. Inui, et al. Intracerebral pain processing in a Yoga Master who claims not to feel pain during meditation. *European Journal of Pain* 2005; 9:581–589.

Does Functional Connectivity fMRI Yield "Real" Data?

18. M. Fox, A. Snyder, J. Zacks, et al. Coherent spontaneous activity accounts for trial-to-trial variability in human evoked brain responses. *Nature Neuroscience* 2006; 1:23–25.
19. M. Fox, A. Snyder, J. Vincent, et al. Intrinsic fluctuations within cortical systems account for intertrial variability in human behavior. *Neuron* 2007; 56:8–9.
20. M. Fox, M. Raichle. Spontaneous fluctuations in brain activity observed with functional magnetic resonance imaging. *Nature Reviews Neuroscience* 2007; 8:700–711.

A Return of the "Magic Mushroom?"

21. R. Griffiths, W. Richards, U. McCann, et al. Psilocybin can occasion mystical-type experiences having substantial personal meaning and spiritual significance. *Psychopharmacology* 2006; 187:268–283. Psilocybin is the active agent of the special "magic mushroom" that native South American tribes used in religious ceremonies.
22. R. Charman. Minds, brains, and communication. *Network Review* 2007; 93:11–15.
23. E. Laszlo. The hypothesis of the Akashic field. *Network Review* 2007; 94:12–16.
24. C. Clarke, M. King. Laszlo and McTaggart—in the light of this thing called physics. *Network Review* 2006; 92:6–11.

In Closing

1. I. Schloegl. *The Zen Way*. London, Sheldon Press, 1977, 116.

Glossary

1. Cf. T. Cleary. *Zen Essence. The Science of Freedom*. Boston, Shambhala, 1989.

Source Notes

In the interest of this shorter third book, readers are spared attributions for many epigraphs, save for the following.

Part III

The 100th Year of Joshu Sasaki-Roshi. Ithaca NY, Cayuga Press, 2007, 88.

The roshi's major emphasis on no-self (*anatta*) does not mean he was unaware of the two other general aspects of existence: its unsatisfactoriness (*dukkha*), and its impermanence (*anicca*). However, these two so-called signs of being were not the immediate realizations in this author's experience of kensho.

Part IV

M. Haverstock. *George Bellows: An Artist in Action.* London, Merrell, 2007, 139. Robert Henri was Bellows's teacher at the New York School of Art, and a founder of the so-called Ashcan School of modern American painting. Henri emphasized a quick, spontaneous approach to oil painting, reminiscent of the Zen approach to creative expression in general.

Index

Allocentric processing (cont.)
terminology related to, 57t
thalamocortical contributions in, 88f, 90
ventral direction of, 59, 61f, 62, 88f
ventral subnuclei of pulvinar in, 90
in visual perception, 55–56
deficits in, 67–69
integration with egocentric processing in, 56–58
Allophilia, 57
Alpha waves
as reverse measure of activation, 162
in visuospatial perceptual tasks, 167–168, 296n11
in word association tasks and insight processing, 162–165, 167
in preparation for tasks, 164–165
relationship with gamma waves, 162–164
Altruistic punishment, 216
Alzheimer's disease, 178
Amaro, Ajahn, 204
γ-Aminobutyric acid nerve cells, 92, 108, 119, 285n6, 285n8
in extinction mechanisms, 234
in internal absorptions, 121
Amygdala, 251–252
in affect labeling, 9
in conflicts with facial expressions, 176–177
anatomy of, 61f
in anger response, 230
definition of, 270
in emotional conflicts, 176–177
in fear response, 224, 229t, 229–230, 231, 307n1
age-related changes in, 241–242
functional connectivity analysis of, 241
in spider phobia, 224, 251
gender differences in responses of, 251
in humor and cartoon viewing, 138
in Implicit Association Test responses, 209–210
in kensho, 179–180
long-term meditative training affecting, 201
in music recognition, 148, 293n8
in psychological well-being, 176, 297n5
in regulation of negative affect, 243, 306n12
Anarchists, 204
Anatta, 87, 117, 120, 193, 219

Anesthesia, functional MRI in, 108, 288n12
Anger, 223
explosive, 230
normal pathway of, 228–229, 229t, 239
recall of, 225
heart rate response in, 225, 302n5
response to facial expression of, 228, 229t, 230
Angular gyrus
anatomy of, 24f, 60f, 88f
as metabolically active region, 71, 195
pulvinar connections with, 89
in self-referential network, 67, 105, 195
in visuospatial neglect, 66–67
and computerized alertness training, 7
Animal studies
on conditioned behaviors, 234
on dopamine system, 199–200, 300n1
on functional MRI in anesthesia, 108, 288n12
on mirror neurons, 76
on music response, 147–148
on nitric oxide, 310n22
on nucleus accumbens, 205–206
on tool use and socially specialized speech, 258–259, 309n6
Anomia, 291n2
Anticipation of event
negative bias and pessimistic attitude in, 207, 301n13
nucleus accumbens in, 206
in spider phobia, anxiety in, 224, 302n1
Anxiety
anticipatory, 224, 302n1
attacks of, 230
insula in, 254, 308nn13–14
Apperception, 281n2
Appetite stimulus, nucleus accumbens response to, 205–206
Archimedes, 129
Aristotle, 193, 194, 223
Artistic talents
in autism, 182
in frontotemporal dementia, 181–182, 298n3
Association tasks in word problems, 159–167. *See also* Word association tasks
Attention, 1–48
age-related changes in, 240, 243
allocentric other-centered perspective in, 55–56

Cerebral blood flow and nitric oxide
production, 260–261, 310nn15–16
Cerebrum, 270
Cessations of experience, 5–6
Ch'an Buddhism, 202, 203, 216
meditation practices in, 52
Chanting, 96
Children and adolescents
allocentric perspective in, 55, 281n1
anger attacks in, 230
brain development in, 212, 219, 301n2
conduct disorder and gray matter volume in,
255–256, 308n23
empathy and intuition in, 211
interpretations of intentions of others by,
212
loss of parent, and depression as adult, 245
pop-out phenomenon in, 35–36, 279n3
problem-solving networks in, 238t
risk-taking behavior in, 205, 300n8
Self and social knowledge in, 74, 283n7
Chinul, Master, 239
Chiyono, 191–192
Christensen, Mark, 27, 278n2
Christianity, meditative traditions in, 11,
276n3
in Catholic contemplative orders, 44–46
Cigarette smoking, insula in addiction to, 255,
308n20
Cingulate cortex
anterior
anatomy of, 25f, 61f
in cognitive conflicts, 172
functions of, 23
in insightful problem solving, 170–171
in lapses of attention, 23
left, in memory of mystical experiences,
45
in loving-kindness-compassion meditation,
41
right, in embodiment, 78
posterior
anatomy of, 25f, 61f, 88f
as metabolically active region, 71
in self-referential network, 105
Cingulate gyrus
anterior
in attention, 20, 179

in cognitive conflicts, 20, 278n13
in depression, 177
in emotional conflicts, 20, 176–177, 179,
278n14, 297n7
in humor and cartoon viewing, 138
in Implicit Association Test responses, 209
in posttraumatic stress disorder, 177
in problem solving and insight, 187
in readiness for word association tasks, 166
in Vipassana meditation, 42
in visuospatial neglect and alertness
training, 7
posterior
in children, 74
in readiness for word association tasks, 166,
167
Cingulo-opercular network, anatomy and
functions of, 238t, 239, 305n1
Clarity
emotional, in long-term meditators, 239–240
perceptual, 27–29, 145
Coan, J., 216, 302n3
Cognition
definition of, 125, 270
moral, 207–208, 210
and motivational drives, 218
social, 74–75, 283n8, 283n11
in children, 74, 283n7
negative aspects of, 210
in schizophrenia, 213–214, 301n1
speed and clarity in, 145
Cognitive-behavioral therapy, 154
Cognitive conflicts
anterior cingulate cortex and gyrus in, 20,
172, 278n13
in interpretation of ambiguous sentences,
171, 172
Coherence
definition of, 270
in meaningful visual images, 135–141, 186
Coleridge, Samuel, 143–144, 146
Colliculus
inferior, 89
superior, 89
in subject/object distinctions, 80
Compassion
differentiated from empathy and intuition,
211–213

DeFontenelle, Bernard, 237
Dehaene, Stanislas, 28, 278n3
Déjà vu phenomena, temporal lobe role in, 133–134, 264, 291n5
DeLuca, C., 106, 287n4
Dementia
  in Alzheimer's disease, 178
  frontotemporal, 139, 292n11
    artistic talents in, 181–182, 298n3
  semantic, 132
Depression
  as adult, after loss of parent during childhood, 245
  biofeedback procedures in, 226, 303n9
  resting state functional connectivity in, 175–176, 297n4
  sadness in, 224
  vagus nerve stimulation in, 173–176, 296–297nn1–2
Desmosthenes, 81
Disgust, 232
  insula in, 232, 253, 254
Disinhibition, 180, 270
Dogen, Master, 49, 64, 198
Dopamine
  animal studies of, 199–200, 300n1
  in nucleus accumbens, 205
  in religious activities, 117, 189–190nn12–13
Dorsal attention, 29, 30, 279n1
  age-related changes in, 243
  anatomy in, 33f
  compared to ventral attention, 31t
  in pop-out phenomenon, 36
  top-down processes in, 30, 31t, 33f, 40t, 47
Drug addiction, 201
  ventral striatum in, 206
Dualism, 79
Dunhuang, Buddhist caves at, 116
Dusek, J., 261, 310n23
Dwelling in tranquility, 5, 274n5

Edison, Thomas, 128, 205
Edwards, T., 260, 309n12
Efficiency in attentional processing
  resource management in, 286n3
  training affecting, 35–39
Egocentric processing, 54–55, 83
  age-related changes in, 243

in assigned tasks, functional MRI during, 101–102
balance with allocentric processing, 109
  reciprocal cycle of spontaneous fluctuations in, 103–108, 112, 187–188
  triggering stimuli affecting, 113, 114
bias toward, 92
compared to allocentric processing, 63t
deactivation of, 111, 114, 118–119
dorsal direction of, 58–59, 60f, 88f
frontoparietal regions in, 99, 101–102, 105
hippocampus in, 96–97
integration with allocentric processing, 56–58, 62–64
let go in meditation, 11
in memory, subconscious processes in, 100
networks in, 82, 105–106
  functional connectivity of, 103
  reciprocal cycle of slow spontaneous fluctuations in, 103–108
parietal lobe in, 65–67, 134–135
  lesions affecting, 65–67
  Self-orientation of networks in, 82
right hemisphere in, 61f, 64, 69, 70t, 282n4
shift to allocentric processing, 92–93
  frequency of spontaneous shifts in, 111, 288n2
  implications of, 93–94
  in kensho, 119
  neuroimaging during, 98–103
  reciprocal cycle of spontaneous fluctuations in, 103–108, 112
in spatial reference, 58–64, 80, 281n4
  in verbal descriptions, 73–74, 283n6
  visual fields in, 115, 289n4
terminology related to, 57t
thalamocortical contributions to, 88f
in vision, 54–55
Einstein, Albert, 135
Eisai, Master, 203
Electroencephalogram (EEG)
  alpha waves in. See Alpha waves
  in children and adolescents, 212, 301n2
  definition of, 271
  in ever-present awareness, 37
  gamma waves in. See Gamma waves
  of resting state networks, 257–258
  theta phase in, 16, 277n6

Electroencephalogram (EEG) (cont.)
  in visual perception, 167–169
    alpha waves in, 167–168, 296n11
    gamma activations and deactivations in,
      168–169
  in word anagram problem-solving, 258
  in word association tasks and insight
    processing, 161–165, 167, 187
    alpha and gamma waves in, 162–164, 167
    in preparation for tasks, 164–165, 295–296n10
Electromyography of facial muscles
  in kensho, 145
  in positive affective responses, 145
Ellenbogen, J., 127, 290n9
Embodied simulation, 77, 283n2
Embodiment, 78, 284nn9–12
  as body ownership, 78, 255, 284n11, 308n17
  definition of, 78
  insula in, 78, 255, 308n17
Emerson, R. W., 204
Emotions, 221–248
  anterior cingulate gyrus in conflicts of, 20,
    176–177, 179, 278n14, 297n7
  and clarity in long-term meditators, 239–240
  covert associations of, 208–210
  daily patterns of changes in, 246–247, 307n1
  labeling of, 9, 276n4
    congruence with facial expressions in, 176–
      177, 297n7
  learning about, 223
  limbic system in, 89, 90
  modulation of, 223–232
    in long-term meditation, 228–232
  and motivational drives, 218
  recalling memory of, 224–225
  suppression of unwanted, 247
  Zen commentary on, 224
Empathy, 77, 283nn4–5
  differentiated from intuition and compassion,
    211–213, 212t
  insula in, 253, 254, 256
  medial prefrontal cortex in, 213–215
  observation of pupil size and perception of
    sadness in, 224, 302n2
Emptiness, 219
  phenomena of, 196
  in satori, 196
  of self, 191

Enlightenment
  behavioral manifestations of, 217–218
  definition of, 271
  freedom in, 204
  insight-wisdom in, 197–198
  in kensho, 125
  of Siddhartha under Bodhi tree, 115–116, 129,
    197, 247–248
Entorhinal cortex in head direction signals,
  259
Epictetus, 51, 281n1
Equipoise, 112
Eternity, 94
Ethical behavior, 4, 202–204
Etkin, A., 176, 179, 297n7, 297n11
Eureka! moment in insight, 129
Evoked (event-related) potentials, 14–16
  in attention blinks, meditative training
    affecting, 7, 275n13
  in attention shifts, 262
  definition of, 271
  in introspection, 15–16
  in response to facial expressions, 240–241
    in happy expressions, 242–243
  in visual perception of bare stimulus, 14–15,
    38
Experiant, definition of, 271
Experience
  cessations of, 5–6
  nondual, selfless mode of, 54
Extinction
  as active form of new inhibitory learning, 234
  of fear, 234, 304nn6–7
    of death, 235
  mechanisms of, 234–235
  in neurology, 304n2
  newer views of, 233–235
  in psychology, 233
  of Self in nirvana, 233
Extrastriate body area in embodiment, 78
Extroversion, 236

Facebook, 51, 281n2
Facial expressions
  in absorptions, 293n3
  age-related changes in responses to, 240–243,
    247
    in fearful expressions, 241

in happy expressions, 242–243
angry, responses to, 228, 229t, 230
event-related potentials in responses to, 240–241, 242–243
fearful, responses to, 36, 176–177, 228–230, 229t, 301n3, 303–304n1
  age-related changes in, 241
  thalamic lesion affecting, 232
functional MRI in responses to, 240–241, 242
happy, responses to, 176–177
  age-related changes in, 242–243
oxytocin affecting interpretation of, 244, 306n2
sad, recognition of, 224, 302n2
vasopressin affecting responses to, 245
Facial muscle electromyography
in kensho, 145
in positive affective responses, 145
Fallshore, M., 191, 299n1
"Far Side" cartoons, 136, 291n6
Fear
of death, 235
extinction of, 234, 304nn6–7
  in fear of death, 235
facial expression of, response to, 36, 176–177, 228–230, 229t, 301n3, 303–304n1
  age-elated changes in, 241
  thalamic lesion affecting, 232
heart rate response in recall of, 225, 302n5
loss in kensho, 179, 180, 207, 230–231, 235
normal pathway of, 228–230, 229t
responses to, 135, 228–230, 291n7
  age-related changes in, 241–242
  amygdala in. See Amygdala, in fear response
  dopamine release in, 205
  functional MRI signals in, 224, 241, 242, 251
  magnetoencephalography in, 242
  subliminal, 242
spider phobia in, 224, 251, 302n1
Figure/ground distinctions, 136
Fiore, S., 191, 299n1
Flashes of insight, 94, 151–152
Fluency in processing, 145
Ford, James, 10, 276n11
Forebrain
left, parasympathetic activity in, 235
right, sympathetic activity in, 235

Foresight, magnetoencephalography studies of, 19
Forgivability judgments, medial prefrontal cortex responses in, 213–215
Fox, M., 29, 103, 104, 105, 262, 267, 279n1, 287n1, 310n24, 312n20
Foyan Quingyuan, 158, 270
Franklin, Benjamin, 215, 228
Fransson, Peter, 106, 287n2
Freedom in enlightenment, 204
Freud, Sigmund, 79, 130, 131, 223, 284n2
Frings, L., 73, 283n4
Frontal cortex
age-related thinning of, meditation affecting, 243, 306n10
lateral, in top-down visual attention, 17
right ventrolateral, in ventral attention system, 31, 31t
superior, in self-referential network, 105
in visuospatial neglect and alertness training, 7
Frontal eye field
anatomy of, 24f, 33f, 60f
in attention, 228
  in dorsal network, 30, 31t
direct stimulation of, 17
in other-referential network, 104
Frontal gyrus
inferior
  anatomy of, 24f, 33f, 60f
  in cognitive control pathway, 232
  in coordination of attention systems, 32
  in lapses of attention, 23, 25, 26
  in loving-kindness-compassion meditation, 42
  in spatial judgments in virtual 3-D environment, 73
middle
  anatomy of, 33f, 60f
  in cognitive control pathway, 232
  in coordination of attention systems, 32
  executive role of, 62
  in humor and cartoon viewing, 138
  in insightful problem solving, 170
  in memory of street navigation, 73
  in Self-centered and other-oriented tasks, 62
superior, in insightful problem solving, 170
in visual processing, 19

Hakuin, Master, 154
Hakuun Yasutani, 53
Hallucinations in internal absorption, 98, 111, 262
Han, Shihui, 135, 291n1
Happiness
  facial expressions of, responses to, 176–177
    age-related changes in, 242–243
  heart rate response in recall of, 225, 302n5
Happo biraki, 38
Harmonic resonances, 144, 145, 146, 147
Head direction signals, 259, 309n7
Heart rate variability, 225, 302–303nn5–10
  in biofeedback procedures, 226–227, 303nn8–9
  in concentrative meditation, 303n10
  and oxytocin levels, 244, 306n1
  in recall of emotions, 225, 302n5
  in slow breathing rate, 226
Heisenberg, Werner, 141
Hempel, H., 39, 279n1
Henri, Robert, 123, 125, 143
Hillis, A., 65, 282n2
Hippocampal formation, 96–97
  in allocentric processing, 73
Hippocampus
  in allocentric and egocentric processing, 96–97
  definition of, 271
  effects of bilateral damage, 80, 284n4
  in humor and cartoon viewing, 138
  in memory, 107, 178, 288n7, 297n9
  in navigation, 259, 309n8
  in response to associative novelty, 134, 291n5
  spatial view cells in, 62
Hölzel, B., 39, 42, 279n1, 280n6
Hongzhi Zhengjue, 191, 299n1
Huang-po, 92, 189, 196
Hui-Neng, 203
Human body
  and body ownership, 78, 255, 284n11, 308n17
  and embodiment. *See* Embodiment
  recognition of, 78
Humor, meaning in, 134, 136–138
  frontotemporal dementia affecting, 139
  vision and language in interpretation of, 134, 138, 291n6
Huxley, Aldous, 146

Huxley, Thomas H., 144
Hypothalamus, 271

I-Me-Mine
  destructuring in kensho-satori, 173
  dissolution in selfless insight, 188
  limbic associations linked to, 93
  and no-self, 117, 193
  restructuring and transformation of, 10, 153
  role of Me in, 200
  and self-referential processing, 100, 110, 117, 120
  and shift toward You-Us-Ours, 240
  susceptibility to spiritual materialism, 52
Ikkyu Sojun, 3, 34, 274n1
Imitation of meaningful acts, PET scans in, 132–133, 291n4
Immanence, 199, 219
Implicit Association Test, 208–211, 288n8
  racial and gender attitudinal biases in, 210–211
  responses to legal and illegal behaviors in, 208–209, 210
Impulsive behaviors, 237
Inclinations
  moral, Implicit Association Test of, 208–211
  nucleus accumbens in, 205–206
  in post-kensho period, 206–207
Incongruence and congruence
  in Implicit Association Test, 208t, 208–211
  in labeling of facial expressions, conflict resolution in, 176–177
Incubation process
  in creativity, unconscious mechanisms in, 155, 295n7
  in insight, 153–158
  restructuring in, 127–128
Induced responses compared to evoked responses, 16, 17t, 48
Infants
  empathy in, 211
  pop-out phenomenon in, 35–36, 279n3
Infarction of thalamus, attentional bias in, 21, 278n16
Inferences
  bihemispheric processing in, 150–151, 151t
  in story comprehension, 150–151, 151t, 294n2

Insight
  Aha! phenomenon in, 128–129, 159, 160
  definition of, 126, 271
  Eureka! moment in, 129
  flashes of, 94, 151–152
  incubation process in, 127–128, 153–158
  in introspection, 110, 153–156
  intuitions on, 125–129
  lotus puzzle as example of, 130
  in matchstick tasks, 183–184
  minor events of, 154–155
  nature of, 123–188
  neuroimaging studies in, 158–173
  ordinary forms of, 125–130, 158–173
  physiological basis of, 125
  preliminary feeling of, 128
  restructuring in, 126–128
    functional MRI during, 170–172
  in schizophrenia recovery, 214
  selfless, 156–157, 158, 289n12
    functional anatomy in, 188
    in kensho, 186, 187
  sequence of excitatory and inhibitory events
    in, 187
  types of processes in, 127, 128
  verbalizations affecting, 150, 294n1
  in word association tasks, 159–167
Insight therapy, 154
Insight-wisdom, 94, 117, 125, 274n5
  in awakening, 197–198
  compared to ordinary factual knowledge, 202
  definition of, 126, 271
  flashes of, 152
  in kensho, 129, 219
  path toward, 189–219
  selfless, 13, 129, 186
  triggering stimuli in precipitation of, 191–192
Instincts and motivational drives, 218
Insula, 253–256
  in addiction to cigarette smoking, 255,
    308n20
  anatomy of, 253
  in anxiety, 254, 308nn13–14
  in depression and vagus nerve stimulation,
    174, 175
  in disgust, 232, 253, 254
  in embodiment or body ownership, 78, 255,
    308n17

  in empathy, 253, 254, 256
  in expectation of aversive taste, 254, 308n15
  functions of, 253–256
  in humor and cartoon viewing, 138
  left, in parasympathetic activity, 236
  in loving-kindness-compassion meditation, 41
  in other-referential network, 104
  right, 235–236
    in sympathetic activity, 236
  in sexual stimulation, 255, 308nn18–19
Integrative body-mind training, 42–43
Intentions
  differentiated from attention, gamma
    frequencies in, 168, 296n14
  interpretations of, 77, 136, 283n3, 292n6
    by adolescents, 212
Internet sites
  habit-forming and addictive behaviors in use
    of, 51, 52
  self-indulgent expression on, 51, 281n3
Interoceptive awareness, 253, 307n8
Interpersonal behaviors, 74
  affiliative, oxytocin in, 244
Intraparietal sulcus
  in dorsal attention network, 30, 31t
  in other-referential network, 104
  posterior
    anatomy of, 24f, 33f, 60f
    in clarity of visual perceptions, 28
    in voluntary attention, 59
Introspection, 74–75
  event-related potentials in, 15–16
  insight in, 110, 153–156
  and self-analysis, 153–154
Introversion, 236
Intuition, 77, 186
  alpha-gamma sequence in, 163
  creative, 163–164
  definition of, 125, 271
  differentiated from empathy and
    compassion, 211–213, 212t
  on insight, 125–129
  minor events of, 154–155
Ippolito, M., 129, 290n13, 290n15
Iriki, A., 258, 259, 309n6

Jackson, Hughlings, 54
Jain, S., 9, 276n5

James, William, 1, 27, 141, 173, 198, 251
Jazz improvisations, deactivations during, 149, 184, 294n11
Jerome, Saint, 244
Jha, A., 39, 280n2
Jones, R., 193, 299n1
Judgments
  and decision-making, ventromedial prefrontal cortex in, 256, 308n24
  empathic, medial prefrontal cortex in, 213–215
  spatial, in virtual 3-D environment, 73
Jung, Carl, 87, 109, 125
Jung-Beeman, Mark, 159, 163, 295n3, 295n8
Just this, 11–13, 199
  ancient uses of, 12, 276n5
  as mantra in meditation, 11–12
Justice, symbolic image of, 112

Kabat-Zinn, Jon, 8, 275nn1–2
Kapur, N., 181, 298n2
Karuna, 213
Kaszniak, A., 239, 305n4
Keats, John, 143
Kenosis, 11
Kensho, 36–37, 48, 57, 62, 178–180
  and absorptions, 121, 139, 285nn7–8
  allocentric processing in, 94, 120
  brief awakenings of, 111
  conscious experience in, 120
  definition of, 126, 197, 271
  dissolution of sense of conflicts in, 179–180
  enlightenment in, 125
  and ethical behavior, 202, 203
  extended stability of visual processing sequences in, 36
  fearlessness in, 179, 180, 207, 230–231, 235
  as imbalance in shifting responses, 111, 152, 188
  and inclinations in post-kensho period, 206–207
  insight in, 129, 186, 187, 219
  meaningful reality in, 139
  memory of, 97
  moonlight phase of, 94
  nitric oxide in, 261
  no-Self in, 117
  as nothing special, 94, 188

  and psychological maturity, 239
  realization of Self as problem in, 153, 173
  release from layers of Self in, 200, 202
  residual representation of self-image in, 93
  selflessness in, 82, 117, 119, 129, 188
  sequence of events in, 137, 292n7
  shift from egocentric into allocentric processing in, 119
  sudden awakenings into, 37
  taste of, 97–98, 115, 286n6
  tests of working hypotheses for, 231–232
  time sense in, 193, 195–196
  trait changes in, 198
  as transient experience, 204
  triggering stimuli in precipitation of, 112, 113, 114, 118, 191
    in upper visual field, 115
  ultimate reality in, 199
  visual phenomena in, 286n4
Kensho-satori, 94, 172–173, 282n4
Kircher, T., 178, 297n9
Klein, S., 282n2
Knoblich, G., 169, 296n1
Knutson, K., 301n2
Koan, 44, 129, 150, 155–156
  definition of, 271
  uses of, 188
Kobori-Roshi, Nanrei, 79, 117, 202, 246, 284n1
Koch, C., 28, 278n4
Korean Zen, 239, 305n2
Kornfield, Jack, 5–6, 275n11
Kounios, J., 159, 258, 295n3, 309n5
Kristeller, J., 9, 276n6
Kuhn, T., 205, 300n6

La Rochefoucald, F., 75
Labeling of affect or emotions, 9, 276n4
  congruence with facial expressions in, 176–177, 297n7
Lachaux, J., 168, 296nn12–13
Language
  episode of hyperfluent processing, 96
  left side of brain specialized for, 47
  and word thoughts affecting no-thought processing, 150–152
Larson, C., 251, 307n1
Larson, Gary, 136
Lateral attention systems, 30, 34, 105

Lateralization
  anatomical, of ventral attention system, 32
  in contralateral bias of dorsal attention
    system, 30
Lau, H., 155, 294n8
Lazar, S., 243, 255, 306n10, 308n22
Leaf hallucination in internal absorption, 98,
  111
Lee, K., 213, 301n1
Left hemisphere
  in allocentric processing, 69, 70t, 282n4
  compared to right hemisphere, 70t, 236
  in problem-solving, 160, 160t, 161t, 172
  lateral view of, 24f, 60f
  in semantic processing, 161t
Leggenhager, B., 78, 284n9
Letting go intervals in meditation, 155
Liberal Buddhism, 10
Liberation in wisdom, 199
Limbic nuclei of thalamus, 90–92, 119, 271
  in kensho, 180
  as metabolically active brain region, 91
Limbic system
  definition of, 271
  in emotions, 89, 90
Lin-Chi I-shuan, 216
Literary Period in China, 156
Living Zen, 13, 203
Locus ceruleus, 252
Loori, J., 152, 294n4
The Lost Chord, 147, 153
Lotus puzzle, insight in, 130
Loving-kindness-compassion meditation, 146–
  147
  functional MRI in, 41–42
Lubart, T., 237, 305n5
Luo, Jing, 158, 159, 169, 295n1, 295n2, 296n1
Luo, Q., 208, 228, 301n1, 303–304n1
Lutz, A., 4, 41, 274n4, 280nn4–5
Lutz, B., 233, 304n1

MacPhillamy, D., 239, 305n3
Magic Eye task, 164, 295n6
Magic mushrooms, 267–268, 312n21
Magnetic resonance imaging, functional (fMRI)
  in affect labeling, 9
    congruence with facial expressions affecting,
      176–177, 297n7

age-related changes in, 177–178, 297n8
  in frontal lobe, 177–178, 243
  in responses to facial expressions, 240–241,
    242
in auditory mirror system, 77
in auditory spatial attention, 20
blood oxygen level-dependent (BOLD)
  signals in, 106, 287n2
  nitric oxide production affecting, 261,
    310n15
in resting conditions, 289n3
in clarity of visual perceptions, 27, 28, 278n2
in concentrative meditation, 41
in daily meditation, 5
in depression, 174–176
  resting state functional connectivity in, 175–
    176, 297n4
  and vagus nerve stimulation, 174–175
in dorsal and ventral attention, 29–32
in egocentric and allocentric decisions, 58
in embodiment, 78
in emotional conflicts, 176–177, 297n7
in empathic and forgivability judgments,
  213–215
in fear response, 224, 241, 242, 251
functional connectivity in, 266–267
  in depression, 175–176, 297n4
humor and cartoons affecting, 134, 137–138,
  291n6
in Implicit Association Test, 208–211
in introspective meditation, 74–75
long-distance interactions of brain networks
  in, 287n4
in loving-kindness-compassion meditation,
  41–42
in music listening and playing, 148–149,
  294n11
in naturalistic audiovisual stimulation, 34
in navigational tasks, 72–73
in post-kensho period, 206–207
precautions in interpretation of, 178
in problem-solving tasks, 159, 160–161, 170–
  172, 295n4
in recall of mystical experience, 44–46,
  280nn1–2
reciprocal cycle of fluctuations in, 103–108,
  287nn1–2
in response to facial expressions, 240–241

Meditation (cont.)
  incremental changes in, 200, 201
  modulation of emotions in, 228–232
  oxytocin levels and response in, 245–246
  plasticity of brain in, 247
  training attention in, 37–38
  trait changes in, 231
  vasopressin levels and response in, 245–246
  loving-kindness-compassion type of, 41–42, 146–147
  mindfulness in, 8–10
    advantages of extended years of practice in, 37–38
    compared to relaxation training, 9, 276n5
  minor insights in, 154–155
  no-thought silent intervals in, 76, 103
  and orientational aspects of attentional processing, 26, 278n4
  and pain sensitivity, 265, 311nn15–16
  perceptual rivalry tests in, 6, 275n12
  for quiet periods of several hours, 5
  receptive. See Receptive meditation
  and seizures, 265–266, 312nn12–14
  Self-imposed discipline of regular practice, 95
  shifts of attention in, 21–26
  top-down and bottom-up forms of attention in, 39–41, 43
  training attention in, 3–7
    advantages of extended years of practice in, 37–38
    and processing efficiency, 38
  transcendental, 227, 265
    and seizures, 265, 312nn13–14
Meditative quiescence, 275n10
Medulla, 272
  vagus nerve origin in, 227
Melatonin, 261, 310n19
Memory
  age-related changes in, 240
  in agnosia, 131, 132–133
  in Alzheimer's disease, 178
  assessment in competency determination, 100–101
  autobiographical, 71, 72
    in quickening episode, 97
    time sense affecting, 193–194
  in déjà vu phenomena, 133–134

  of emotions
    heart rate response in, 225, 302n5
    in sad episodes, 224–225
  of kensho experience, 97
  metabolically active brain regions in, 82
  mirror neurons in, 76, 77
  of mystical experience, functional MRI monitoring in, 44–46
  in navigational tasks, 72–73, 282n3
  of negative events, reappraisal in, 175
  nitric oxide in, 260, 309n12
  object-location associations in, 260, 309n11
  of positive and negative events, 240
  prospective, 194, 299n3
  relational, 127, 130
  resource management and data disengagement in, 286n3
  Self-centered
    subconscious processes in, 100
    thalamocortical interactions in, 91–92
  and sleep, 127–128, 290nn9–10
  temporal lobe functions in, medial, 285n4
  true and false recollections in, 142, 293n3
  in virtual 3-D environment tasks, 73
Meta-awareness, 10
Metabolic activity in brain
  medial distribution of, 30
  in memory, 82
  PET scans of, 60f–61f, 71, 91, 99, 282n1
  in resting conditions, 70–76
    baseline function in, 98–99, 102, 104, 286n1
Metabotropic receptors, 108
Methylphenidate response, compared to psilocybin response, 267–268
Meynert basal nucleus, 194
Midbrain
  in humor and cartoon viewing, 138
  in subject/object distinctions, 80
Miller, Bruce, 181, 182, 298n3
Mind-reading, oxytocin affecting, 244, 306n2
Mind-wandering thoughts, 102
Mindfulness, 8–10
  of bodily sensations, 9
  in cognitive therapy, 154
  internal experience of, 8
  long-term benefits of, 10
  in meditation, 8–10

Networks in brain (cont.)
  long-distance interactions of, 268, 287n4
  in problem-solving, 238t, 238–239
  psychophysiological responses in, 257–
    258
  reciprocal cycle of slow spontaneous
    fluctuations in, 103–108
  resting state, 257–258
Neuroticism, 236
New Buddhist Psychology, 10
New Yorker magazine cartoons, 137, 291n6,
    292n8
Newton, Isaac, 129
Nielson, L., 239, 305n4
Niki, K., 159, 295n2
Nirvana
  evolving views of, 233–234
  first taste of, 5
Nitric oxide, 260–261
  animal studies on, 310n22
  and cerebral blood flow, 260–261, 310nn15–
    16
  and inhibitory activity in thalamus, 261,
    310n17
  in kensho, 261
  in memory, 260, 309n12
  in relaxation response, 261, 310n23
3-Nitrotyrosine, 261, 310n21
No-Self, 87, 117, 120, 193
No-thought awareness, 150–152, 153–154
Non-I state, 97, 120
Nondual experience, selfless mode of, 54
Not-knowing, 204
Nucleus accumbens, 117
  animal studies of, 205–206
  in anticipation of event, 206
  dopamine in, 205
  redefining inclinations in, 205–206
  response to positive and aversive stimuli,
    205–206

Oates, Joyce Carol, 282n2
Object-centered perception, 55–56, 281n2. *See
    also* Allocentric processing
  integration with Self-centered point of view,
    56–58
  temporal lobe lesions affecting, 65

Object consciousness, 54
Object-location associations, memory of, 260,
    309n11
Object/subject distinctions, 80
Observations in mindfulness of bodily
    sensations, 9
Obsessive-compulsive disorder, 235, 305n10
Occipital lobe, visual processing in, 15
  in inferior cortex, 34
Occipito-temporal region responses in visual
    perception of bare stimulus, 14
Olendzki, Andrew, 11, 276n1
Olfactory pathway, 285n8
Omniself, 101
Oneness, 77–78, 93, 94, 284n7
Openness to experience, 236, 237
Operculum, frontal, 254
  in humor and cartoon viewing, 138
Opposing functions, balance of, 109–117. *See
    also* Balance of opposing functions
Orbital cortex, right inferior, in recall of
    mystical experiences, 45
Orbitofrontal cortex, 256–257
  in decision-making, 256, 308nn26–27
  interactions with nucleus accumbens, 205
  lateral, in visual attention, 18, 18t
  medial
    in recall of mystical experiences, 45
    in visual attention, 18t
  in sexual stimulation, 256–257, 309nn28–29
Orgasm
  correlation between insula activation and
    self-reports on quality of, 255, 308nn19
  orbitofrontal cortex in, 256, 309n28
Origins of Self, 49–83
Ospina, M., 13, 276n8
Ota, Hisaaki, 65, 281–282n1
Other
  and allocentric processing, 55–56, 83. *See also*
    Allocentric processing
  knowledge on, in normal development, 74
  physiological balance with Self, 93–94
  and Self/other distinctions
    right inferior parietal lobule in, 196, 300n5
    subcortical contributions to, 79–81
    temporal lobe networks oriented toward, 82
  value placed on, compared to Self, 54

Other-referential processing, 55–56, 83. *See also* Allocentric processing
  balance with Self-relational functions, 180
  deactivations in, 99–100
  network in, 103–105
    reciprocal cycle of slow spontaneous fluctuations in, 103–108
  shift from self-referential form to, 98–103
Ott, U., 39, 279n1
Out-of-body experiences, 264
Overconditioned attitudes, striking at the roots of, 202–207
Oxytocin, 244–245, 306nn1–5, 310n22
  in affiliative interpersonal behaviors, 244
  and cortisol levels, 244–245, 306n3
  and interpersonal trust, 245, 306nn4–5
  in long-term meditative training, 245–246

Pain sensitivity, meditation affecting, 265, 311nn15–16
Panic attacks, 230
Paquette, V., 43, 44, 280n1
Parahippocampal gyrus, 96
  anatomy of, 25f, 61f
  in memory, 178
    of street navigation, 72
  in naturalistic audiovisual stimulation, 34
  in spatial judgments in virtual 3-D environment, 73
  spatial view cells in, 62
Parahippocampal region activation in indoor settings, 116
Paralimbic regions, 272
Paranormal phenomena, quantum theories on, 268
Parasympathetic activity
  left forebrain in, 235
  left insula in, 236
Parietal cortex
  medial posterior, in children, 74
  posterior, in visual attention, 18, 18t
Parietal lobe
  in children, 74
  in egocentric processing, 65–67, 134–135
    Self-orientation of networks in, 82
  in meaningful experiences, 134–135
  in time sense, 194–195

  in visual processes, 18, 18t
    and clarity of perceptions, 28
    neglect in lesions of, 64, 65–67, 184–185, 298–299n13
    in top-down processes, 17
Parietal lobule
  inferior
    in allocentric processing, 73, 104
    in egocentric processing, 65, 102
    in recall of mystical experiences, 45
    in Self/other discriminations, 196, 300n5
    in time processing pathway, 194–195
  medial, in Self-referential functions, 102
  medial superior
    anatomy of, 25f
    in shifts of attention, 32, 279n3
  superior
    in allocentric processing, 73
    anatomy of, 24f, 88f
    in egocentric processing, 58–59, 60f, 67
    lateral posterior nucleus interactions with, 90
    in memory of street navigation, 72
    in recall of mystical experiences, 45
    as somatosensory association area, 58–59
Parieto-occipital cortex, in insight processing in word association problems, 162, 167
Pascal, Blaise, 143
Passingham, R., 155, 294n8
Path of Zen, 48, 95
  deactivations in, 75
  insightful awakenings in, 153
  silent illumination in, 43
Pattern recognition, temporal lobe functions in, 62, 132
Pavlov, Ivan, 233–234
Peak experiences, 37, 38, 44, 125, 172, 197
  in natural outdoor settings, 113–115
  as transient state, 204
Peirce, Charles S., 144, 293n1
Peptides, 244–246
  oxytocin, 244–245, 306nn1–5
  vasopressin, 245–246, 306–307n6
Perceptual rivalry, meditation affecting, 6, 275n12
Peroxynitrite, 261
Persinger, M., 263, 311n4

Person of the Year award in 2006 from *Time* magazine, 51–52
Personal life stories, memory of, 71, 72
  in quickening episode, 97
  time sense affecting, 193–194
Personality traits, 236–237
Pessimism in anticipation of event, 207, 301n13
  fearlessness of kensho affecting, 207
Phenomenal consciousness, 15, 29
Plasticity of brain, 37, 42, 259
  in animal studies, 258
  long-term meditative training affecting, 247
Polich, J., 13, 276n7
Pop-out phenomenon, 35–36, 279n3
Porter, Adelaide, 147
Positive resonance, 226
Positron emission tomography scans
  deactivations in, 75
  in embodiment, 78
  in imitation of meaningful acts, 132–133, 291n4
  metabolically active brain regions in, 60f–61f, 71, 91, 99, 282n1
  in reading or recitation of Twenty-third Psalm, 46
  in resting conditions, 60f–61f, 71, 99, 118, 282n1
Postcentral gyrus, right inferior, in viewing coherent meaningful images, 136
Posttraumatic stress disorder, 177, 234–235, 304–305nn8–9
Pragmatism, 198
Prajna, 197, 274n5
  definition of, 126, 272
Preattentive processing, 28, 29, 35
  in meaning, 139–141
  in pop-out phenomenon, 35–36
  in response to fearful face, 229
Precentral sulcus, inferior, anatomy of, 24f
Preconscious processing in visual perception, 28–29, 278n3
Precuneus, 252
  anatomy of, 25f, 61f, 88f, 252, 307n4
  in attention-deficit hyperactivity disorder, 252, 307n7
  in auditory attention, 252
  in children, 74

  in egocentric processing, 73, 252
  functions of, 252, 307n4
  in humor and cartoon viewing, 137
  in lapses of attention, 24
  lateral posterior nucleus interactions with, 90
  in memory, 252
    of street navigation, 72
  as metabolically active region, 71, 252
  Self-referential role of, 73, 105, 252
  in visuospatial processing, 252
    alertness training affecting, 7
    in virtual 3-D environment, 73
Prefrontal cortex
  anterior medial
    anatomy of, 25f
    in stereotyped attitudes, 210, 211
  comparison of medial and lateral region responses, 19, 277n10
  in creative problem-solving, 195, 298n14
  dorsal lateral
    anatomy of, 24f
    in attention shifts, 20
    in stereotyped attitudes, 210–211
    in visual attention, 18, 18t
  dorsal medial
    anatomy of, 25f
    in social cognition, 75
    in Vipassana meditation, 42
  medial
    anatomy of, 61f
    in attention shifts, 20
    in empathic and forgivability judgments, 213–215
    in extinction mechanisms, 234
    in introspective meditation, 74–75
    as metabolically active region, 71
    in recall of mystical experiences, 45
    in Self descriptions by children, 74
    in self-referential network, 102, 105
    subdivisions of, 61f
  orbital medial, anatomy of, 25f
  in reading, gamma band activities in, 168, 296n13
  in true and false recollections, 142, 293n3
  unconscious activation of, 155, 294n8
  ventral lateral, in visual attention, 18, 18t
  ventral medial, 256–257
    anatomy of, 25f

in attention shifts, 20
in decision-making and judgment, 256, 308n24
in depression, 174, 175
gender differences in functions of, 256, 308n25
in regulation of negative affect, 243, 306n12
Premotor cortex, mirror neurons in, 76
Presence, sense of, 262–263
in transcranial application of magnetic fields, 262–263, 311n4, 311nn1–2
Pretectal nucleus, anterior, 89, 92
Problem-solving
Aha! phenomenon in, 128–129, 159, 160
electroencephalography during, 161–165
Eureka! moment in, 129
flexible approach to, 205
functional MRI during, 159, 160–161, 170–172, 295n4
incubation process in, 127–128
insightful, 125–130, 158–173
in lotus puzzle, 129–130
in matchstick tasks, 183–184
maturation of networks involved in, 238t, 238–239
prefrontal cortex in, 195, 298n14
preparation and readiness for, 164–167, 169
and problem-finding, 153
restructuring of problem in, 126–128, 170–172
right hemisphere in
compared to left hemisphere, 160, 160t, 161t, 172
in uncertainty and ambiguities, 195, 298n14
in visuospatial tasks, 136
in word association problems, 160
types of processes in, 127
visuospatial
alpha rhythms in, 167–168, 296n11
egocentric and allocentric decisions in, 58
meditation experience affecting performance in, 39–41
right hemisphere in, 136
in word anagrams, electroencephalography in, 258
in word association tasks, 159–167, 187
Proprioception, 135
Prospective memory, 194, 299n3

Psalm 23, PET scans during reading or recitation of, 46
Psalm 121, 116, 289n6
Psilocybin, 267–268, 312n21
Pulvinar of thalamus, 87–90
bidirectional role of, 87
connections with angular gyrus, 89
dorsal, 88f, 89–90
subnuclei in, 89–90, 119
and emotional processing of limbic system, 89
in kensho, 37
in pop-out mechanisms, 36
in recognition of fearful facial expressions, 232
in spatial attention, 89
in subject/object distinctions, 80
ventral, 88f, 90, 120
subnuclei in, 89, 90
Punishment, altruistic, 216
Pupil size and sad facial expressions, 224, 302n2

Quantum theories on paranormal phenomena, 268
Questioning in Zen, 47
Quickenings, 95–96, 97
in meditative retreats, 215
Quiet periods, 5–6

Racial biases detected in Implicit Association Test, 210–211
Raichle, M., 70–71, 75, 98, 267, 282n1, 283n13, 286n1, 312n20
Reading
prefrontal cortex gamma band activities in, 168, 296n13
of Psalm 23, PET scans during, 46
Reality
age-related changes in view of, 237
as art theme in frontotemporal dementia, 181
Self as overriding authority on, 53
ultimate, 145, 199
value systems for, 143–146
virtual, 143
spatial judgments in, 73
Reappraisal, 175, 297n3

Receptive meditation, 3–4, 5, 259
  compared to concentrative meditation, 4t
  shift from concentrative meditation to, 41, 43
  shift to concentrative meditation from, 8
Reflective consciousness, 15
Relaxation, simple body, compared to
    mindfulness meditation, 9, 276n5
Relaxation response, 7, 8, 275n14
  nitric oxide production in, 261, 310n23
Religious experiences
  interpretation of mystical experience as, 263,
    311n3
  in reading or recitation of Twenty-third
    Psalm, PET scans during, 46, 280n3
  remembering of, functional MRI during, 44–
    46, 280nn1–2
  in seizures, 264, 311n7
Remote word association tasks, 159–160
Respiration
  breathing rate in, 225–226, 302–303n7
    in biofeedback procedures, 226–227, 303n11
    slow, psychophysiological changes in, 225–
      226
  JUST THIS mantra in, 11–12
Resting conditions
  active brain metabolism in, 70–76
  baseline functions in, 98–99, 102, 104, 286n1
  electroencephalography of networks in, 257–
    258
  functional connectivity of networks in, 106–
    107, 267, 287–288n6
    in depression, 175–176, 297n4
  functional MRI in, 118, 267
    in depression, 175–176, 297n4
  incubation process and insight in, 127–128
  intrinsic network fluctuations in, 111, 289n3
  PET scans in, 60f–61f, 71, 99, 118, 282n1
Restructuring and transformation, 10–11
  in insight, 126–128
    functional MRI during, 170–172
    incubation process in, 127–128
    types of processes in, 127
Reticular nucleus, 81, 89, 92, 284n5, 285nn6–7
  definition of, 272
  firing properties of, 92, 108, 285n7
  inhibitory influence of, 108, 119, 121, 288n9
    nitric oxide affecting, 261

Retreats, meditative, 95
  alertness of advanced meditators after, 39,
    40–41
  effects on attentional blink, 7, 275n13
  flashes of insight in, 151–152
  mirrors avoided in, 52
  reflection and objectivity in, 110
  rigorous, 215–216
Retrosplenial cortex
  anatomy of, 25f, 61f, 88f
  in memory, 74
    of street navigation, 73
  as metabolically active region, 71
  in other-referential functions, 73–74
  in self-referential network, 105
  in spatial judgments in virtual 3-D
    environment, 73
Reverberi, C., 184, 298n8
Revonsuo, A., 162, 195n6
Reward-seeking behaviors, 205–206, 300n11
Rickard, N., 260, 309n12
Riddles, word hints and problem solving in,
  187
Right hemisphere
  in attention, 47, 160
  compared to left hemisphere, 70t, 236
    in problem-solving, 160, 160t, 161t, 172
  in egocentric processing, 61f, 64, 69, 70t,
    282n4
  lateral view of, 33f
  medial view of, 25f, 61f
  in problem-solving
    compared to left hemisphere, 160, 160t, 161t,
      172
    in uncertainty and ambiguities, 195, 298n14
  in visuospatial tasks, 136
  in word association tasks, 160, 161, 162–163
  in semantic processing, 161t
Rinzai Zen, 158, 191, 202, 216
Risk-taking behavior in adolescents, 205,
  300n8
Ronci, Seido Ray, 117, 290n14
Rosenbaum, R., 72, 282n3
Roshi, definition of, 272
Rousseau, Jean Jacques, 213
Route skills in navigation, 259–260, 309n9
Rumiati, R., 132, 291n4
Russell, Bertrand, 228

Sadness, 224–225
  facial expression in, 224, 302n2
  recall of, 224–225
    heart rate response in, 225, 302n5
Sage wisdom, 198, 199, 236, 244
St.-Pierre, L., 263, 311n4
Salience, definition of, 272
Samadhi, 274n5
Sarinopoulos, I., 254, 308n15
Sasaki-Roshi, Joshu, 85, 155
Sati, 10
Satori, 94, 111, 197
  definition of, 272
  emptiness during, 196
  trait changes in, 198
  unexpected sensory stimulus as trigger of, 112
Sawyer, K., 153, 294n1
Sayadaw, Mahasa, 5
Schizophrenia, social cognition in, 213–214, 301n1
Schloegl, Irmgard (Myokyo-ni), 27, 81, 87, 223, 224, 247, 268, 278n1, 284n6
Schooler, J., 150, 191, 192, 294n1, 299n1, 299n3, 299n6
Sdoia, S., 115, 289n4
Seely, W., 139, 292n11
Seizures, 264–266
  and meditation, 265–266, 312nn12–14
  and mystical experiences, 264–265
  temporal lobe, 264, 265, 311nn7–11
Self
  and egocentric processing, 54–55, 83. *See also* Egocentric processing
  and embodiment, 78, 284nn9–12
  extinction of, in nirvana, 233
  identification with mother in Chinese culture, 283n10
  with initial capital letter, 81–82
  and introspection, 74–75
  knowledge on, in children, 74, 283n7
  layers of, 199–202
    I-Me-Mine in, 200
    release from, 200, 202
  loss of, in awakening, 81
  number of dictionary entries for, 53
  in oneness, 78
  origins of, 49–83

and other distinctions
    right inferior parietal lobule in, 196, 300n5
    subcortical contributions to, 79–81
  as overriding authority on reality, 53
  parietal lobe cortical networks oriented toward, 82
  physiological balance with other, 93–94
  psychic, 91
  and *Time* magazine 2006 Person of the Year award, 51–52
Self-analysis, 153–154
  functional MRI during, 75
Self-centered point of view, 54–55
  egocentric processing in. *See* Egocentric processing
  integration with other-centered perspective, 56–58
  in memory, subconscious processes in, 100
  parietal lobe lesions affecting, 65
Self-referential processing. *See also* Egocentric processing
  during assigned tasks, functional MRI during, 101–102
  deactivation of, 111, 114, 118–119
  frontoparietal regions in, 99, 101–102, 105
  let go in meditation, 11
  network in, 105–106
    functional connectivity of, 103
    reciprocal cycle of slow spontaneous fluctuations in, 103–108
  shift to other-referential form, 93, 98–103
Self-relational functions, 71–74
  balance with other-relational functions, 180
  in children, 74, 283n7
  thalamocortical interactions in, 91–92
Self-worship in mirror use, 52
Selfless mode of nondual experience, 54
Selflessness, 85–121
  deactivation in, 92
  effects of repeated major sudden shifts into, 93–94
  of kensho, 82, 117, 119, 129, 188
  in ordinary insight, 156–157
  path toward, 95–98, 110
Selfothering, 58, 59, 72, 74
Semantic processing
  interactive components of, 161, 161t
  in word association tasks, 159–167

Subconscious activities, 284n2
  in creative thoughts, 155
Subcortical mechanisms
  inhibitory, 92–93
  in Self/other distinctions, 79–81
Subject consciousness, 54
Subject/object distinctions, 80
Subliminal processing in visual perception, 28,
    278n3
Substance abuse, 201
  ventral striatum in, 206
Suchness, 219
Sullivan, Arthur, 147, 293n4
Sung period in China, 156
Supramarginal gyrus
  anatomy of, 24f, 60f
  in other-referential network, 104
Surgical patients, response to music of, 148,
    293n9
Suzuki, Daisetz, 205
Suzuki, Shunryu, 204
Sympathetic activity
  right forebrain in, 235
  right insula in, 236
Synchronization, definition of, 272
Syzygy, 113

Ta-hui, Master, 180
Tang, Y., 42, 280n7
Tang dynasty, 156, 216, 224
Tao Te Ching, 150
Taoist beliefs, 109, 173
Taylor, Jill, 152, 294n5
Temporal area, middle
  anatomy of, 24f, 33f, 60f
  in egocentric processing, 195
Temporal cortex
  in allocentric processing, 69
  in recall of mystical experiences, 45–46
  in self-referential network, 105
  social concepts represented in, 145, 293n4
  in viewing coherent meaningful images, 136,
    186
Temporal gyrus
  inferior, anatomy of, 24f
  middle, in recall of mystical experiences, 46
  right anterosuperior, in word association
    tasks, 161

superior
  in allocentric processing, 60f, 69, 131
  in out-of-body experiences, 264
Temporal lobe, 146–152
  agnosia in damage of, 131–133
  in allocentric processing, 59, 61f, 62
    defects in, 65, 67–69
    distant early warning orientation in, 133
    and kensho, 131
    other-orientation of networks in, 82
  anatomy of, 33f
  auditory language functions in, 150–152
  in déjà vu phenomena, 133–134, 264, 291n5
  frontotemporal dementia in degeneration of,
    181–182
  in meaningful experiences, 131–134, 136, 186,
    187–188
    in déjà vu phenomena, 133–134
    distant early warning orientation of, 133
  medial
    in active goal-directed behaviors, 284n3
    deactivation of, 284n3
    in déjà vu phenomena, 134
    memory functions of, 142
    in visual coding of subject/object distinc-
      tions, 80
  in music perception and interpretation, 146–
    149
  in out-of-body experiences, 264
  in pattern-recognition, 62, 132, 142
  posterior
    in other-referential network, 104
    in readiness for word association tasks, 166
  in recall of mystical experiences, 45–46
  in seizures, 264, 265, 311nn7–11
  in self-referential network, 105
  social concepts represented in, 145, 293n4
  and thalamus connections, 285n4
  in visual processing, 15
    agnosia in damage of, 131–133
    and clarity of perceptions, 28
    neglect in lesions of, 64–65, 67–69
  in word association tasks, 161, 162, 166
Temporal sulcus
  posterior superior
    anatomy of, 24f
    in loving-kindness-compassion meditation,
      41

Temporal sulcus (cont.)
superior
anatomy of, 33f
in empathy and insight, 212
in humor and cartoon viewing, 137–138
as interface in temporal lobe and parietal
lobe interactions, 146
posterior part of, 142, 292n1
in processing of semantic messages, 142
Temporo-occipital responses in visual
perception of bare stimulus, 14
Temporoparietal junction, 278n2
anatomy of, 24f, 33f, 60f
in embodiment, 78
as interface in temporal lobe and parietal lobe
interactions, 146
right
deactivation in visual search, 26, 278n3
in inferences on intentions, 136
in lapses of attention, 25, 26
in loving-kindness-compassion meditation,
41
in shifts of attention, 262
in ventral attention system, 31, 31t, 32,
279n2
Thalamus, 87–92
γ-aminobutyric acid nerve cells in, 92, 285n6,
285n8
anterior nucleus of, 88f, 91, 119
in attentive skills, 21, 278n16
cortical connections of, 119
in egocentric and allocentric processing, 88f,
90
deactivation of nuclei in, 93
dorsal, 90–92, 119
frontal lobe interactions with, 81
functions of, 48
infarction of, attentional bias in, 21, 278n16
inhibition of, 92–93
lateral dorsal nucleus of, 88f, 91, 119
lateral posterior nucleus of, 88f, 90, 119
limbic nuclei of, 90–92, 119, 271
in kensho, 180
as metabolically active brain region, 91
medial dorsal nucleus of, 88f, 91, 119
pulvinar of. See Pulvinar of thalamus
in Self-relational memories, 91–92
in shifts of attention, 82, 107–108

and temporal lobe connections, 285n4
ventral nuclei of, 119, 120
Theravada school of Buddhism, 216
Theta phase in EEG, 16, 277n6
Thich Nhat Hanh, 228, 262
Thompson, R., 246, 306–307n6
Thoreau, Henry, 95, 202
Threats, social regulation of neural response
to, 216, 302n3
Tianyi Yihuai, 192
Time, sense of, 193–196
autobiographical, 193–194
frontal lobe in, 193–194
in kensho, 193, 195–196
parietal lobe in, 194–195
Time magazine 2006 Person of the Year award,
51–52
Tool use by monkeys, and socially specialized
speech, 258–259, 309n6
Top-down processes, 34
acquisition of skills in, 43
anatomy in, 33f, 47
in dorsal attention system, 30, 31t, 33f, 40t, 47
in external absorptions, 110
gamma wave responses in, 277n5
in lapses of attention, 23
in meditation, 39
in visual attention, 17–18, 19, 28–29, 277n7,
277n11
as voluntary, 47
and goal-directed, 277n1
and intentional, 29, 35
Touch perception
overactivity of, 96
skin receptors and parietal lobe in, 135
Training attention, 3–7. See also Attention,
training of
Trait, definition of, 272
Tranel, D., 193, 299n1
Tranquility, 5, 274n5
dwelling in, 5, 274n5
Transcendental meditation, 227
and pain sensitivity, 265
and seizures, 265, 312nn13–14
Transcortical connections, 81
Transcranial magnetic stimulation, 195, 196
sensed presence in, 262–263, 311nn1–2,
311n4

Trust, oxytocin affecting, 245, 306nn4–5
Truth
  dynamic aspects of, 141–143
  value systems for, 143–146
Tsarikiris, M., 255, 308n17
Tsuchiya, N., 28, 278n4
Tweney, R., 129, 290n13, 290n15
Twin studies, 224–225, 302n4

Uddin, L., 196, 300n5
Unity and oneness, 77–78
Unselfconscious behavior, 43
Urry, H., 243, 306n12
User-Generated Generation, 52

Vagus nerve
  functions associated with, 247
    sensory and motor, 303nn11–12
  origin in medulla, 227
  in respiratory and heart rate variability, 226–227
  stimulation in depression, 173–176, 296–297nn1–2
Value systems for truth, beauty, and reality, 143–146
Vandenbulcke, M., 291n3
Vandiver, Willard D., 217, 302n1
Vasopressin, 245–246, 306–307n6
  gender differences in influences of, 245, 306n6
  in long-term meditative training, 245–246
  and response to facial expressions, 245
Ventral attention, 29, 30–32, 279n1
  in alertness and environmental monitoring, 48
  anatomy in, 33f
  bottom-up processes in, 31, 31t, 33f, 40t, 42, 47, 48
  compared to dorsal attention, 31t
  in pop-out phenomenon, 36
Vestergaard-Poulson, Peter, 227, 303n13
Vincent, J., 107, 288n7
Vipassana meditation
  effects on attentional blink, 7, 275n13
  functional MRI in, 42
Virtual reality, 143
  spatial judgments in, 73
Visual agnosia, 131–133, 186, 291n2

Visual association areas, 15, 132, 136
Visual awareness negativity, 14, 15
Visual cortex
  in top-down visual attention, 17, 23
  in visual agnosia, 132
Visual fields
  lower, 115
  upper, 115, 120–121
    in spiritual awakening, 115–116
Visual perception
  allocentric processing in, 55–56
    deficits in, 67–69
    integration with egocentric processing, 56–58
  attentional blinks in, 38
  in autism, 182–183
  of bare stimulus, event-related potentials in, 14–15, 38
  clarity in, 27–29
  conscious processing in, 28, 278n3
  dominant eye in, 100, 120
  egocentric processing in, 53, 54–55
    deficits in, 65–69
    integration with allocentric processing, 56–58
  electroencephalography in, 167–169
    alpha rhythms in, 167–168, 296n11
    gamma activations and deactivations in, 168–169
  in frontotemporal dementia, 181–182
  gist mechanisms in, 28–29
  internal experience of, 15–16
  in kensho, 286n4
  lapses of attention in, 22–26
  meaning in
    and agnosia, 131–133
    in coherent visual images, 135–141
    in humor, 134, 136–138
  object-centered, 55–56, 281n2
    integration with Self-centered perspective, 56–58
  preconscious processing in, 28–29, 278n3
  recurrent impulses in, 15
  rivalry between images in, attention training affecting, 6
  sequences during top-down attention in, 17–18, 19, 277n7, 277n11
  subliminal processing in, 28, 278n3